The Care Homes Guide

The Care Homes Guide

THE INDEPENDENT GUIDE TO
CHOOSING A CARE HOME IN
THE SOUTH-WEST OF ENGLAND

crimson

This edition first published in Great Britain 2008 by
Crimson Publishing, a division of Crimson Business Ltd
Westminster House
Kew Road
Richmond
Surrey
TW9 2ND

A catalogue record for this book is available from the British library.

ISBN 978-1-85458-406-9

Printed and bound in Turkey by Mega Printing

Contents

Finding the right care

Today, almost half a million people in the UK live in care homes. Finding the right care home can often be a daunting task. With almost 1,600 in the south-east of England and 1,300 in the south-west, how do you go about finding the right one? How will you know that you or your loved ones will be well cared for? If you are searching for care for a relative, you will also feel a responsibility to meet their personal preferences, and ensure they are happy.

ASSESSING YOUR OPTIONS

Beginning the process

It is never easy to make the decision to move into a care home. Many are reluctant to leave their own homes and familiar surroundings and fear they will lose their privacy and independence by moving into residential care. Although the situation is undeniably difficult, more often than not, the decision to move can have a positive effect. Many elderly or disabled people struggle with household tasks such as doing the laundry, cooking, shopping or paying the bills. It can be a relief not to have to worry about coping with the difficulties of daily living.

Depending on the situation, it is sometimes best to plan for the future by looking for an appropriate care facility, so that you will be more prepared when the time comes to making a decision. The introduction to this book aims to guide you through each step of finding care for an elderly relative.It is always useful to make some enquiries and chat to friends and relatives about the different options available. Your GP and local council will also provide you with information about the different types of care available.

Care assessments

Care assessments are an evaluation of a person's individual needs, usually carried out by an occupational therapist, and organised by the local council. From this meeting, you will glean a better idea of the type of care your relative's needs, and therefore, where to begin looking. The assessment will also determine whether your relative is eligible for council funding. Based on their income, a Financial Assessment Officer will decide whether they are entitled to funds to assist with nursing or residential care.

Everyone is entitled to a free care assessment irrespective of their financial situation. The therapist will assess the difficulties your relative may be experiencing at home and try and find a way to help and support them. For example, if they are having difficulty with carrying the shopping or cleaning the home, then they may be entitled to home care help. Other services in the home might include the provision of disability equipment and adaptations to the home or the therapist may help your relative consider the option of day care and care homes. The main aim of the assessment is to provide your relative with the best support possible and to ensure that they are not putting themselves at risk by living on their own.

If your local council agrees that your relative is eligible to move into a care home, then they may receive some financial help, which would go towards the cost of the care home fees. (Please see *How to fund care* for more details on funding.)

If you or your relative is unhappy with the result of the assessment, you are fully entitled to make a complaint to your local council. The Citizens Advice Bureau also provides guidance about how to make a complaint of this nature.

Once a person's needs are assessed, then the necessary steps are put in place to ensure that their personal wishes have been taken into account. This is put into a document known as a 'care plan'. As people's health needs are likely to change over time, it is important that the care plan is reassessed and reviewed on a regular basis. If at any time you or your relative feel like you would like a reassessment, contact your local council.

To make an appointment to have a care assessment, contact your local council. Please see the *County contact list* at the back of this book.

Types of care homes

There are many different types of care homes. Some simply cater for elderly residents, while others specialise in looking after those who need specific nursing care, such as those with disabilities or mental illnesses.

Terminology:
Care homes (previously known as residential homes)
Care homes with nursing (previously known as nursing homes)

Care homes

A care home is designed to provide care and security within a comfortable setting. It can be a relief not to have to worry about bills or running your own home and most residents enjoy the safety of being in a secure environment. Residents are not expected to cook, make their own beds, clean, do their laundry or do any housework – these tasks are carried out by the care assistants in the home.

Each resident has their own bedroom and bathroom which they are usually allowed to decorate themselves. Some homes offer shared accommodation. This is a less expensive option for an individual, and ideal for married couples wanting to remain together.

Most residents in care homes are quite active and mobile and need minimal assistance in carrying out day-to-day tasks. This means that there is no in-house nursing staff to provide medical assistance. However, there are care assistants on hand to help with personal care and many homes have a district nurse who visits when necessary.

In instances where residents fall ill, they have to be moved to a care home with nursing where they can receive the best medical care. Sometimes this move is upsetting for residents until they adjust to their new surrounings. It is worth considering the long-term when initially deciding on a care home – it is often a good idea to find a home that has both a residential wing and a nursing wing, so that if care needs increase, your relative will not have to change homes entirely.

Care homes with nursing

A care home with nursing is for people who are less mobile and need a higher level of care than those in a care home. Although the residents may be infirm, for the most part, they do not require hospitalisation but would be unable to care for themselves if they were to stay on their own homes.

These homes provide full-time highly qualified medical staff consisting of doctors and duty nurses who are on hand to assist with medical and other health needs.

Dual registered homes

Some homes offer both nursing and residential care. This means that in the event of illness, your relative would not have to endure the upheaval of being moved to a medical facility. This type of home is ideal for those who think that their level of care may change in the future, or for couples who have different health care needs.

Temporary stay/respite care

Many care homes reserve space for those who would only like to stay a short period of time. This option might appeal to those who have been ill and need some extra help in order to recover. If there is a carer involved, this is also a good way to give the carer a break if they both have been through a particularly difficult time.

This sort of home does not usually provide nursing care but everyone admitted is fully supervised. Respite care also allows you to assess what it is like to be in a care home without committing to it long-term.

Specialist care

Some care homes offer different levels of care and specialise in catering for specific illnesses including: dementia, Alzheimer's, Parkinson's, Huntington's, schizophrenia and depression. These homes have medical staff who are especially trained to deal with patients with these disabilities.

Caring for those with Alzheimer's and dementia

Discovering that loved ones are ill is always devastating and, depending on the stages of the disease, it can be difficult to care for them at home. Your doctor may recommend a clinic that specialises in the care of those with Alzheimer's or dementia. It can become increasingly difficult and distressing for the carer to cope with the more advanced stages of forgetfulness and odd behaviour. If you are a carer in this position and are finding it difficult to manage, the social services department within your local council will be able to advise you about different types of care. They should also provide you with a list of appropriate homes that would best suit your relative's needs.

Elderly Mentally Infirm (EMI) home

An Elderly Mentally Infirm (EMI) home typically cares for residents with dementia and Alzheimer's disease. Registered Mental Nurses (RMNs) are on duty at all times and are fully qualified to ensure that the residents are cared for and treated with respect and dignity. Doctors are also on hand to monitor the progress of the patients and prescribe medication where necessary.

Many of these homes run activities such bingo, cards or chess, and bring the residents out on day trips. Some even provide memory boxes and sensory gardens, which help to stimulate the senses. Usually, friends and relatives are allowed to visit at any time of the day.

Care homes for mental disorders

These are homes that specialise in caring for elderly residents with illnesses such as depression or schizophrenia. As with EMIs, the staff are fully trained to handle people with this sort of illness and provide them with a high level of care. Usually, a Community Psychiatric Nurse (CPN) pays frequent visits to the care home to examine the residents and monitor their progress.

Palliative care

If it is not appropriate for the patient to return home or go into a hospice, some care homes offer places for terminal or palliative care. Palliative care focuses on reducing the symptoms of the patient to relieve any pain and suffering and improving the quality of life.

Staff that care for the terminally ill provide physical, psychological, practical and spiritual support for the patient. They are also trained in dealing with bereavement and will help to support family members through this sad time.

This is a particularly difficult time for friends and family and you might feel you could benefit from some extra emotional support. The British Association for Counselling and Psychotherapy (0870 443 5252; www.bacp.co.uk) is the professional body for counsellors who should be able to provide you with comfort and advice.

Alternatives to care homes

The decision to move into a care home is not an easy one. It is best to consider all alternative options before making a final decision. There are many options available to those who would prefer not to move into a care home:

Staying in your own home

Many people choose to stay in their own homes rather than moving into a care home. Remaining in your own home is ideal for those who are still relatively healthy and active and feel that they would like to retain their independence.

If your relative does not want to move into a care home, your local council has a duty of care to ensure that they are comfortable, provide them with support and make their life as easy as possible. This might involve organising home help to assist them with personal care such as bathing, as well as helping with the shopping. Your relative can also choose to have meals delivered to their homes via a 'meals on wheels' service, which saves them the effort of preparing their own meals.

Often, the elderly are also given an option of a community alarm which is activated by pressing a button; this alerts a response centre which answers alarm calls any time of the day or night. Sometimes referred to as a 'lifeline', this button can be added to their phone or worn around their neck; whatever is more convenient for them. Once the response centre are alerted, they will contact your relative's next of kin to let them know there is a problem.

Sheltered housing/retirement housing

This option may appeal if your relative wishes to lead a more independent life and does not require the level of care provided by care homes. If they are over the age of 60 (single or in a couple) they are eligible to apply to most sheltered housing schemes. Typically, the scheme includes the provision of self-contained flats or bungalows, especially equipped to service the needs of the residents. There are also communal areas and some schemes even offer group activities.

There is a scheme manager (sometimes called a warden) who usually lives on the premises or nearby and can usually be contacted through an alarm system. The manager's responsibility is to keep in regular contact with the residents, check that they are comfortable, liaise with relatives or doctors where necessary and be there in case of an emergency. The manager is not there to carry out duties like shopping or cleaning, but it is worth remembering that residents can still apply for other services such as meals on wheels and home help.

Whether buying or renting their flat, residents are still obliged to pay a service charge that covers maintenance (garden, building repairs etc) and the cost of the onsite scheme manager. It is essential to verify what is and isn't included in the service charge as this can vary from scheme to scheme, for example, costs for electricity, phone etc may not be covered by the service charge. You might find it helpful to ask for a record of previous service charges and check if there have been any sudden increases in the past.

Extra care (assisted living) housing

In the last few years, new schemes have been set up to assist the needs of frailer, older people. This can be an ideal option for those who are unable to live on their own but, again, do not require the high level of care available in a care home. Like sheltered housing, the accommodation offered consists of mostly flats and bungalows and has the same communal areas, living rooms, dining rooms etc. However, with extra sheltered housing, there are usually a greater variety of communal facilities, for example, hobby rooms and health and fitness areas. There is also a number of onsite staff that provide domestic support such as preparing meals and helping with personal care.

The Commission for Social Care Inspection (CSCI)

The Commission for Social Care Inspection (CSCI) was created by the Health and Social Care (Community Health and Standards Act) 2003, as a means of promoting best practice, regulating, inspecting and reviewing all aspects of adult social care in England. Launched in 2004, the commission annually reports these findings to the government in a document called *The State of Social Care in England*, which is also available to the public.

Prior to the CSCI, the regulation of social care had been carried out by several different organisations including the Social Services Inspectorate (SSI) and the National Care Standards Commission (NCSC). The CSCI incorporated all these organisations and now acts as a single, independent body for the inspection of all the social care services in England, bringing with it a much-needed organised approach.

The CSCI works with local councils to ensure they are providing the highest quality services to members of the community and meeting the needs of different groups of people. The commission gives each council a rating and if they fall short of the expected standards, they are penalised.

The commission also inspects adult social care services and vets those who apply to run these services. They are also responsible for the treatment of the residents in care homes to ensure they are not at risk of abuse; a policy which is called 'protection of vulnerable adults' (POVA).

In 2008, the CSCI will also begin the process of rating care homes, awarding stars (from 0–3) to those that meet the right standards. This will make it a lot easier to choose a care home and assess the quality of care services in different areas. The introduction of the star system will be a gradual process, and this book pre-empts the government's selection (see *How to use this book* for more detail).

The commission assesses the care homes on a number of areas including the facilities, accommodation, communal space, overall care and services, and generally ensures that the needs of the residents are fully met. If the adult social care services fail to meet the national minimum standards, the CSCI has, by law, the right to impose the appropriate conditions. In the event that the care homes fail to improve and meet these conditions, then the CSCI has the legal right to shut them down.

Care home inspections

Care home inspectors from the CSCI carry out thorough inspections of all registered care homes periodically The number of inspections made depends on the quality of care measured in the last report. If a home exceeds standards, the next inspection will be more infrequent than for a home that does not reach the required standards or where the inspectors are not happy with certain aspects of the running of the home.

During the inspection, the inspectors will spend time with the care home managers to go through their records and files relating to the daily operations of the home. Residents' care plans will be checked and medication records examined. They will also tour the home, chat to residents and observe them to assess their well-being. The inspector also monitors the staff while they are on duty to ensure they are treating the residents with the highest quality of care. When they have collated this information, they feed it back to the care home manager for further discussion.

CSCI reports

The CSCI create full reports based on these inspections that can be accessed online at www.csci.org.uk. We have used these reports, and interviewed each home, to provide you with a summarised, easily accessible list of the main information about each home. This includes contact details for the home, and information on the home's building, location and outdoor areas. See *How to use this book* for more details of what is included in this guide. Once you have cross-referenced the homes you are interested in, it is a good idea to then look at their reports and read some additional information about the home.

In addition to the information in this guide, you may want to read about:

- What kind of care the home offers residents. It is a good idea to check the number of beds the home has available for dementia, for example.
- The admissions process. The inspectors make sure this process it is as smooth as possible. The report will also specify how thorough care plans are and the efficiency of staff.
- How the staff interact with the residents and if the inspector believes the residents are treated with respect.
- Staffing levels and if there is a need to increase the level of staff.
- How the staff maintain residents' accounts and that files are organised and up to date If there should be additional staff training
- How the meals are presented and if they are based on a healthy balanced diet
- Whether the inspector has notes any improvements that the care home needs to make in time for the next inspection. At the following inspection, the care home will be assessed on how well they made these improvements.
- Information on the cleanliness of the care homes.
- Health and safety standards of the home.

HOW TO USE THIS BOOK

How we chose the homes included in our listings

Our choice of care homes has been based on the findings of the CSCI reports. Our team of researchers have only selected the care homes that have been considered by the CSCI to have met or exceeded government standards. Those who fell short of these standards at the time of the report have not been included in this book.

Understanding the information

Aabletone

Manager: Mary Nayakandi
Owner: Cedar Care Homes Ltd
Contact: Waltham House,
Stoke Park Road, Stoke Bishop,
Bristol BS9 1JF
☎ 0117 9682097
@ mimal@cedarcarehomes.com
🖱 www.cedarcarehomes.com

Aabletone is a period Cotswold-stone house near the Durdham Downs. It is next door to botanical gardens, and the home's grounds contain a cedar tree which is more than 100 years old. The home arranges a residents meeting every three months to allow residents to voice their opinions on any issues they may have. The home also has an activities coordinator who arranges daily activities such as armchair aerobics. Outings are offered to the residents and the home has its own minibus for transport.

1 Registered places: 42
2 Guide weekly rate: £472–£650
3 Specialist care: Nursing, respite
4 Medical services: Podiatry, dentist, optician, physiotherapy
5 Qualified staff: Undisclosed

Home details
Location: Rural area, 3.2 mile from Bristol
Communal areas: Lounge, dining room, conservatory, garden
6 Accessibility: *Floors:* 2 • *Access:* Lift • *Wheelchair access:* Good
7 Smoking: ✗
8 Pets: At manager's discretion
9 Routines: Flexible

Room details
Single: 31
10 Shared: 9
11 En suite: 33
12 Facilities: TV point, telephone point

13 Door lock: ✗
14 Lockable place: ✗

Services provided
Beauty services: Hairdressing
15 Mobile library: ✗
16 Religious services: ✗
17 Transport: Minibus
Activities: *Coordinator:* ✓ • *Examples:* Armchair aerobics, games
Outings: ✓
18 Meetings: ✓

Key

 nursing care

 wheelchair access

 no smoking

 pets allowed

 transport facility

General information

1. **Registered places:** Number of beds registered with CSCI. If the registered places does not equal the number of rooms, some shared rooms may have become single occupancy.
2. **Guide weekly rate:** The home's approximate weekly rate. These change annually in April/March and vary depending on the amount of care needed. Please contact the homes for their most up-to-date rates.
3. **Specialist care:** All of the homes care for 'old age'. Other care denotes any specialist care the home is registered to offer. These include: nursing care, dementia care, respite beds, palliative care, terminal care, physical disability, sensory impairment and learning disability. Each home will have a certain number of beds dedicated to the specialist care. Please contact the homes for details of this. If there is no specialist care, the home is purely a residential home. Some homes provide additional care to their registered categories: whether the home can provide the care you need is at the discretion of the home manager.
4. **Medical services:** Services that residents can access in the home; in-house visits organised. Most homes organise transport to local facilities, but this is not usually included in the weekly fee.
5. **Qualified staff:** The CSCI requirement is that 50% of staff must be qualified to NVQ level 2. The percentage of staff trained is included if this information was available.

Home details

6. **Accessibility:**Access: If 'None', there is no assisted access upstairs. This may not be appropriate for those in wheelchairs or the frail.
   Wheelchair access:
   Good: All rooms and communal areas are accessible in a wheelchair. The home has a lift.
   Limited: Wheelchair access may only be on the ground floor as there is no lift, or some areas may be accessed by steps.
   None: Cannot accommodate wheelchairs.
7. **Smoking:** Smoking is allowed inside care homes in designated areas. The areas must be clearly signposted and separate from the main lounge. Many homes are non-smoking or have a designated area outside.
8. **Pets:** Indicates whether residents' pets can live permanently in the home. Many managers will allow smaller pets such as budgies but not larger pets (this is signalled by 'At manager's discretion').
9. **Routines:** This indicates the home's daily routine. Most homes offer a flexible routine with some structure built in, eg set mealtimes. For homes that care for a large number of high-dependency residents, the routine may be more structured.

Room details

10. **Shared:** Either two single beds or one double bed (for couples).
11. **En suite:** The CSCI definition of en suite includes a basin and toilet, not necessarily a shower or bath.
12. **Facilities:** Indicates if rooms have a TV or telephone installed, or a TV point or telephone point for residents to bring their own appliances.
13. **Door lock:** All residents should have the choice of having a lock on their door, unless their risk assessment suggests otherwise.
14. **Lockable place:** All rooms should have a lockable facility to store valuables. 'Yes' indicates that there is a lockable place in residents' rooms. Some homes have a communal safe instead.

Services provided

15. **Mobile library:** Indicates whether a mobile library visits regularly. 'Library facilities' is used if the home has other facilities, such as its own library.
16. **Religious services:** Details any religious services that occur at the home – specifically, organised services or visits. All homes must make arrangements to meet residents' spiritual needs, so homes that do not offer religious services at the moment will organise this on an individual basis.
17. **Transport:** Some homes have their own transport, in which they take residents on outings or to appointments. Some will share transport with a nearby home, others order taxis or use dial-a-ride.
18. **Meetings:** In some homes, residents meet regularly to discuss the daily life of the home and raise any issues with the staff. These are sometimes called Residents Tenants' Associations, but many are more informal. Topics covered often include their likes and dislikes on the menu and activities they would like to repeat or new activities they would like to try. Where there are a large number of residents with dementia, or where residents are too frail, homes often organise regular relatives' meetings instead, as a forum to raise any issues and keep them informed about events at the home.

Frequently used terms

Residents: Those who live in care homes are often called 'service users'. Throughout the guide we have called them 'residents'.
Undisclosed: This information was either not available as it was subject to change or the homes would not divulge this information.
Pets As Therapy: www.petsastherapy.org. Pets As Therapy is a national charity now in its 25th year. It organises visits of assessed/vaccinated PAT Dogs and PAT Cats with registered volunteers to care homes, often providing comfort, companionship and therapy.

We have also only included homes that offer 'old age' care. Many offer other types of care as well, such as specialist dementia care, but all are equipped for elderly care.

Our researchers have spoken with each care home listed in this book to make sure the information we have provided is up-to-date and relevant to you.

The book is designed to help you quickly find essential information about a home, and be able to cross-reference this with other homes in the region. When you come to think about your priorities when looking for a home (discussed more in *How to choose a home*) you will be able to check if the home meets all your criteria. Read more about how to use the information in this book on in *Understanding the information*.

Regional concerns

This book is split into counties. In many cases, people prefer to move to a home near to the area they live in or where they already know some of the residents. For many, being located near to their relatives is an important consideration. Some even take this opportunity to move to the coast or to somewhere they have always wanted to live.

HOW TO FUND YOUR CARE

Most of us think financially as far as retirement and don't consider that we may need extra funds to pay for our care or the care of others. It is during a difficult time that your relative is faced with having to pay for care and the information provided can appear confusing.

Funding statistics
- More than 60% of residents in care homes have some or all of their fees paid by their local authority.
- 95,000 people in residential and nursing homes fund their own care.
- 32% of people in care homes are paying for their own care fees with little or no support from the state.

(source: Laing & Buisson UK Market Survey 2006)

Due to the nation's rising life expectancy, the government no longer pays for the increasing cost of caring for the elderly. There is a cost, whether you receive care at home or move into a care home. As the average care home costs between £20,000 and £30,000 a year, finding the funds can be a daunting prospect and a major cause for concern.

The cost of a home can
depend on:
- The level of care you need
- The size of the home
- The facilities of the home

Usually, the basic fees cover:
- Accommodation
- Care
- Bed linen, towels etc
- Meals
- Laundry
- Heating

Government funding

The National Health Service and Community Care Act 1990, enforced in 1993, shifted the funding responsibility from the Department of Health to the social services department within local councils. In England, under this act, you are eligible to receive help with your care and accommodation if you have savings and assets of less than £21,000.

Although the government no longer pays wholly for care, there are still a number of benefits that your relative could be entitled to. You can find out more about their rights by contacting your local council. They will arrange a member of social services to meet with your relative to assess their situation and establish the type of care they need. See the *Care assessment* section on page vii.

Financial assessment

Based on the findings of your relative's care assessment carried out by your social services representative, a financial assessor will visit them to carry out a means test to evaluate their income. This will include:

- State pension
- Allowances (including disability allowance)
- Investments
- Savings
- Stocks and shares
- Other properties (if you own more than one)

Do they qualify?

Depending on this financial assessment, the local council will either contribute towards the costs of your relative's care or they may have to pay for it themselves. If their assets exceed £21,000, then they will have to fund the entire amount of fees themselves. If they are in a position to fund their own care for a certain amount of time, but know they will struggle to finance it at a later date, then their local council is obliged to assist them, but only up to a certain amount. Thus, it is worth reviewing their finances to establish if they can afford longer-term care.

They are entitled to some financial assistance from the State if the value of their total amount of assets falls below £21,000. However, they will still have to provide a large amount of their income towards their care. You may also find that the allowance provided by the State does not cover the fees required by your relative's chosen care home. In this case, a relative is permitted to contribute to the fees provided they can prove that they will be able to continue with the ongoing payments.

Property

There may be a number of reasons where the financial assessor would exclude your relative's property from their evaluation, for example, if their house is occupied by:

- A family member or spouse
- A relative over 60 years of age
- A child under the age of 16

Similarly, if they choose to receive care in their own home, their house will not be taken into consideration when it comes to evaluating their assets.

Joint savings and investments

The assessment does not include a spouse's sole assets but if they have joint savings and investments, it will be assumed that they each own half of the assets and this will be included when it comes to making a financial assessment.

Gifted assets

If they decide to 'gift' some of their assets, make sure they get the proper financial advice. If they have gifted assets and then attempt to claim state benefit, they may be accused of 'deprivation of assets' and their local council may still include the value of these assets as part of the financial assessment.

If you are seeking independent advice, always make sure the firm you use is a member of the FSA. Check their website www.fsa.gov.uk

Care in your own home

If your relative qualifies for care at home, their local council will provide them with a set amount of money through direct payments to contribute towards their care. Receiving care at home used to be free but some local councils do charge for the service so it is best to check the rates first. The payments also may not cover the cost of the care and your relative may be required to contribute some of their own income towards home help.

State benefits

Regardless of whether your relative does or doesn't qualify for funding, everyone is entitled to some welfare benefits:

Attendance allowance

This allowance is a tax-free benefit for those over 65 who are physically or mentally disabled and need help with personal care such as bathing, dressing, eating or assistance getting around their home. This benefit is rarely subject to a financial assessment and, therefore, usually applies to all those that qualify, irrespective of their financial circumstances.

The rate provided very much depends on the level of care required. For example, lower rates are paid if your relative only needs supervision and assistance either during the day or night. However, if your relative needs help throughout the day and night, they are paid a higher amount.

Disability living allowance (DLA)

This is a tax-free benefit for people under 65 who are physically and mentally disabled and need help with personal care or assistance with mobility. Again, the rates vary depending on the required level of care.

Registered nursing care contribution

The NHS now pays for nursing care if a resident is covering the entire cost of staying in a care home. This means that self-funded residents no longer have to pay the extra cost of receiving nursing care while they are living in a care home.

Self-funding your care

If your relative is paying for their own care, then you will need work out their own personal finances. There is no doubt that self-funding is expensive and requires a detailed overview of what they can afford.

You can start the process by:

- Evaluating their assets, including savings and investments
- Finding out how much money is annually generated by their assets
- Assessing how their assets can generate extra income and for how long.

It can be confusing to work out how to pay for long-term care over a number of years without running out of money and it is best to get some financial advice so you can assess the options.

Care Fee Annuity

If your relative doesn't wish to sell off all their assets to cover their long-term care, they may wish to consider purchasing a Care Fee Annuity. This involves paying a lump sum to an annuity provider who will guarantee a tax-free set amount towards care fees provided it is paid directly to the care home. The exact amount is determined by the provider and can vary widely depending on the annuity provider and circumstances.

When assessing the annuity, they will take into account:

- Age
- State of health
- Expected longevity of life.

Based on the above, they will make a decision on how much income to provide during your relative's stay in a care home. This option can be ideal for those who want to invest some of their capital but don't want to sell off all their assets. However, bear in mind that the annuity stops at the point of death and there is no compensation in the event of remaining monies. One way of ensuring against this loss is by purchasing a life assurance option, which guarantees a return of an agreed percentage of the lump sum. However, be aware that adding life assurance will increase the cost of the annuity.

Investing capital

Your relative may have a large amount of capital that they would like to invest in order to generate more income. However, no matter how financially experienced you may be, this can be a risky business as you are subject to the volatility of the financial markets. It can also take a long period of time before investments pay off so it is important to cater for that time when your relative will need to access to your funds. If your relative would like to invest some capital, then a financial adviser can help you to structure a portfolio and perhaps spread the capital across a range of low-risk investments.

Equity release scheme

There are different types of schemes available, but they are all based on loaning you money based on the value of your house. With house prices rising in many areas in the UK, many have found that the value of their home has doubled in price. Releasing cash from property is a popular option for retired people who still want to live in their home and have an income for it.

Generally, a company will assess the value of the house and then pay a set amount per month or sometimes even a lump sum. Many people use the lump sum to make alterations or improvements to their home to enable them to live comfortably in the long term.

The company will then reclaim the money by selling the house after death or if your relative decide to sell it. Generally, to be eligible for an equity release scheme you need:

- To be between 55 and 70 years of age
- To have a property worth at least £30,000 to £40,000
- To be a freeholder (although this can differ from scheme to scheme).

However, it is important to do your homework before entering into a scheme like this, as there can be some major pitfalls. For example, if your relative does enter into an equity release scheme, the company will eventually reclaim their money by selling their house. This means that they will not be able to leave their house as inheritance.

Depending on the value of their home, it might also mean that they do not qualify for State benefits. Therefore, it is essential that you or your relative seeks proper legal and financial advice before making the decision to enter into a scheme like this.

Deferred payment scheme

This is an option for those who are moving into residential care and do not wish to sell their homes. Alternatively, this scheme may also appeal to those who are moving into residential care but are unable to sell their homes quickly enough to pay for their care fees.

Under a deferred payment scheme, the local council may be able to give your relative an interest-free loan by taking a legal charge on their property; for example, they might take over the mortgage. The idea is that the loan would help to pay for care home fees. It is also based on the condition that the council reclaims the money after death by selling the home. They can also reclaim the loan if you decide to terminate the agreement or your relative sells the house. You can qualify for the scheme if:

- Your situation has been assessed by your local council and they agree that you require residential or nursing care
- Your home is of enough value to cover the fees of your stay in the care home
- You are able to pay a weekly contribution.

Again, there can be advantages and disadvantages to this option. While the loan is interest-free, it may affect the value of your relative's property. This means that when the property is sold, there may not be a large amount of inheritance left for family. Additionally, some councils do not offer this scheme or they only agree to pay a low amount which might not meet your relative's needs. Your relative may also be required to contribute a weekly amount based on their assets and income. It is best to check out the options with your local authority to find out how they operate the scheme, if available.

Other funding options

Renting out property

If your relative is not living in their own home and receiving care in a care home, then you may wish to consider letting out their property. You would have to ensure that the amount is enough to cover the mortgage (if applicable) and the care home fees. This option is appealing for those who would like to keep a property that may increase in value over time. It also means the family would be able to inherit the property after your relative's death.

However, there is no guarantee that the property will always be tenanted so it is important to have funds set aside for this potential situation. Be aware that you will still have to pay maintenance charges and buildings insurance and the rental income will be subject to income tax.

Charities
Many charities also provide useful information and some run care homes and offer full-time support for those with disabilities.

Financial assistance from friends and family
There are many ways for family to contribute towards care: they could either pay directly into your relative's account or help pay money towards other funding options such as a Care Fee Annuity.

Practicalities of paying

Self-funding
If residents are self-funding (ie paying for the care home themselves) then paying by direct debit is probably one of the most convenient ways of paying the fees. Many homes prefer fees to be paid on a monthly basis so it is worth checking with the home what date the money will be coming out of your relative's account. Make sure the date is convenient and works with the availability of finances.

Power of attorney
Your relative may wish to appoint a power of attorney to handle their financial affairs in the event that their health declines. Relatives are able to pay for care on their behalf if their power of attorney to do so.

You should ensure your relative appoints someone that they trust completely. Since 2007, you are now able to appoint someone to also make decisions about your health and general welfare, as well as looking after your legal and financial affairs.

It is relatively inexpensive to set up a power of attorney and it gives your relative reassurance that their affairs are being handled by someone that they trust. Without a power of attorney, the decisions about their finances and other matters rest with the Court of Protection which can involve higher costs and other added complications.

Contributions from social services
If care is being paid for partly by yourself or you relative and partly by social services, then social services will make their financial contributions directly to the care home. It is up to you to arrange with the care home how you or your relative will pay the remainder of the fees.

HOW TO CHOOSE A HOME

If, after your relative's care assessment, you both make the decision to move them into a care home, then it is important to know how to go about finding a home and organising the move.

The first step is to contact the social services department within your local council. Social services will send you all types of information about care homes, including a list of all the care homes in your area. However, be aware that it is entirely up to you what kind of home you choose as your local council is not permitted to recommend a particular home.

Choosing care for a relative

Choosing a care home for a relative is never an easy task. There is so much to consider and it is important to ensure your relative is given the best care possible. The first thing to do is to sit down with your relative and write down the following essential facts:

- Full name
- Date of birth
- Address
- Past profession
- Your relation to them

- Medications
- Medical history
- Mobility/wheelchair-dependent
- Doctor's name

A great concern of most people is that they will choose a home that their relative does not like or becomes unhappy with your decision. To ensure you meet your relative's needs and preferences, you might find it helpful to discuss the following areas with your relative and ask them some questions to help determine the type of care they are looking for:

Food and drink

- Does your relative have any food or drink intolerances or allergies?
- Do they need a special diet? For example, if your relative has diabetes or suffers from obesity, they will need to be on a very strict diet.
- What sort of food preferences do they have?
- Are they able to eat on their own?

Mobility

- Are they able to walk without assistance?
- Are they able to use the toilet on their own?
- Would they benefit from handrails on the walls of the bedroom and bathroom?
- Is there enough space for them to move around?

Speech

- What is their speech like? Is it clear enough to understand?

Hearing

- What is the extent of your relative's hearing problems?
- Do they use sign language? If so, it is important to ensure that the staff are also skilled in this area.
- Do they use a hearing aid? If so, note down the type of hearing aid and the sort of batteries it uses.

Sight

- Do they have difficulties with their sight?
- Do they use glasses? How many pairs do they have?
- What kind of prescription do they use?
- If your relative has a guide dog, does the home cater for pets?
- Is there any reading material available for the sight-impaired such as documents and literature printed in Braille?

Personality

Personality is very important in deciding which sort of care home is most suitable for your relative. If they are outgoing, then they may enjoy a wide range of social activities. Similarly, if they are a more private person who values peace and quiet, they may prefer a library or a garden on the premises.

The following questions are useful to keep in mind when assessing your relative's personality:

- What sort of person is your relative?
- Does he/she still have an active mind?
- What kind of hobbies would they enjoy?
- What kind of people do they get on best with?

Spiritual needs

- Does your relative have any religious preferences or spiritual needs?

Hobbies

- What kind of hobbies or activities does your relative enjoy?
- What kinds of facilities should the care homes offer that would fit their needs?

Be sure to make notes from talking with your relative, and take these with you when visiting homes as they will be useful when talking to the managers or matrons of them. The answers to these questions will give you a guide to make sure a home covers all your relative's needs.

Placement agencies

There are a growing number of agencies that assist in finding the right care home for you. This involves conducting a thorough interview with those considering residential care. Based on the interviews, the agency will look for the home that best fits your criteria.

There is a fee for this service and the agency consultants do work on a commission basis, so their advice may not be impartial. Some agencies charge a fee for providing information that is freely available elsewhere. The agencies can save you time and worry, but it is best to do your homework before approaching placement agencies to ensure you are getting value for money.

Know your priorities

It really important to take time to think about what your relative would like and expect from a care home. They might prefer to move to a care home that is near friends and family, or choose one that allows pets. Their personal preferences are very important and having a clear idea of what these are before you begin your search will help to ensure that their needs are fully met.

Everybody will have different priorities when choosing a care home. Some will want to be near the centre of town; others will want a quiet lounge; others, a large garden where they can help in. For many, the deciding factors come down to cost and location. It is a good idea to write down these priorities and number them. Keep referring to this list throughout the process.

Remember, you are not just choosing a place to live – you are choosing a home.
The people are just as important as the place.

The categories below are a few examples of points you may want think about – everyone will have different preferences, you need to work out what your relative's are. The considerations are numerous, so take time to think about all aspects of daily life.

Size of the home

Larger homes often have better facilities, and a choice of communal areas; while smaller homes will often have a homely feel. It is not always as black and white as this: many large homes have a great atmosphere, and small homes can have ample communal space. Often it is better to consider the type of home your relative would like, without considering its size.

Single or shared rooms

Is it very important for you to have your own room, or would you consider sharing if other aspects of the home were suitable?

Purpose-built/conversions

Many care homes have been converted from older, grander buildings such as manor houses. These buildings can look beautiful and are usually set in large grounds. The cost of staying in one of these homes is higher as it takes a lot of money to run such a large estate. Also, the accommodation might not be as modern as it would be in newer builds. If the care home is situated far outside a city, public transport may be a problem. As these homes are larger, they can hold a greater number of residents. These buildings usually have many floors and can be quite spread out. If you have difficulty with mobility, do take these points into consideration if you are thinking about moving into a large, country estate. Care homes that have been purpose-built for elderly residents are more modern and usually lower in cost. Many have fully functioning lifts and modern facilities.

Location

There are some very picturesque homes in wonderful rural settings; there are also care homes in the centre of towns. Think about the location your relative would like. Do they love the countryside and fresh air or do they value being able to pop to the shops or meet friends independently for a coffee? A large consideration is the availability of public transport around the home, and if the home has its own transport.

Do your homework

There are probably a number of nursing homes in your area – some that you have heard have good reputations, some that you don't know anything about. This is when this book becomes invaluable, as, when researched, the homes included all met CSCI standards. The information in this guide will give you a good grounding for your research.

Once you have established your budget, care needs and priorities, you can begin your search. Begin by going through the listings in this book and choosing the homes that meet your list of priorities. Don't restrict yourself to only looking at care homes in your local area; also check out the ones a little farther afield. Consider homes in the surrounding counties, or ones with good transport links.

This is when your numbered priorities list will come in useful: the reality is you may have to compromise on some of your choices. If you have decided that your home must have a garden, you may not be able to be as near to town as you would like. Keep your priorities in mind when looking through the homes.

Short-listing the homes

Jot down your top 10 or 20 homes. With this list, you can conduct some further research into the homes that you and your relative like the sound of.

Gathering a few brochures together always helps to narrow down the number of suitable choices. Begin by acquiring all 10–20 brochures and then decide on a shortlist. Be aware that the information in these brochures can sometimes be limited or out of date or the photos may not be an accurate representation of the size of the bedrooms or dining rooms etc, so it is best to visit the homes to get a feel for them first-hand.

Visiting care homes

Preparation
Before you pay a visit to the care homes of your choice, call first and speak to the care manager or matron. Ask if there is room currently available at the care home or if there is a waiting list and double-check if they can cater for your relative's needs. If you don't already have the brochure of that particular care home, then ask them to send you one.

If you are satisfied that the care home may be a suitable option, then make an appointment with the care manager to further discuss your relative's needs.

Visiting the home
Try not to visit too many care homes in one day. It can be an exhausting and an emotionally draining experience and with so many details to remember, it is easy to become confused and forget what each of them has to offer.

On your first visit, take your relative's list of priorities with you and ensure that you are armed with as much information about your relative as possible, including the answers to the questions in *Choosing care for a relative*.

Typically, you will be given a tour of the premises so try to note down as much detail as possible about each home. Notice whether each home meets your priorities, and make notes of distinguishing features. This will really help when you are looking back at your visit, trying to remember which home had the lovely water feature in the garden! Things to keep in mind are as follows:

First impressions
First impressions do count. Think about the presentation of the home from the exterior.
Are the gardens well maintained?
Is the driveway swept?
Assess how you are greeted as you walk in. *Are you given a warm welcome or are you ignored?*

Staff

Are the staff friendly and polite?

Observe how the staff treat the residents. Have a chat with some members of the staff and see if you can find out what they think of their own working environment. Discontented staff can have a negative impact on the residents. Staff should be warm, respectful, good humoured, calm and sensitive towards the residents. Residents should always feel comfortable in approaching staff with any problems and staff should support the residents to the best of their ability.

Are the staff fully qualified?

The CSCI requires that 50% of staff working in care homes are fully qualified to National Vocational Qualification (NVQ) level 2 status. Ask for this information when you are visiting care homes. We have indicated whether a home meets the standard in this guide, but bear in mind that the percentage of qualified staff can change dramatically if staff leave, or if unqualified staff pass their NVQ. Many care homes also conduct in-house training on 'Abuse in the Care Home' to learn about how to protect vulnerable residents from abuse. Find out what kind of staff training each care home offers.

Other training

If your relative suffers from a mental illness such as dementia or Alzheimer's, ask the care manager if the staff keep up-to-date about any medical progress in these areas and if they undergo any further training on how to handle residents with these type of illnesses.

What are the staffing levels like?

Ask to see a copy of the staff rota and check how many staff are on duty at night and during the day. If the care home is in the process of hiring new staff, ask about their recruitment policy and procedures. Usually all new staff are subject to mandatory induction training which includes fire drills, manual handling and health and safety.

Fees

Find out exactly what the fees cover. Are there extra fees for:

- Single room
- En suite
- Refreshments for visitors
- Services like hairdresser, chiropodist
- Outings
- Laundry
- Prescriptions
- Visits from the GP

The residents

Do the residents seem healthy and happy?

What is the general atmosphere like?

Note how the staff and residents interact with each other. Depending on what you see, you might want to consider making a surprise visit on another occasion to make sure that you get a realistic view of the care home.

Try and have a chat with a few of the residents to gauge their opinions on the care home and their general environment. Ask the residents to describe an average day in the home.

Accommodation

Are the rooms clean?

Make sure you thoroughly inspect the bedrooms, bathrooms and all communal areas to ensure that they have been cleaned to a high standard and that they smell nice and fresh.

Are the bedrooms big enough?

The size of the rooms vary from home to home. Check the size of the room and ensure that it is a comfortable size for your relative. The CSCI have a minimum size a single and shared room must be: you will see in the report if there are any rooms that are too small. Bear in mind, a room may meet government standards but still feel too small if you have a lot of furniture!

Can your relative bring in their own furniture?

Most homes will allow you to bring in your furniture from home provided it is in good shape (no woodworm etc). However, some bedrooms can be quite small and there may not be enough space for larger items of furniture.

Do residents have to bring their own appliances?

Some care homes will have already furnished the bedrooms with a telephone and television. However, if they don't provide these appliances, check that there are the right electrical points in the rooms so you can connect your own electrical equipment.

Can the rooms be personalised and decorated according to the resident's wishes?

Moving to an entirely different setting can be a traumatic affair. Being surrounded by familiar items from home can help with the adjustment period. Check with the care home to ascertain exactly what kinds of items you can bring. Some care homes do permit the bedroom to be repainted; at task which is usually carried out by their own maintenance man. Some homes even make a point of redecorating before a new resident arrives.

Are there en suites available?

Again, the provision of en suite bathrooms can vary from home to home. Remember that 'en suite' might not mean a fully equipped bathroom, but simply a basin and a toilet. In some care homes, the bedrooms do not have an adjoining bathroom as there is not enough space. Some residents prefer communal bathrooms as they are usually very large and they are easier to manoeuvre through.

Accessibility and space

What is accessibility like?

Are there enough handrails to make it easier to get around?

Many homes have excellent access, due to the high percentage of wheelchair-users. Check that there is assisted access on the ground floor as well as the upper floors. If you are quite frail and has difficulty with stairs, then ensure the home has a lift. If there is no lift on the premises, check if the staff help to assist the residents when they wish to get to the upper floors.

Is there proper wheelchair access?

If you use a wheelchair, check and see if the care home can accommodate it. Again, some care homes may not have a lift and may only allow for ground floor wheelchair access. Check that the route to the bedroom you are looking at is also accessible – even if a home has a lift, there may be a few steps up to a room.

Is there enough inside and outside space?

If you use a wheelchair, ensure that there is enough room to move around comfortably. The amount of space also depends on your personality. If you value your privacy, you will appreciate as much space as possible and may like a care home with a large garden or well-stocked library.

Meals

What's the menu like?

Ask to see a copy of the menu. Usually, this will change on a daily basis so request the week's menu to get a comprehensive idea of what kind of food is being served. Ask about the ingredients and produce they use. If you are used to organic food and home cooking, check with the care home manager or matron if this is available.

If possible, have a chat with the chef and ensure that he can prepare meals to suit special dietary requirements and personal preferences. In some care homes, the chef regularly meets with the residents to get their feedback on the meals provided and some even attend the residents meetings.

Does the food/drink look, taste and smell good?

Most homes are happy to let you try the food. Make sure it is presented nicely, tastes fresh and smells appealing. Ensure your cup of tea or coffee is hot (rather than lukewarm) and the milk is fresh.

Rules

What are the rules of the home?

Many care homes are very flexible but they will still have a number of rules, mostly concerning the personal safety of their residents.

Rules on pets

The decision to allow pets is usually at the manager's discretion. Many homes allow small pets such as budgies but it is more difficult to find a care home that permits larger pets to live in with the resident. If you having difficulty finding a care home that allows larger pets, then check with the care manager if a relative is able to bring the pet when they visit.

Access to GP and other services

Will you still have access to a GP?

This very much depends on where the care home is located. If it is near your relative's home, then it is likely that the local GP will make visits to the care home. However, if the care home is situated elsewhere, the likelihood is your relative will have to change to a local practice. The care manager should be able to advise you on this matter.

Will there be visits from a hairdresser, chiropodist, physiotherapist and dentist?

Many care homes organise weekly appointments with people from the above professions and a list of these services is included in the information in the book. You need to find out how often these services occur and if there is an extra cost. These services usually benefit residents and need to be taken into account when choosing a care home.

Entertainment and activities

What kind of entertainment is available in the care home?

We have included some example activities that homes partake in. While visiting the home, ensure you ask for a complete list of activities and entertainment that is organised.

Many care homes consult with the residents about their preferences in entertainment and activities. Depending on the feedback, the staff will draw up a monthly timetable and post it in communal areas so residents and their visitors are aware of any upcoming planned activities and events. Check with the care home if they draw up a schedule of events and ask if you can see their most recent one.

Ask the care manager if they have any photos of past events that you can take a look at.

Exercise activities are usually held daily in most care homes. It is essential that the residents keep mobile (where possible) and do a certain amount of gentle physical exercise. However, do check with your relative's GP to ensure that these exercises are suitable.

If gardening is a preference, are residents allowed to get involved in gardening?

Some homes have lovely gardens, and many let residents help with gardening. An increasing number of homes, especially purpose-built homes, have raised flowerbeds so that wheelchair-users can also participate in gardening.

Are church services organised at the home or do the residents have to travel to where the service is taking place?

This is often a very important consideration. Many homes offer an in-house service, but these are sometimes only once a month. If your relative would like to attend a service more regularly, or if it is important to attend a specific denomination, make sure there is a service nearby and that there is transport available.

Facilities

What are the facilities like?

Most care homes will have communal rooms where the residents can gather together and watch television or play games. Check the chairs are comfortable and whether the communal rooms are pleasant places to sit. Some homes have spectacular views from their lounges, which is much appreciated by residents.

Cleaning services

Do the care homes have laundry services?

The majority of care homes have an in-house laundry where they wash and dry clothes and return them to the residents' rooms. They do not usually have dry cleaning facilities and may ask for an extra charge for this service.

How often are the bedrooms cleaned and linen changed?

Transport

Does the home have its own transport?

Many care homes have a minibus or people carrier to bring the residents to local places of interest or on shopping trips. Most residents enjoy the change from their own environment and like to experience new things. The information in this guide will tell you whether transport is available. It is a good idea to ask how frequently the transport is used, to go on outings etc.

If not, what is the public transport like?

Ask about local bus services, dial-a-ride and any council-run transport services for older people. This is especially important if your relative wants to retain some independence.

Is there a trolley shop?

Some residents in care homes may be physically unable to partake in shopping excursions. If this is the case, then many care homes offer a weekly shopping trolley which contains useful items that the residents can purchase. Check with the care home if they have a trolley like this available and ask for a list of the items and prices offered.

The daily routine

What is the daily routine?

Try and get a sense of what takes place during a typical day at the home. Depending on the type of home, the routine will either be flexible or structured. Generally, mealtimes are usually set, but it is useful to find out how the residents fill their days. Check what happens if residents miss their meals or 'stray' from the routine.

Resident's charter

Most homes have a resident's charter which sets out the rights of the resident during their stay in the care home. Usually, this charter is on display in the home; if you can't see it, ask for a copy to review. Sometimes the charter is on the care home website. The charter includes information on the rights and privileges that residents are entitled to and outlines the standards and quality of services provided by the care home.

Typically, the charter would include the following with regards to the rights of the residents:

- To observe the residents' right to privacy
- To encourage and maintain independence of the residents
- To be treated with courtesy, dignity and respect
- To be provided with appetising food according to their diet and personal wishes
- To be given the opportunity to pursue new hobbies and activities
- The right to complain about any aspect of the home and its services without fear of reprisal
- To have full information about his/her health
- To have individual preferences and personal wishes taken into account
- To always have access to own room whenever they want
- To rise and go to bed any time they wish
- To manage their own finances
- To freely choose how to spend their day
- To be free to worship and attend religious services

Registration and insurance certificates

The CSCI are responsible for registering all facilities that provide personal and nursing care. If the care home meets the required standards, they will be granted a certificate of registration which should be displayed on the wall of the care home. Insurance certificates should also be exhibited prominently. Look out for both while you are touring the home.

Options for visitors

As relatives (and others) will most likely be regularly visiting, you and your relative will need to know some information about the following:

Car parking

Assess the car-parking situation and ensure that there is either space within the grounds of the care home or nearby. Some care homes are situated on busy roads and sometimes there can be very little room to park.

Public transport

If the care home is in the middle of the countryside, the public transport may not be too frequent. Check and see if there are regular buses or trains to the care home.

Visiting hours

Make sure you find out what times of the day people are able to visit. Some homes have an open-door policy, in that they allow visitors any time of the day. However, depending on the home, there might be restrictions around visiting hours so it is best to check this out.

The second visit

Once you have visited a few care homes and created a short list of those that you think might appeal, ask your relative to come with you on a second round of visits so you can gauge their opinion. This is important as it includes your relative in the decision-making process and will help them adjust to the idea once they become familiar with the types of homes available. It is also important to get a second opinion as they may notice things you may not have.

Make sure you have all your questions prepared for the care managers you are seeing so you can address any concerns you both may have.

After your second visit

If you and your relative cannot decide between homes and like one or more, check if your relative can stay for a day or two so they can get a feel for the environment. If there is a waiting list on the care home of your choice, check with social services and see if they can assist you. The care manager or matron of the care home can also visit your relative at home to ensure that they are a suitable candidate for the home and will also check if they can afford the fees. They will also advise you on the fees involved when reserving a room. If everything goes well, then your relative might decide to move into one of the care homes.

MOVING HOME AND SETTLING IN

Preparing for the move

Moving into a care home can be a very stressful experience. In the months prior to the move, it is important that you keep informed about everything to do with the home and include your relative in every decision you make. You can also take your relative on several visits to the care home so they become a bit more familiar with their surroundings. It is also helpful for you and your relative to have frequent chats with the manager of the care home and the staff to ensure that all your questions are answered.

Packing

If you are helping a relative pack for the move, be aware that this can be quite a big job and needs careful organisation before transporting belongings to their new home. Assess how much space there is in your relative's new bedroom for furnishings, equipment and clothes.

Clothing

There may only be a small single wardrobe available in the bedroom so do not pack too many items of clothing. It is important to choose a combination of warm and light clothes, even in the summer. Many elderly people feel cold even when it's warm outside and need appropriate clothing on hand to make them feel comfortable. At the beginning of each season, do check that your relative has the appropriate clothes for the weather ahead. Make sure that all the clothes are suitable for a commercial washing machine and tumble dryer.

Labelling

It is essential that you mark every item your relative is bringing to the care home as they can get lost or go missing very easily. You can mark clothes by sewing on name labels or using a marking pen. Do check these labels regularly as sometimes they can come off or become faded after the clothes are washed repeatedly. Some care homes order labels for the residents' clothing so check with the care manager if they offer that facility.

Apart from marking clothes, it is very important to label all other belongings. If your relative is bringing in their own electrical appliances such as a television, radio or portable/mobile phone, make sure they are labelled appropriately.

You will also need to mark any medical equipment your relative may be bringing with them. For example, if they have dentures, there are dentists that can label them. However, this can incur a charge that varies from dentist to dentist. Do shop around to find the most reasonable fee for carrying out this work.

If your relative has a hearing aid, there should be enough space to mark their name. If not, then store it in a container that is marked clearly. Similarly, make sure spectacles are also labelled appropriately.

Your relative might also be bringing in walking aids such as a Zimmer frame, walking stick or wheelchair. Their name can be painted on to the back of the wheelchair but it is trickier to mark smaller items such as walking sticks etc. In this case, you should either carefully paint their name on or use sticky labels. Marking all their belongings will make it significantly easier for the staff to return any missing items to your relative.

Toiletries

Remember to also pack some toiletries. The care home will provide some of these, so check with them first before packing. There is no need to pack six months' worth of toiletries. There will be facilities to buy toiletries, such as a trolley shop or trips into town.

Moving day

Ensure your relative has a friend or relative on hand to help on moving day. Bear in mind they will need all the support they can get on the day of the move. Make sure you or someone else is available to bring your relative to the care home or at least be there when they arrive. It can be a traumatic experience and it will help your relative to have a familiar face around. Staff will help to answer any questions you both may have and then assist your relative by unpacking their belongings and settling them into their new bedroom. They may also be introduced to some of the other residents.

Admissions process

This can be a difficult time and it is important that the admissions process is as smooth as possible and that the staff are kind, comforting and supportive of their new residents.

The care home should provide you with a contract of terms and conditions on admission which your relative will have to sign. They will also explain how the residents' care is assessed and evaluated.

Care plans

On the day of admission, the care manager will discuss your relative's needs, create a care plan to include their requirements and make sure they are carried out. Care plans are personalised for each resident and include a list of their social care, cultural, personal and health needs. Each plan should also contain a medication profile that details prescriptions and include details of any medicinal side effects.

The care home manager will also ask about your relative's daily routine and likes and dislikes. Friends and family should also be consulted during the creation of the care plan to give their input. Photographs may also be taken to include in their file. Care plans should be checked regularly to ensure that the needs of the residents are being met and updated to include any changes in their requirements.

End of life care plans

After a period in the care home, your relative may wish to establish their wishes relating to palliative care and the provisions they would like to be made. This is a very difficult subject to discuss but the care home staff are trained in this area and should advise you and your family appropriately and treat the matter with the sensitivity it deserves.

Preparing for your arrival

The staff should have prepared your relative's bedroom in anticipation of their arrival to the care home. The room should be clean with fresh sheets on the bed and towels in the bathroom, if it is an en suite room. Each room should have a fully functioning call bell, which the staff will ensure is in working order before your relative arrives. They should also ensure that a jug of fresh water is placed within reach of the bed.

Make sure that this preparation has been done before your arrival and also ensure that any of your relative's belongings, such as furniture etc have been arranged appropriately in the room.

Staff in the care home

It can be confusing and emotional to be surrounded by so many new faces, especially if your relative has been used to living alone. Try to visit as many times as you can prior to the move so your relative gets to know some of the staff. This will help them adjust more quickly to the environment if they are greeted by a familiar face on moving day.

In most care homes, the staff will wear a uniform which is traditionally navy blue.

Once you have moved

Culture shock

Adjusting to a new environment can be difficult to begin with. Your relative may not be used to being surrounded by so many other people and might also find it hard to adapt to the routine of the care home. They may also miss the familiarity of home and well-known surroundings.

The adjustment period can be difficult for all involved, especially family that visit. Your relative might be withdrawn and upset for the first while and might feel self-conscious about needing help with bathing or dressing. During your visits with your relative, it is important to encourage them to adopt a more positive attitude and try and lift their spirits as much as possible. You can help with the settling in period by:

- Visiting your relative as often as you can
- Encouraging other friends and family to also visit frequently
- Giving them all the contact details for their closest friends and family
- Hanging a calendar on their bedroom wall marked with significant occasions
- Putting photos and messages on their wall
- Bringing in meaningful gifts to cheer them up
- Taking them out for walks or short trips
- Bringing in their pet if the care home permits it
- Chatting to them about how they are feeling and offering comfort and advice.

It will take time for your relative to settle in but after a period, you may notice that they are more contented and may even be enjoying the experience of meeting new people and taking part in the different activities.

Changing routine

Depending on your relative's situation, they will most likely have settled into their own routine according to their lifestyle. They might have risen at a certain time every morning and prepared meals at the time of day that suited them best. Care homes do have a routine but it is a flexible one. The residents can to go to bed whenever they wish and rise at their preferred time in the morning. Mealtimes are generally at set times but some care homes also serve the meals in the residents' bedrooms if they prefer.

For the most part, residents have the freedom to do as much or as little as they wish on every given day. Some care homes impose a set time for bathing and washing etc. As many of the residents need help with their personal care, it can be helpful to know what day this will be taking place. Most care homes have specialist baths which are designed to make the experience as easy and comfortable as possible. A member of staff will always be on hand to help with getting in and out of the bath.

Resolving problems

There might be instances where your relative may feel uncomfortable about certain aspects of the care home and wish to air their grievances. This could be anything from noise volume to complaints about the staff or the meals. Some care homes hold weekly meetings to discuss any issues that the residents may have. Minutes might also be taken and circulated to the families of the residents to keep them up to date on any new decisions.

If your relative would prefer to talk privately about their problem, the best thing would be for you or your relative to have a chat with the care manager about the problem. If the problem persists then you can also write a letter to the proprietor explaining the nature of your complaint and why you feel it needs to be addressed. Most care home managers are willing to listen when you do have a grievance and it is always best to air your complaint as early as possible so it can be resolved quickly.

Quality assurance

Care homes are required to enforce a formal quality assurance system to accurately assess the needs of the residents, gather feedback and act on it if necessary. This might come in the form of surveys and comment cards which the residents and their relatives will be asked to complete. It is not compulsory to fill out these forms but it is an excellent way for the care home to assess the level of satisfaction with regards to the services they offer.

Visiting protocol

Taking your relative out

You may wish to take your relative out for lunch, bring them shopping or even take them back to your home for the day. Make sure you notify the care manager of your intentions and ask about any medication you might need for your relative while they are away from the home.

If you choose to take your relative and others from the care home on an outing, make sure your car is insured to cover all your passengers. If it is a special occasion, such as your relative's birthday, Christmas etc, inform the care home and let them know of your plans to take them out. It is always best to check with the care home about the most suitable times of day to pick up your relative and to let them know what time you will return.

Holiday

You may wish to bring your relative away on holiday. In this case, you must inform the care manager at least one month prior to the trip. Let them know how long you will be away, your contact details at your destination and the dates of your absence.

Meals

You may wish to have a meal with your relative during your visit. It is best to call ahead and let the home know that you are planning to stay for the meal. Some homes do not impose a charge for the meals, but there are homes that put the cost of the meal onto the resident's account. When you are looking around for suitable care homes, confirm what their policy is on accompanying your relative for meals.

Other visitors

There may be a number of people who would like to pay a visit to the home to see your relative. Some might be friends and may be elderly themselves. Therefore, it is important that their visit is made as comfortable as possible. Most care homes will provide visitors with free cups of tea and biscuits, but do confirm what sort of refreshments they offer and if there is a cost involved.

Other information

Telephone calls

Most care homes will have pay phones available to make calls to friends and family. These phones may be fixed to the wall or will be brought around on a trolley to cater for residents with mobility problems. The bedrooms will generally not have telephones already installed and it might be expensive for to set this up. They also may not need a telephone in their room if they only make calls a couple of times a week.

Some homes offer a facility whereby the resident can make calls from their own room through the care home's switchboard and the price of the calls charged to their account. If this is a facility that may appeal to your relative, make enquiries during your visits to the care home.

If you do decide to install a telephone for your relative, it is best to take into account the following:

- Does your relative have a hearing problem? If so, telephone providers can supply a phones that amplify the sound to make it easier for your relative to receive the call.
- Does your relative have failing sight? There are telephones available for the visually impaired that are equipped with large buttons, extra-bright ring flashers and Braille keypads.
- Payment for the calls will be made from a private account between your relative and a telecommunications company, so the care home will not be involved in the payment of the bills.

Mobile phones

If you are considering purchasing a mobile phone for your relative, then check with the care home first. Depending on the type of care home, some may forbid the use of mobiles in case they interfere with sensitive medical equipment.

TV licence

If your relative wishes to take their own TV into the care home, then they will have to purchase a TV licence. However, if they are over 75 years of age, then they no longer have to pay this fee.

Useful contacts

Please see page 299 for a list of useful contacts for councils, financial and medical advice and further information about care homes.

Action plan

When faced with the prospect of going into a care home, the process can be daunting and rather confusing. We have broken it down into 10 steps which will help you on the way to finding the right care for you or your relative. Details of how to go about each step are found in the relevant sections of this introduction.

- ☐ Care assessment
- ☐ Care home or other care options?
- ☐ What are your care needs? (nursing/dementia etc)
- ☐ Are you eligible for council funding?
- ☐ With or without funding, what is your budget?
- ☐ What are your priorities?
- ☐ Shortlist 10–20 homes
- ☐ Request their brochures/look up reports
- ☐ Visit a few homes; visit top 2 or 3 again
- ☐ Make a decision and reserve a place

Aabletone

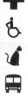

Manager: Mary Nayakandi
Owner: Cedar Care Homes Ltd
Contact: Waltham House, Stoke Park Road, Stoke Bishop, Bristol, BS9 1JF
) 0117 9682097
@ mimal@cedarcarehomes.com
⌐ www.cedarcarehomes.com

Registered places: 42
Guide weekly rate: £472–£650
Specialist care: Nursing, respite
Medical services: Podiatry, dentist, optician, physiotherapy
Qualified staff: Undisclosed

Home details

Location: Rural area, 3.2 miles from Bristol
Communal areas: Lounge, dining room, conservatory, garden
Accessibility: *Floors:* 2 • *Access:* Lift • *Wheelchair access:* Good
Smoking: In designated area
Pets: At manager's discretion
Routines: Flexible

Room details

Single: 31
Shared: 9
En suite: 33
Facilities: TV point, telephone point

Door lock: ✗
Lockable place: ✗

Services provided

Beauty services: Hairdressing
Mobile library: ✗
Religious services: ✗
Transport: Minibus
Activities: *Coordinator:* ✓ • *Examples:* Armchair aerobics, games
    Outings: ✓
Meetings: ✓

Aabletone is a period Cotswold stone house near the Durdham Downs. It is next door to botanical gardens, and the home's grounds contain a cedar tree which is more than 100 years old. The home arranges a residents meeting every three months to allow residents to voice their opinions on any issues they may have. The home also has an activities coordinator who arranges daily activities such as armchair aerobics. Outings are offered to the residents and the home has its own minibus for transport.

Amerind Grove

Manager: Daisy Matthews
Owner: BUPA Care Homes Ltd
Contact: 124–132 Raleigh Road, Ashton, Bristol, BS3 1QN
) 0117 9533323
@ AmerindGroveALL@BUPA.com
⌐ www.bupacarehomes.co.uk

Registered places: 150
Guide weekly rate: Undisclosed
Specialist care: Nursing, dementia, palliative care, respite, terminal care
Medical services: Podiatry, physiotherapy
Qualified staff: Undisclosed

Home details

Location: Residential area, 4 miles from Bristol centre
Communal areas: 5 lounges, 5 dining rooms, hairdressing salon, kitchenette, garden
Accessibility: *Floors:* 1 • *Wheelchair access:* Good
Smoking: In designated area
Pets: ✓
Routines: Flexible

Room details

Single: 150
Double: 0
En suite: 0
Facilities: TV point, telephone point

Door lock: ✓
Lockable place: ✗

Services provided

Beauty services: Hairdressing
Mobile library: ✓
Religious services: ✓
Transport: ✓
Activities: *Coordinator:* ✓ • *Examples:* Arts and crafts, singalongs
    Outings: ✓
Meetings: ✗

Situated in a quiet residential area of Bristol, Amerind Grove is on a local bus route and within walking distance of local shops. This purpose-built home has been designed to meet the needs of elderly residents. It comprises five separate houses, each with its own character. Four provide nursing care and one dementia care. Each house has a lounge, conservatory and dining area, and access to attractive gardens and patio areas. All bedrooms are single occupancy. Daily activities include reminiscence therapy, gardening, games and bingo, and trips to local places of interest.

Blenheim House

Manager: Evelyn Tiu
Owner: Desai Care Homes
Contact: 16–18 Blenheim Road,
Durdham Down, Bristol, BS6 7JW
☎ 0117 9739459
@ blenheimhouse@cedarcarehomes.com
🖰 www.cedarcarehomes.com

An older property located in a quiet residential area, Blenheim House is a few minutes' walk from local amenities and the Downs. The home employs an activities coordinator who arranges a wide range of activities according to the residents' wishes. These include one-to-one sessions and outings to the local pub.

Registered places: 34
Guide weekly rate: Undisclosed
Specialist care: Nursing
Medical services: Podiatry, dentist, optician, physiotherapy
Qualified staff: Meets standard

Home details
Location: Residential area, 2.5 miles from Bristol
Communal areas: Lounge/conservatory, dining room
Accessibility: *Floors:* 3 • *Access:* Lift • *Wheelchair access:* Good
Smoking: ✗
Pets: At manager's discretion
Routines: Flexible

Room details
Single: 28
Shared: 6
En suite: 0
Facilities: None

Door lock: ✗
Lockable place: ✓

Services provided
Beauty services: Hairdressing
Mobile library: ✗
Religious services: ✗
Transport: ✗
Activities: *Coordinator:* ✓ • *Examples:* One-to-one sessions *Outings:* ✓
Meetings: ✗

Bradley House

Manager: Elisabeth Laycock
Owner: Elisabeth Laycock
Contact: High Street,
Shirehampton, Bristol, BS11 0DE
☎ 0117 9235641
@ elisabeth.bradleyhouse@
btopenworld.com

Bradley House is a listed Georgian building with many period features. The home is located in a residential area, approximately six miles from Bristol. The large garden has several patio areas and a barbecue. A large vegetable garden and greenhouse provide fresh produce for residents' consumption during most of the year. The activities coordinator arranges a variety of group activities such as card games but also encourages the residents' own hobbies on a one-to-one basis.

Registered places: 10
Guide weekly rate: Undisclosed
Specialist care: Respite
Medical services: Podiatry
Qualified staff: Exceeds standard: 100% at NVQ level 2

Home details
Location: Residential area, 6 miles from Bristol
Communal areas: Lounge, dining room, conservatory, garden
Accessibility: *Floors:* 3• *Access:* Lift • *Wheelchair access:* Good
Smoking: ✗
Pets: ✓
Routines: Flexible

Room details
Single: 30
Shared: 0
En suite: 28
Facilities: TV point

Door lock: ✓
Lockable place: ✓

Services provided
Beauty services: Hairdressing
Mobile library: ✗
Religious services: ✗
Transport: ✗
Activities: *Coordinator:* ✓• *Examples:* Card games, gardening *Outings:* ✗
Meetings: ✓

Registered places: 26
Guide weekly rate: £339–£610
Specialist care: Day care, dementia, respite
Medical services: Podiatry, dentist, optician, physiotherapy
Qualified staff: Exceeds standard: 70% at NVQ level 2

Home details
Location: Residential area, 2.5 miles from Bristol
Communal areas: 2 lounges, dining room, conservatory, garden
Accessibility: *Floors:* 4 • *Access:* Lift • *Wheelchair access:* Good
Smoking: ✗
Pets: ✓
Routines: Flexible

Room details
Single: 24
Shared: 1
En suite: 23
Facilities: TV point

Door lock: ✓
Lockable place: ✓

Services provided
Beauty services: Hairdressing
Mobile library: ✗
Religious services: ✗
Transport: ✗
Activities: *Coordinator:* ✓ • *Examples:* Bingo, cookery
  Outings: ✓
Meetings: ✓

Carlton Mansions

Manager: Sugandhva Jadeja
Owner: Acegold Ltd
Contact: 8 Apsley Road,
Clifton, Bristol, BS8 2SP
☏ 0117 9734394

A Victorian property located in a residential area of Bristol near amenities, Carlton Mansions offers a wide range of meals available and everything is home cooked. The home also caters for special diets. Meals can be served either in the dining room, or be delivered to one of the residents' rooms, so that they can dine in privacy if they wish. The home itself is very clean and well furnished. The home has an activities coordinator who arranges outings for the residents as well as internal activities such as cookery and chair aerobics.

Registered places: 26
Guide weekly rate: £765–£950
Specialist care: Nursing, physical disability, respite, terminal care
Medical services: Podiatry, occupational therapy, physiotherapy
Qualified staff: Exceeds standard: 77% at NVQ level 2

Home details
Location: Residential area, 4 miles from Bristol
Communal areas: Lounge, dining room, library, garden
Accessibility: *Floors:* 3• *Access:* Lift• *Wheelchair access:* Good
Smoking: Undisclosed
Pets: Undisclosed
Routines: Flexible

Room details
Single: 24
Shared: 1
En suite: 15
Facilities: TV point, telephone point

Door lock: ✗
Lockable place: ✗

Services provided
Beauty services: Hairdressing, aromatherapy
Mobile library: Library facilities
Religious services: ✓
Transport: ✗
Activities: *Coordinator:* ✓• *Examples:* Arts and crafts• *Outings:* ✓
Meetings: ✓

Druid Stoke Nursing Home

Manager: Amanda Durbin
Owner: BUPA Care Homes Ltd
Contact: 31 Druid Stoke Avenue,
Stoke Bishop, Bristol, BS9 1DE.
☏ 0117 9688111
🖰 www.buapcarehomes.co.uk

Close to the Downs, Druid Stoke Nursing Home is situated in one of Bristol's nicest residential areas. Looking out onto an attractive garden, terrace and pond, the building has been purpose-designed to offer bright, comfortable, homely accommodation. In addition to the terrace, there is a lounge and dining room. The activities coordinator is kept busy organising social events and joining in with a variety of craftwork and hobbies enjoyed by residents.

Druid Stoke Residential Home

Manager: Karen Hunt
Owner: BUPA Care Homes Ltd
Contact: 29 Druid Stoke Avenue, Stoke Bishop, Bristol, BS9 1DE
☎ 0117 9681854
🖱 www.bupacarehomes.co.uk

Close to Clifton and the Downs, Druid Stoke House is minutes away from excellent shopping, entertainment and open spaces. The home comprises of a listed Georgian building and a new contemporary wing. There are several lounges, dining rooms and a library. Summer garden parties, in-house entertainment, lunch, shopping and theatre trips and coach parties are some of the optional events organised by the activities coordinator.

Registered places: 36
Guide weekly rate: £610–£800
Specialist care: Respite
Medical services: Podiatry, dentist, optician, physiotherapy
Qualified staff: Meets standard

Home details

Location: Rural area, 4 miles from Bristol
Communal areas: 2 lounges, 2 dining rooms, library, patio and garden
Accessibility: *Floors:* 3 • *Access:* Lift • *Wheelchair access:* Good
Smoking: ✗
Pets: ✗
Routines: Structured

Room details

Single: 33
Shared: 0 | **Door lock:** ✓
En suite: 30 | **Lockable place:** ✓
Facilities: TV point, telephone point

Services provided

Beauty services: Hairdressing, aromatherapy
Mobile library: Library facilities
Religious services: Monthly Communion service
Transport: ✗
Activities: *Coordinator:* ✓ • *Examples:* Games, videos, quizzes
  Outings: ✓
Meetings: ✓

Field House

Manager: Francaise Miles
Owner: Bristol Care Homes Ltd
Contact: Blakeney Road, Horfield, Bristol, BS7 0DL
☎ 0117 9690990
@ fran.fieldhouse@btconnect.com
🖱 www.bristolcarehomes.co.uk

Field House is a purpose-built home that sits close to a range of shops. The home has its own minibus, which is used to transport residents to places of interest. Visits to the nearby town are also regularly arranged. Family and friends are always welcome within the home. The home has its own shop, so that residents can buy items conveniently. The home also possesses its own hairdressing salon, which proves useful for the residents. A kitchenette is available on both floors and residents can make snacks here.

Registered places: 54
Guide weekly rate: £625–£675
Specialist care: Nursing
Medical services: Podiatry, optician
Qualified staff: Undisclosed

Home details

Location: Rural area, 3 miles from Bristol
Communal areas: 2 lounges, 2 dining rooms, conservatory, hairdressing salon, patio and garden
Accessibility: *Floors:* 2 • *Access:* Lift • *Wheelchair access:* Good
Smoking: Undisclosed
Pets: Undisclosed
Routines: Undisclosed

Room details

Single: 49
Shared: 5 | **Door lock:** ✗
En suite: 3 | **Lockable place:** ✗
Facilities: TV, telephone point

Services provided

Beauty services: Hairdressing
Mobile library: ✗
Religious services: ✗
Transport: Minibus
Activities: *Coordinator:* ✓ • *Examples:* Exercise sessions
  Outings: ✓
Meetings: ✗

Registered places: 76
Guide weekly rate: £635–£705
Specialist care: Nursing, dementia
Medical services: Podiatry, dentist, optician
Qualified staff: Exceeds standard: 75% at NVQ level 2

Home details
Location: Residential area, 3 miles from Bristol
Communal areas: 2 lounges, dining room, library, computer facilities, chapel, garden
Accessibility: *Floors:* 2 • *Access:* Lift • *Wheelchair access:* Good
Smoking: ✗
Pets: ✗
Routines: Flexible

Room details
Single: 76
Shared: 0   Door lock: ✓
En suite: 76   Lockable place: ✓
Facilities: TV point, telephone point, computer point

Services provided
Beauty services: Hairdressing, hydrotherapy
Mobile library: Library facilities
Religious services: Daily service, weekly Communion service
Transport: Minibus and car
Activities: *Coordinator:* ✗ • *Examples:* Arts and crafts, music and movement, relaxation sessions • *Outings:* ✓
Meetings: ✓

The Garden House

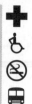

Manager: Donna McDermott
Owner: St Monica Trust
Contact: Cote Lane,
Westbury-on-Trym, Bristol, BS9 3TW
📞 0117 9494000
🖱 www.stmonicatrust.org.uk

Situated on a large estate bordering the Downs, The Garden House is a purpose-built property that is also home to a dementia unit called The Sundials. The home has a chapel in the grounds that is used for concerts and plays as well as religious services. There is also a hydrotherapy pool which is used for physiotherapy. The home has introduced a television link where residents may view the home's services through a link on their televisions. As well as holding their own meetings, residents are invited to The Garden House's monthly Resident's Liaison Meetings.

Registered places: 29
Guide weekly rate: £471–£600
Specialist care: Nursing
Medical services: Podiatry, optician
Qualified staff: Exceeds standard

Home details
Location: Residential area, 2.5 miles from Bristol
Communal areas: Lounge, dining room, conservatory, garden
Accessibility: *Floors:* 3 • *Access:* Lift • *Wheelchair access:* Good
Smoking: ✗
Pets: At manager's discretion
Routines: Flexible

Room details
Single: 7
Shared: 15   Door lock: ✗
En suite: 5   Lockable place: ✓
Facilities: TV point, telephone point

Services provided
Beauty services: Hairdressing
Mobile library: ✗
Religious services: ✗
Transport: ✗
Activities: *Coordinator:* ✗ • *Examples:* Arts and crafts, exercise
    Outings: ✗
Meetings: ✓

Glenavon House

Manager: Denise Worgan
Owner: Gemleigh Ltd
Contact: 22 St John's Road,
Clifton, Bristol, BS8 2EZ
📞 0117 9734232
@ glenavonhouse@tiscali.co.uk

A detached Victorian property, Glenavon House is situated in Clifton, close to local shops and Clifton station, where there are regular trains into the centre of Bristol. With five places available for individuals between 50 and 65 years of age, the home may offer younger residents one-to-one sessions as part of the home's activities programme. The residents select the timetable of activities. The home also has a conservatory and a garden for residents to relax in.

Gracelands

Manager: Rosemarie Hancock
Owner: Rosemarie Hancock
Contact: 443 Fishponds Road,
Fishponds, Bristol, BS16 3AP
) 0117 9653019
@ rosie@rosie6.wanadoo.co.uk

A small property, situated in a residential area three miles from Bristol, Gracelands is on a bus route and in close proximity to shops and amenities. As a result of the home's size, the activities coordinator is able to conduct one-to-one sessions with the residents. The home also has a garden for the residents to relax in, in the warmer months.

Registered places: 6
Guide weekly rate: £359
Specialist care: Mental disorder
Medical services: Podiatry, optician
Qualified staff: Fails standard

Home details
Location: Residential area, 3 miles from Bristol
Communal areas: Lounge, dining room, garden
Accessibility: *Floors:* 2 • *Access:* Stair lift • *Wheelchair access:* Good
Smoking: ✗
Pets: ✓
Routines: Flexible

Room details
Single: 6
Shared: 0
En suite: 2
Facilities: TV

Door lock: ✓
Lockable place: ✗

Services provided
Beauty services: Hairdressing
Mobile library: ✗
Religious services: ✗
Transport: ✗
Activities: *Coordinator:* ✓ • *Examples:* One-to-one sessions *Outings:* ✗
Meetings: ✗

Hartcliffe Nursing Home

Manager: Ruth Andrews
Owner: Methodist Homes for the Aged
Contact: Murford Avenue,
Hartcliffe, Bristol, BS13 9JS
) 0117 9641000
@ home.hcl@mha.org.uk
⌒ www.mha.org.uk

A purpose-built home in a suburban location, Hartcliffe Nursing Home aims to offer a homely atmosphere for residents. Although the home is run by Methodist Homes for the Aged, those of any or no faith are welcomed. The home has two gardens: a large area with lawns, plants and so on and a smaller, secluded, paved garden. The home arranges a residents meeting every two months to allow residents to voice any issues they may have.

Registered places: 66
Guide weekly rate: From £597
Specialist care: Nursing, physical disability, respite
Medical services: Podiatry, optician, physiotherapy
Qualified staff: Meets standard

Home details
Location: Residential area, 5 miles from Bristol
Communal areas: 4 lounges, 2 dining rooms, 2 gardens
Accessibility: *Floors:* 2 • *Access:* Lift • *Wheelchair access:* Good
Smoking: In designated area
Pets: ✗
Routines: Structured

Room details
Single: 64
Shared: 1
En suite: 66
Facilities: TV point, telephone point

Door lock: ✗
Lockable place: ✓

Services provided
Beauty services: Hairdressing
Mobile library: ✓
Religious services: Monthly church service
Transport: ✗
Activities: *Coordinator:* ✓ • *Examples:* Arts and crafts, bingo, musical entertainment • *Outings:* ✗
Meetings: ✓

Registered places: 15
Guide weekly rate: £388–£398
Specialist care: Day care, respite
Medical services: Podiatry, dentist, optician
Qualified staff: Undisclosed

Home details
Location: 2 miles from Hengrove
Communal areas: Lounge, dining room, garden
Accessibility: *Floors:* 2 • *Access:* Lift • *Wheelchair access:* Limited
Smoking: In designated area
Pets: At manager's discretion
Routines: Flexible

Room details
Single: 15
Shared: 0
En suite: 8
Facilities: TV point, telephone point

Door lock: ✓
Lockable place: ✓

Services provided
Beauty services: Hairdressing.
Mobile library: ✓
Religious services: Weekly Catholic Communion service, monthly
    Baptist Communion service
Transport: ✗
Activities: *Coordinator:* ✗ • *Examples:* Exercise, games, musical
    entertainment • *Outings:* ✓
Meetings: ✓

Hengrove Lodge Retirement Home

Manager: Margaret Osbourne
Owner: Mr and Mrs Staniforth
Contact: 29 Petherton Road,
Hengrove, Bristol, BS14 9BX
☎ 01275 833006

Hengrove Lodge is situated in a quiet area of Hengrove, and within a mile's radius of both the local comprehensive school as well as a number of shops. Hengrove Lodge has an attractive patio garden at the rear of the house, accessed through the car park by way of a flowered archway. Run as a family business, the home's proprietors can often be seen at the home joining in the various activities, such as singalongs.

Registered places: 64
Guide weekly rate: £339–£500
Specialist care: Nursing, day care, respite
Medical services: Podiatry, dentist, dietician, optician, physiotherapy
Qualified staff: Undisclosed

Home details
Location: Residential area, 2 miles from Bristol centre
Communal areas: 3 lounges, 2 dining room, computer facilities,
    garden
Accessibility: *Floors:* 2 • *Access:* Lift • *Wheelchair access:* Good
Smoking: In designated area
Pets: ✓
Routines: Flexible

Room details
Single: 53
Shared: 3
En suite: 54
Facilities: TV point, telephone point

Door lock: ✓
Lockable place: ✓

Services provided
Beauty services: Hairdressing, aromatherapy, beautician, manicures,
    massage
Mobile library: ✓
Religious services: Weekly church service, fortnightly Communion
    service
Transport: ✗
Activities: *Coordinator:* ✓ • *Examples:* Bingo, men's group,
    quizzes • *Outings:* ✓
Meetings: ✓

Honeymead Care Home

Manager: Isla Nicholson
Owner: Mimosa Healthcare
Contact: 183 West Street,
Bedminster, Bristol, BS3 3PX
☎ 0117 9535829
@ honeymead@mimosahealthcare.com
🖱 www.mimosahealthcare.com

A modern, red-bricked and purpose-built home, Honeymead is situated 100 yards from local amenities in the main Bedminster area, while a bus service passing in front of the home can take more adventurous residents into the centre of Bristol. There are easily accessed attractive gardens and a seating area in a secure and private setting. The home advocates a flexible visiting policy and holds relative meetings monthly. There is designated visitors' parking by the home's front entrance.

John Wills House

Manager: Angela Healey
Owner: St Monica Trust
Contact: Jessop Crescent,
Westbury Fields, Westbury-on-Trym,
Bristol, BS10 6TU
✆ 0117 3773700
🖰 www.stmonicatrust.org.uk

Situated in Westbury Fields Retirement Village, one of the first of its kind in the UK, John Wills House is part of a community of over 200 older people. The village is set in a 12-acre site, with buildings surrounding a village green and cricket pitch. The home shares its building with a pub called the Cricketer's. The home has meetings for the residents twice a month and has an activities coordinator who arranges a range of activities and outings. These include art sessions and musical entertainment.

Registered places: 60
Guide weekly rate: Undisclosed
Specialist care: Nursing, dementia, physical disability, respite
Medical services: Podiatry, physiotherapy
Qualified staff: Exceeds standard: 84% at NVQ level 2

Home details
Location: Residential area, 5.5 miles from Bristol
Communal areas: Lounges, dining room, garden
Accessibility: *Floors:* 2 • *Access:* Lift • *Wheelchair access:* Good
Smoking: ✗
Pets: ✗
Routines: Flexible

Room details
Single: 60
Shared: 0
En suite: 60
Facilities: TV point, telephone point

Door lock: ✓
Lockable place: ✓

Services provided
Beauty services: Hairdressing, aromatherapy
Mobile library: ✗
Religious services: Weekly Anglican service
Transport: ✗
Activities: *Coordinator:* ✓ • *Examples:* Art, musical entertainment
Outings: ✓
Meetings: ✓

Patron House

Manager: Emma-Louise Marshall
Owner: Ablecare Homes
Contact: 212 Stoke Lane,
Westbury-on-Trym, Bristol, BS9 3RU
✆ 0117 9682583
@ www.ablecare-homes.co.uk

A modern detached house that is part of the Ablecare Homes group, Patron House is a family-run home that is located a few minutes' walk from local village amenities and on a bus route to the centre of Bristol. With a homely style that offers a quiet lounge as an alternative to the TV room, the room leads into a patio and the home's attractive gardens. The home's surroundings feature an array of flowers and shrubs. Although the home has generally good wheelchair access, steps at the back of the home provide some restrictions.

Registered places: 12
Guide weekly rate: £425–£550
Specialist care: Day care, emergency admissions, respite
Medical services: Podiatry, dentist, optician, physiotherapy
Qualified staff: Fails standard

Home details
Location: Residential area, 3 miles from Bristol
Communal areas: 2 lounges, dining room, patio and garden
Accessibility: *Floors:* 2 • *Access:* Stair lift • *Wheelchair access:* Limited
Smoking: ✗
Pets: ✗
Routines: Flexible

Room details
Single: 10
Shared: 1
En suite: 11
Facilities: TV, telephone point

Door lock: ✓
Lockable place: ✓

Services provided
Beauty services: Hairdressing, beautician
Mobile library: Library facilities
Religious services: Monthly Anglican Communion service
Transport: ✗
Activities: *Coordinator:* ✓ • *Examples:* Arts and crafts, bingo, visiting entertainers • *Outings:* ✓
Meetings: ✓

Registered places: 17
Guide weekly rate: £410–£480
Specialist care: None
Medical services: Podiatry, dentist, optician
Qualified staff: Exceeds standard: 90% at NVQ level 2

Home details
Location: Village location, 6.5 miles from Bristol
Communal areas: 2 lounges, dining room, conservatory, garden
Accessibility: *Floors:* 2 • *Access:* Lift • *Wheelchair access:* Good
Smoking: In designated area
Pets: ✓
Routines: Flexible

Room details
Single: 15
Shared: 1 En suite: 14
Facilities: TV point, telephone point

Door lock: ✓
Lockable place: ✓

Services provided
Beauty services: Hairdressing
Mobile Library: ✓
Religious services: Fortnightly Methodist service, monthly Anglican
  Communion service
Transport: ✓
Activities: *Coordinator:* ✓ • *Examples:* Bingo, reminiscence therapy
  Outings: ✓
Meetings: ✓

Penhill Residential Home

Manager: Barbara Ann
Owner: Stephen Ann
Contact: 81 Station Road,
Shirehampton, Bristol, BS11 9TY
☎ 0117 9822685
@ jon@penhill.com
🖰 www.penhill.com

Built in 1926, Penhill Residential Home is located in the small village of Shirehampton, close to a train station and a library. With gardens which feature a fishpond, well-stocked flowerbeds and a pergola, residents often choose to spend time outside during warmer weather. The home has introduced a new system where information on activities and menus can be accessed through a selected channel on their televisions. There is a TV room containing a large screen plasma TV with a surround sound system.

Registered places: 68
Guide weekly rate: From £560
Specialist care: Nursing, palliative care, physical disability
Medical services: Podiatry, dentist, optician, physiotherapy
Qualified staff: Exceeds standard: 70% at NVQ level 2

Home details
Location: Residential area, 2 miles from Bristol
Communal areas: 4 lounges, 2 dining rooms, chapel, garden
Accessibility: *Floors:* 2 • *Access:* Lift • *Wheelchair access:* Good
Smoking: In designated area
Pets: ✗
Routines: Flexible

Room details
Single: 60
Shared: 4
En suite: 64
Facilities: TV point, telephone point

Door lock: ✓
Lockable place: ✓

Services provided
Beauty services: Hairdressing, reflexology
Mobile library: Library facilities
Religious services: Weekly Catholic Mass, monthly Anglican service
Transport: Minibus
Activities: *Coordinator:* ✓ • *Examples:* Musical entertainment
  Outings: ✓
Meetings: ✓

Riversway Nursing Home

Manager: Angela Glover
Owner: Riversway Care Ltd
Contact: Crews Hole Road,
St George, Bristol, BS5 8GG
☎ 0117 9555758
@ riversway@btconnect.com

Riversway Nursing Home is situated in a residential area, occupying a riverside site. With a large garden that has raised flowerbeds, the surroundings are picturesque and are taken advantage of in the weekly outings the home offers during the summer. As well as a monthly residents meeting the home has a newsletter it sends out approximately twice a year. The home also has a chapel and its own library facilities.

Rose Villa

Manager: Julia Slocombe
Owner: Philip and Julia Slocombe
Contact: 167 Talbot Road,
Brislington, Bristol, BS4 2NZ
☎ 0117 9721608

Rose Villa is a Grade II listed building situated in its own grounds. The home has a walled garden containing a fishpond and a lawn. It is a five-minute walk to the nearest shops and two and a half miles to Bristol. The home has its own car for transport and arranges daily activities for the residents such as reminiscence therapy and bingo.

Registered places: 10
Guide weekly rate: Up to £460
Specialist care: Day care, dementia, mental disorder
Medical services: Podiatry, dentist, optician
Qualified staff: Meets standard

Home details
Location: Residential area, 2.5 miles from Bristol
Communal areas: Lounge, dining room, garden
Accessibility: *Floors:* 2 • *Access:* Lift • *Wheelchair access:* Limited
Smoking: ✗
Pets: At manager's discretion
Routines: Flexible

Room details
Single: 9
Shared: 0
En suite: 5
Facilities: TV

Door lock: ✓
Lockable place: ✓

Services provided
Beauty services: Hairdressing, aromatherapy
Mobile library: ✓
Religious services: ✗
Transport: Car
Activities: *Coordinator:* ✗ • *Examples:* Bingo, reminiscence therapy
　　Outings: ✗
Meetings: ✗

Rosedale House

Manager: Julie Edwards
Owner: Ann Rogers
Contact: 163 West Town Lane,
Brislington, Bristol, BS14 9EA
☎ 0117 9714991

Situated in a residential area, Rosedale House is on a main bus route to Bristol. The home is located approximately three miles from Bristol city centre. The home's gardens contain a pond. There are also two lounges for the residents to enjoy. The home has its own transport and arranges for a Communion service to take place once a month. The residents also benefit from daily activities such as arts and crafts and visiting entertainers.

Registered places: 23
Guide weekly rate: Undisclosed
Specialist care: None
Medical services: Podiatry, optician, physiotherapy
Qualified staff: Meets standard

Home details
Location: Residential area, 3 miles from Bristol
Communal areas: 2 lounges, dining room, conservatory, garden
Accessibility: *Floors:* 3 • *Access:* Lift and stair lift
　　Wheelchair access: Good
Smoking: ✗
Pets: At manager's discretion
Routines: Flexible

Room details
Single: 23
Shared: 0
En suite: 6
Facilities: TV point, telephone point

Door lock: ✓
Lockable place: ✓

Services provided
Beauty services: Hairdressing
Mobile library: ✓
Religious services: Monthly Communion service
Transport: Car
Activities: *Coordinator:* ✗ • *Examples:* Arts and crafts, bingo, visiting entertainers • *Outings:* ✗
Meetings: ✗

Registered places: 17
Guide weekly rate: £400–£535
Specialist care: None
Medical services: Podiatry, optician, physiotherapy
Qualified staff: Fails standard

Home details

Location: Residential area, 3 miles from Bristol
Communal areas: Lounge, dining room, garden
Accessibility: *Floors:* 3 • *Access:* Stair lift • *Wheelchair access:* Good
Smoking: ✗
Pets: At manager's discretion
Routines: Flexible

Room details

Single: 17
Shared: 0
En suite: 17
Facilities: TV point, telephone point

Door lock: ✓
Lockable place: ✓

Services provided

Beauty services: Hairdressing
Mobile library: ✓
Religious services: ✗
Transport: Minibus
Activities: *Coordinator:* ✗ • *Examples:* Musical entertainment, painting, quizzes • Outings: ✗
Meetings: ✓

Rosewood House

Manager: Jane Bowman
Owner: Ablecare Homes
Contact: 55 Westbury Road,
Westbury-on-Trym, Bristol, BS9 3AS
) 0117 9622331
@ sam.hawker@blueyonder.co.uk

Situated in a residential suburb and complete with attractive gardens that include a fishpond, Rosewood House is within walking distance of the nearest shopping centre. The home occupies a location which offers good access to the Downs. The home has its own minibus to transport residents and offers a range of daily activities such as painting and quiz sessions. There are also regular residents meetings.

Registered places: 42
Guide weekly rate: Undisclosed
Specialist care: Nursing, respite
Medical services: Podiatry, dentist, optician, physiotherapy
Qualified staff: Meets standard

Home details

Location: Urban area, 3 miles from Bristol
Communal areas: 2 lounges, dining room, patio and garden
Accessibility: *Floors:* 4 • *Access:* 2 lifts • *Wheelchair access:* Good
Smoking: In designated area
Pets: Undisclosed
Routines: Flexible

Room details

Single: 34
Shared: 4
En suite: Undisclosed
Facilities: TV

Door lock: ✗
Lockable place: ✗

Services provided

Beauty services: Hairdressing, aromatherapy, manicures
Mobile library: ✓
Religious services: ✓
Transport: ✓
Activities: *Coordinator:* ✓ • *Examples:* Bingo, singalongs
Outings: ✓
Meetings: ✓

Saville Manor Nursing Home

Manager: Mrs Defai
Owner: Cedar Care Home Ltd
Contact: Saville Road,
Sneyd Park, Bristol, BS9 1JA
) 0117 9687412
@ savillemanor@cedarcarehomes.com
⌂ www.cedarcarehomes.com

A converted older property, Saville Manor is located in a residential area of north Bristol. The home boasts views of the Bristol Downs. The home has an activities coordinator as well as a lounge assistant, both of whom are available to assist the residents. The daily activities include games and arts as well as outings. The home has its own transport and arranges for visits from a mobile library. There are religious services available as well as services such as hairdressing and manicures.

Stokeleigh Residential Home

Manager: Tracy Bird
Owner: Hartford Care Ltd
Contact: 19 Stoke Hill,
Stoke Bishop, Bristol, BS9 1JN

📞 0117 9684685
@ stokeleigh@hartfordcare.co.uk
🖰 www.hartfordcare.co.uk

Set in large grounds in a residential area close to the picturesque Downs area, Stokeleigh Residential Home is also a few hundred yards from Westbury Park. The home employs a part-time maintenance man who ensures everything is kept in working order. The home also has a dedicated activities coordinator who arranges a variety of activities for residents such as flower arranging and visiting entertainers. There are also outings for residents to partake in.

Registered places: 30
Guide weekly rate: £467–£650
Specialist care: Day care, respite
Medical services: Podiatry, dentist, optician
Qualified staff: Meets standard

Home details
Location: Residential area, 3.5 miles from Bristol
Communal areas: Lounge, dining room, conservatory, garden
Accessibility: *Floors:* 4 • *Access:* Lift • *Wheelchair access:* Good
Smoking: In designated area
Pets: ✗
Routines: Flexible

Room details
Single: 30
Shared: 0
En suite: 30
Facilities: TV point, telephone point

Door lock: ✓
Lockable place: ✓

Services provided
Beauty services: Hairdressing
Mobile library: ✓
Religious services: Monthly Anglican Communion service
Transport: ✗
Activities: *Coordinator:* ✓ • *Examples:* Flower arranging, skittles, visiting entertainers • *Outings:* ✓
Meetings: ✓

Stokeleigh Lodge

Manager: Dawn Sherwood
Owner: Lyn Farrall-Miles
Contact: 3 Downs Park West,
Westbury Park, Bristol, BS6 7QQ

📞 0117 9624065
@ Dawnsherwood22@yahoo.co.uk

Backing on to Durdham Downs and permitting beautiful views, Stokeleigh Lodge is situated very close to local facilities including a supermarket, bookshop and antique shop. The home's mature gardens feature flowerbeds and well-established trees and shrubs. The home has its own transport for outings and arranges a Communion service once a month. The activities coordinator also arranges daily activities such as arts and crafts and musical entertainment.

Registered places: 17
Guide weekly rate: £364–£593
Specialist care: Respite
Medical services: Podiatry, dentist, optician
Qualified staff: Exceeds standard: 70% at NVQ level 2

Home details
Location: Residential area, 2.5 miles from Bristol
Communal areas: Lounge, dining room, conservatory, garden
Accessibility: *Floors:* 3 • *Access:* Stair lift • *Wheelchair access:* Good
Smoking: ✗
Pets: ✗
Routines: Flexible

Room details
Single: 17
Shared: 0
En suite: Undisclosed
Facilities: TV point, telephone point

Door lock: ✓
Lockable place: ✓

Services provided
Beauty services: Hairdressing
Mobile library: ✓
Religious services: Monthly Communion service
Transport: Car
Activities: *Coordinator:* ✓ *Examples:* Arts and crafts, reminiscence *Outings:* ✓
Meetings: ✓

Registered places: 24
Guide weekly rate: £348–£415
Specialist care: Dementia, respite
Medical services: Podiatry, dentist, optician, physiotherapy
Qualified staff: Undisclosed

Home details

Location: Village location, 3 miles from Bristol
Communal areas: 3 lounges, dining room, garden
Accessibility: *Floors:* 3 • *Access:* Lift • *Wheelchair access:* Good
Smoking: ✗
Pets: ✗
Routines: Structured

Room details

Single: 20
Shared: 2
En suite: Undisclosed
Facilities: Telephone

Door lock: ✓
Lockable place: ✓

Services provided

Beauty services: Hairdressing
Mobile library: ✗
Religious services: ✗
Transport: Minibus
Activities: *Coordinator:* ✗ • *Examples:* Entertainment • *Outings:* ✓
Meetings: ✗

The Worthies

Manager: Shaun Locke
Owner: The Worthies Residential Care Home Ltd
Contact: 79 Park Road, Stapleton, Bristol, BS16 1DT
☏ 0117 9390088
🖰 www.worthiescarehome.com

The Worthies is in the village of Frenchay, approximately three miles from Bristol. It is a family-run home with pleasant grounds and mature trees. The Worthies offer social activities such as house parties, themed meals and visiting musicians. It also has its own minibus, meaning regular outings are offered. The home has three lounges for residents to relax in as well as a separate dining room.

Registered places: 21
Guide weekly rate: £380–£500
Specialist care: Emergency admissions, respite
Medical services: Podiatry, dentist, optician
Qualified staff: Exceeds standard: 80% at NVQ level 2

Home details

Location: Residential area, 4.5 miles from Bristol
Communal areas: 3 lounges, dining room, garden
Accessibility: *Floors:* 2 • *Access:* Lift • *Wheelchair access:* Good
Smoking: ✗
Pets: At manager's discretion
Routines: Flexible

Room details

Single: 21
Shared: 0
En suite: 18
Facilities: TV point

Door lock: ✓
Lockable place: ✓

Services provided

Beauty services: Hairdressing
Mobile library: ✓
Religious services: ✗
Transport: ✗
Activities: *Coordinator:* ✗ • *Examples:* Arts and crafts, exercise
   Outings: ✓
Meetings: ✓

Whitelodge Care Home For The Elderly

Manager: Karen Notton
Owner: Quality Care Homes Ltd
Contact: 101 Downend Road, Fishponds, Bristol, BS16 5BD
☏ 0117 9567109

Set back from Downend Road in its own grounds, Whitelodge Care Home is situated in a residential area of Fishponds across the road from local amenities. Whitelodge has spacious lawned gardens with an ornamental pond. The home has been awarded a four-star environmental health award for their 'high standards of food hygiene'. The home also arranges daily activities and regular outings to entertain the residents.

Amberley House Care Home

Manager: Lindsay Pugh
Owner: Dove Care Homes Ltd
Contact: The Crescent,
Truro, Cornwall, TR1 3ES
☎ 01872 271921
@ Amberley1@btconnect.com

Situated in a quiet residential area, approximately 10 minutes' hilly walk from the centre of Truro, Amberley House Care Home is also located close to shops, a post office and other amenities. There are three floors and access is via a stair lift or stairs, therefore there is limited access for wheelchair users.

Registered places: 30
Guide weekly rate: £440–£670
Specialist care: Nursing, physical disability
Medical services: Podiatry, optician, physiotherapy
Qualified staff: Undisclosed

Room details
Single: 16
Shared: 6
En suite: 1
Facilities: TV point

Door lock: ✗
Lockable place: ✗

Home details
Location: Residential area, in Truro
Communal areas: Lounge, garden
Accessibility: *Floors:* 3 • *Access:* Stair lift • *Wheelchair access:* Limited
Smoking: ✗
Pets: At manager's discretion
Routines: Structured

Services provided
Beauty services: Hairdressing, hand massage
Mobile library: ✗
Religious services: ✗
Transport: ✗
Activities: *Coordinator:* ✓ • *Examples:* Bingo, singalongs, *Outings:* ✗
Meetings: ✗

Antron Manor Care Home

Manager: Kenneth Rogers
Owner: Kenneth Rogers
Contact: Antron Hill,
Mabe Burnthouse,
Penryn, Cornwall, TR10 9HH
☎ 01326 376570
@ rogerswsl@aol.com

Antron Manor Care Home is set in an acre of landscaped gardens. The home is located in a village three miles outside of Penryn. The home has three lounges and a conservatory for residents to relax in. There is also a garden for residents to enjoy in the warmer months. There is a Communion service once a month and daily activities such as bingo and musical entertainment.

Registered places: 16
Guide weekly rate: £360–£420
Specialist care: Day care, respite
Medical services: Podiatry, hygienist, optician, physiotherapy
Qualified staff: Undisclosed

Home details
Location: Village location, 3 miles from Penryn
Communal areas: 3 lounges, 3 dining rooms, conservatory, garden
Accessibility: *Floors:* 2 • *Access:* Stair lift • *Wheelchair access:* Good
Smoking: ✗
Pets: At manager's discretion
Routines: Structured

Room details
Single: 15
Shared: 1
En suite: 16
Facilities: TV point, telephone point

Door lock: ✓
Lockable place: ✓

Services provided
Beauty services: Hairdressing
Mobile library: ✓
Religious services: Monthly Communion service
Transport: Car
Activities: *Coordinator:* ✗ • *Examples:* Armchair aerobics, bingo, musical entertainment • *Outings:* ✗
Meetings: ✓

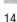

Registered places: 18
Guide weekly rate: £310
Specialist care: Day care, respite
Medical services: Podiatry, hygienist, optician, physiotherapy
Qualified staff: Meets standard

Home details

Location: Rural area, 1 mile from Callington
Communal areas: Lounge, dining room, bar, garden
Accessibility: *Floors:* 1 • *Wheelchair access:* Good
Smoking: ✗
Pets: At manager's discretion
Routines: Flexible

Room details

Single: 18
Shared: 0
En suite: Undisclosed
Facilities: TV point, telephone point

Door lock: ✓
Lockable place: ✗

Services provided

Beauty services: Hairdressing
Mobile library: ✓
Religious services: Monthly Communion service
Transport: ✗
Activities: *Coordinator:* ✗ • *Examples:* Musical entertainment, reminiscence • *Outings:* ✗
Meetings: ✗

Appleby Lodge

Manager: Janice Rider
Owner: Appleby Rest Homes Ltd
Contact: 157 Launceston Road, Kelly Bray, Callington, Cornwall, PL17 8DU
☎ 01579 383979

Appleby Lodge is a purpose-built home with a landscaped garden. It is situated a five-minute walk from local amenities including a pub, post office and shops. Before admission to the home, many of the people have lived locally in the area. Therefore, some people already know the staff and have a good relationship with them. The home also arranges a range of daily activities such as reminiscence sessions.

Registered places: 13
Guide weekly rate: £300–£340
Specialist care: Day care, respite
Medical services: Podiatry, dentist, optician
Qualified staff: Exceeds standard: 60% at NVQ level 2

Home details

Location: Village location, 3 miles from St Ives
Communal areas: 2 lounges, dining room, garden
Accessibility: *Floors:* 2 • *Access:* Stair lift • *Wheelchair access:* Good
Smoking: In designated area
Pets: ✗
Routines: Flexible

Room details

Single: 9
Shared: 2
En suite: 2
Facilities: None

Door lock: ✓
Lockable place: ✓

Services provided

Beauty services: Hairdressing
Mobile library: ✓
Religious services: Monthly Anglican Communion service
Transport: Car
Activities: *Coordinator:* ✗ • *Examples:* Visiting entertainers *Outings:* ✓
Meetings: ✗

Ar-lyn

Manager: Peter Oxley
Owner: Peter Oxley
Contact: Vicarage Lane, Lelant, St Ives, Cornwall, TR26 3JZ
☎ 01736 753330

Set in its own secluded gardens, Ar-lyn is a large property close to the river Hale. The home is located in a village approximately three miles from St Ives. The home's acre of gardens plays host to a variety of small animal enclosures and aviaries. The home has its own car for outings and arranges other activities such as visiting entertainers. There is an Anglican Communion service once a month and the home also arranges for a mobile library to visit the home.

Atlantis

Manager: Catherine Brailey
Owner: Steven and Catherine Brailey
Contact: Polperro Road,
Polperro, Cornwall, PL13 2JE
) 01503 272243
@ atlantis.care@btconnect.com

A detached home set in large grounds, Atlantis permits spectacular views of the surrounding countryside and distant sea. Due to the variation in resident needs, part of the home is kept secure for safety reasons with keypads at the door. The home has three lounges and a garden for residents to socialise in, and organises various activities such as music and movement and clothes shows.

Registered places: 20
Guide weekly rate: £380–£420
Specialist care: Day care, dementia, mental disorder
Medical services: Podiatry, dentist, optician
Qualified staff: Exceeds standard: 62% at NVQ level 2

Home details
Location: Rural area, 1.2 miles from Polperro
Communal areas: 3 lounges, dining room, garden
Accessibility: *Floors:* 2 • *Access:* Stair lift • *Wheelchair access:* Good
Smoking: In designated area
Pets: ✗
Routines: Flexible

Room details
Single: 16
Shared: 2
En suite: 8
Facilities: TV point, telephone point

Door lock: ✓
Lockable place: ✗

Services provided
Beauty services: Hairdressing, massage
Mobile library: ✓
Religious services: Monthly Anglican Communion service
Transport: Car
Activities: *Coordinator:* ✗ • *Examples:* Music and movement, singalongs, clothes show • *Outings:* ✗
Meetings: ✗

Averlea

Manager: Beverley Easdon
Owner: David and Julia Evely
Contact: Fore Street,
Polgooth, St Austell, Cornwall, PL26 7BP
) 01726 66892

Located in the centre of Polgooth, Averlea has good ties with the local community and is a few minutes' walk from a local shop and post office. There is a residents meeting held once a month to give residents the opportunity to voice any opinions they may have. The home also organises an Anglican Communion service twice a month. On a regular basis the home arranges activities such as bingo to entertain residents.

Registered places: 14
Guide weekly rate: From £300
Specialist care: Dementia, respite
Medical services: Podiatry, dentist, optician
Qualified staff: Exceeds standard: 100% at NVQ level 2

Home details
Location: Residential area, 2.5 miles from St Austell
Communal areas: Lounge, dining room, garden
Accessibility: *Floors:* 2 • *Access:* Stair lift • *Wheelchair access:* Good
Smoking: In designated area
Pets: ✓
Routines: Flexible

Room details
Single: 13
Shared: 1
En suite: 1
Facilities: TV point, telephone point

Door lock: ✓
Lockable place: ✓

Services provided
Beauty services: Hairdressing
Mobile library: ✗
Religious services: Fortnightly Anglican Communion service
Transport: ✗
Activities: *Coordinator:* ✗ • *Examples:* Bingo, games • *Outings:* ✗
Meetings: ✓

Registered places: 29
Guide weekly rate: £400–£450
Specialist care: Day care, dementia, mental disorder,
    physical disability, respite
Medical services: Podiatry, dentist, optician
Qualified staff: Exceeds standard: 95% at NVQ level 2

Home details
Location: Rural area, 0.5 miles from North Petherwin
Communal areas: 2 lounges, dining room, conservatory, garden
Accessibility: *Floors:* 2 • *Access:* Stair lift • *Wheelchair access:* Good
Smoking: ✗
Pets: ✓
Routines: Structured

Room details
Single: 29
Shared: 0 | Door lock: ✓
En suite: 29 | Lockable place: ✓
Facilities: TV point, telephone point

Services provided
Beauty services: Hairdressing
Mobile library: ✗
Religious services: Fortnightly Methodist service,
    Anglican Communion service every 3 weeks
Transport: ✗
Activities: *Coordinator:* ✗ • *Examples:* Arts and crafts, bingo, cooking
    Outings: ✓
Meetings: ✗

Beaumont Court

Manager: Sally Julian
Owner: Wentworth Healthcare Ltd
Contact: North Petherwin,
Launceston, Cornwall, PL15 8LR
☎ 01566 785350

Set in its own grounds, Beaumont Court is located in the picturesque Cornish countryside, on the outskirts of a village. The nearest town, Launceton, is seven miles away and residents enjoy trips to the seaside at Bude, 13 miles away. The home also arranges regular activities in the home, such as bingo and arts and crafts sessions. The home also arranges a variety of religious services for residents to partake in.

Registered places: 30
Guide weekly rate: Undisclosed
Specialist care: Nursing, physical disability
Medical services: Podiatry, dentist
Qualified staff: Exceeds standard: 68% at NVQ level 2

Home details
Location: Residential area, 0.5 miles from Liskeard
Communal areas: Lounge, 2 dining rooms, patio
Accessibility: *Floors:* 2 • *Access:* Stair lift • *Wheelchair access:* Limited
Smoking: ✗
Pets: Undisclosed
Routines: Undisclosed

Room details
Single: 25
Shared: 2 | Door lock: ✗
En suite: 0 | Lockable place: ✓
Facilities: TV point

Services provided
Beauty services: None
Mobile library: ✗
Religious services: ✗
Transport: People carrier
Activities: *Coordinator:* ✗ • *Examples:* Arts and crafts, quizzes
    Outings: ✓
Meetings: Undisclosed

Beech Lawn Nursing & Residential Home

Manager: Julie Weale
Owner: Beech Lawn Care Home Ltd
Contact: Higher Lux Street,
Liskeard, Cornwall, PL14 3JX
☎ 01579 346460

Beech Lawn is a listed property with a purpose-built extension situated near the centre of Liskeard in a quiet residential area. At the rear of the home there is a sheltered courtyard patio with pleasant seating areas. A range of activities is organised for residents and trips into the centre of town are made regularly. The home has its own people carrier to transport residents.

The Beeches

Manager: Marian Rich
Owner: Peter and Lesley Pool
Contact: St Georges Road,
Hayle, Cornwall, TR27 4AH
☏ 01736 752725
@ peterpool@thebeechescornwall.co.uk
🖰 www.thebeechescornwall.co.uk

The Beeches is a Grade II listed Georgian building set in one acre of landscaped gardens. The home is located in the centre of Hayle, offering easy access to local amenities. The home has a residents meeting once a year to discuss any issues the residents may have. There are weekly Communion services in the home and the activities coordinator arranges a varied programme which includes bingo and musical entertainment.

Registered places: 28
Guide weekly rate: £525–£625
Specialist care: Nursing, respite, physical disability
Medical services: Podiatry, dentist, optician
Qualified staff: Exceeds standard: 57% at NVQ level 2

Home details

Location: Residential area, 0.5 miles from Hayle
Communal areas: Lounge, dining room, conservatory, garden
Accessibility: *Floors:* 2 • *Access:* Lift • *Wheelchair access:* Good
Smoking: ✗
Pets: At manager's discretion
Routines: Flexible

Room details

Single: 22
Shared: 3
En suite: 25
Facilities: TV point, telephone point

Door lock: ✓
Lockable place: ✓

Services provided

Beauty services: Hairdressing
Mobile library: ✗
Religious services: Weekly Communion service
Transport: ✗
Activities: *Coordinator:* ✓ • *Examples:* Bingo, games, musical entertainment • *Outings:* ✗
Meetings: ✓

Benoni Nursing Home

Manager: Janice Mason
Owner: Benoni Nursing Home Ltd
Contact: 12 Carrallack Terrace,
St Just, Cornwall, TR19 7LW
☏ 01736 788433
@ kenowcare@aol.com

Benoni Nursing Home is located in a residential area, approximately one mile from St Just. The home has an activities coordinator who arranges various activities, which are suitable to the age and general infirmity of the residents. These activities include bingo, exercises and one-to-one sessions. Visitors are always welcome and they visit regularly throughout the day.

Registered places: 21
Guide weekly rate: £350–£550
Specialist care: Nursing, dementia, physical disability, respite
Medical services: Undisclosed
Qualified staff: Meets standard

Home details

Location: Residential area, 1 mile from St Just
Communal areas: Undisclosed
Accessibility: *Floors:* 3 • *Access:* Lift • *Wheelchair access:* Limited
Smoking: ✗
Pets: ✗
Routines: Flexible

Room details

Single: 15
Shared: 3
En suite: Undisclosed
Facilities: None

Door lock: ✗
Lockable place: ✗

Services provided

Beauty services: Hairdressing
Mobile library: ✗
Religious services: ✗
Transport: ✗
Activities: *Coordinator:* ✓ • *Examples:* Bingo, exercise to music *Outings:* ✗
Meetings: Undisclosed

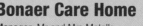

Registered places: 31
Guide weekly rate: £345–£515
Specialist care: Nursing, day care, palliative, physical disability, respite
Medical services: Podiatry, dentist, optician
Qualified staff: Undisclosed

Home details
Location: Residential area, in Hayle
Communal areas: 2 lounges, dining room, conservatory, library/
music room, garden
Accessibility: *Floors:* 2 • *Access:* Lift • *Wheelchair access:* Good
Smoking: In designated area
Pets: ✓
Routines: Flexible

Room details
Single: 25
Shared: 3
En suite: 0
Facilities: TV

Door lock: ✗
Lockable place: ✗

Services provided
Beauty services: Hairdressing
Mobile library: Library facilities
Religious services: Monthly Communion service
Transport: ✗
Activities: *Coordinator:* ✗ • *Examples:* Arts and crafts, bingo, music
therapy, visiting entertainers • *Outings:* ✓
Meetings: ✓

Bonaer Care Home

Manager: Mr and Mrs Metalle
Owner: Mr and Mrs Metalle
Contact: 17 Station Hill,
Hayle, Cornwall, TR27 4NG
☏ 01736 752090

Well-placed to deliver views of Hayle Estuary and St Ives bay, Bonaer Care Home is a five-minute walk from the town's shops, banks and post office and next to the railway station. In Bonaer's gardens there is a fishpond and a rabbit also lives on the premises. Employing flexible visiting rights, residents are encouraged to maintain good links with the community, also enjoying frequent in-house entertainment from local choirs and drama groups. Although only having approximately one outing a year, the home offers a comprehensive in-house activities programme.

Registered places: 38
Guide weekly rate: Undisclosed
Specialist care: Dementia, mental disorder
Medical services: Undisclosed
Qualified staff: Undisclosed

Home details
Location: Residential area, 0.5 miles from St Ives
Communal areas: Undisclosed
Accessibility: *Floors:* 3 • *Access:* Lift and stair lift
Wheelchair access: Good
Smoking: ✗
Pets: ✗
Routines: Undisclosed

Room details
Single: 38
Shared: 0
En suite: Undisclosed
Facilities: None

Door lock: ✗
Lockable place: ✗

Services provided
Beauty services: Hairdressing
Mobile library: ✗
Religious services: Monthly Anglican visits
Transport: ✗
Activities: *Coordinator:* ✓ • *Examples:* Cream tea, singalongs
Outings: ✓
Meetings: ✗

Carrick Lodge

Manager: Trudy Izatt
Owner: Ronald Cottam
Contact: Belyars Lane,
St Ives, Cornwall, TR26 2BZ
☏ 01736 794353

In an elevated position, Carrick Lodge gives residents views of the bay. The home is located in a residential area, half a mile from St Ives. There is a designated activities coordinator at the home. The activities take place on a regular basis and include cream tea afternoons and exercise sessions. Residents are also taken on walks in the local area.

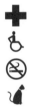

Castle Hill House

Manager: Carol Edwards
Owner: Castle Hill House Ltd
Contact: Castle Hill,
Bodmin, Cornwall, PL31 2DY
☏ 01208 73802
@ carol@castlehillhouse.net
🖥 www.castlehillhouse.net

A grand older-style property, Castle Hill House is set in its own grounds in a quiet residential area of Bodmin. The home's location permits beautiful views of the surrounding countryside. Building works are taking place to add an extension, including a conservatory, to Castle Hill House. The home has a residents meeting every three weeks and the daily activities programme include painting and gardening. The home also has its own transport.

Registered places: 20
Guide weekly rate: £455–£500
Specialist care: Nursing, day care, dementia, mental disorder, physical disability, respite
Medical services: Podiatry, dentist, optician
Qualified staff: Meets standard

Home details
Location: Residential area, 0.5 miles from Bodmin
Communal areas: Lounge, dining room, garden
Accessibility: *Floors:* 2 • *Access:* Lift • *Wheelchair access:* Good
Smoking: ✗
Pets: ✓
Routines: Flexible

Room details
Single: 14
Shared: 3
En suite: 0
Facilities: TV point, telephone point

Door lock: ✓
Lockable place: ✓

Services provided
Beauty services: Hairdressing
Mobile library: ✗
Religious services: Weekly Anglican service, monthly Anglican Communion service
Transport: Car
Activities: *Coordinator:* ✓ • *Examples:* Painting, Pets As Therapy
Outings: ✗
Meetings: ✓

Cathedral View Nursing Home

Manager: Mrs Gilbert
Owner: Cathedral View Ltd
Contact: Kenwyn Church Road,
Truro, Cornwall, TR1 3DR
☏ 01872 222132

Located on the same site as its sister home Cathedral View Residential Home, Cathedral View Nursing Home is a purpose-built home set in two acres of land. With one lounge dedicated to quiet, the other has a piano and patio doors opening onto the home's attractive gardens. With an extensive activities programme that includes one-to-one sessions, Cathedral View Nursing Home also provides residents with outings which are covered by the standard fee and allow residents to venture further from the home's grounds, should they wish.

Registered places: 26
Guide weekly rate: Undisclosed
Specialist care: Nursing, physical disability
Medical services: Podiatry, dentist, optician, physiotherapy
Qualified staff: Undisclosed

Home details
Location: Residential Area, 0.75 miles from Truro
Communal areas: 2 lounges, dining room, garden
Accessibility: *Floors:* 2 • *Access:* Lift • *Wheelchair access:* Good
Smoking: ✗
Pets: ✓
Routines: Flexible

Room details
Single: 18
Shared: 4
En suite: 10
Facilities: TV point, telephone point

Door lock: ✗
Lockable place: ✗

Services provided
Beauty services: Hairdressing.
Mobile library: ✗
Religious services: Monthly Communion service
Transport: ✗
Activities: *Coordinator:* ✓ • *Examples:* Art group, sewing group
Outings: ✓
Meetings: ✓

Registered places: 34
Guide weekly rate: Undisclosed
Specialist care: Day care, dementia, mental disorder, respite
Medical services: Podiatry, dentist, optician, physiotherapy
Qualified staff: Undisclosed

Room details
Single: 30
Shared: 2
En suite: 9
Facilities: TV point, telephone point

Door lock: ✗
Lockable place: ✗

Home details
Location: Residential Area, 0.75 miles from Truro
Communal areas: 2 lounges, dining room, conservatory, garden
Accessibility: *Floors:* 3 • *Access:* Lift • *Wheelchair access:* Good
Smoking: In designated area
Pets: ✓
Routines: Flexible

Services provided
Beauty services: Hairdressing.
Mobile library: ✗
Religious services: Monthly Communion service
Transport: ✗
Activities: *Coordinator:* ✓ • *Examples:* Art group, exercise sessions
   Outings: ✓
Meetings: ✓

Cathedral View Residential Home

Manager: Mrs Gilbert
Owner: Cathedral View Ltd
Contact: Kenwyn Church Road,
Truro, Cornwall, TR1 3DR
☏ 01872 240974

Located on the same site as its sister home Cathedral View Nursing Home, Cathedral View Residential Home is a listed building set in two acres of land. With attractive gardens that include a water feature and outdoor bench, Cathedral View Nursing Home also has two spacious lounges and a number of seating areas throughout the home. For the purpose of quality assurance, residents are sent a questionnaire on an annual basis.

Registered places: 34
Guide weekly rate: £385–£420
Specialist care: Dementia, mental disorder, respite
Medical services: Podiatry, dentist
Qualified staff: Meets standard

Home details
Location: Rural area, 3.5 miles from Bodmin
Communal areas: 3 lounges, dining room, garden
Accessibility: *Floors:* 2 • *Access: Stair lift* • *Wheelchair access:* Good
Smoking: ✗
Pets: At manager's discretion
Routines: Flexible

Room details
Single: 32
Shared: 1
En suite: 28
Facilities:

Door lock: ✓
Lockable place: ✓

Services provided
Beauty services: Hairdressing
Mobile library: Library facilities
Religious services: Monthly Communion service
Transport: ✗
Activities: *Coordinator:* ✗ • *Examples:* Arts and crafts, exercise,
   skittles • *Outings* ✓
Meetings: ✓

Clann House Residential Home

Manager: Julia Frape
Owner: Susan and John Clarkson
Contact: Clann House Residential Home,
Clann Lane, Lanivet, Cornwall, PL30 5HD
☏ 01208 831305
@ Julia.frape@btconnect.com

Clann House is located in a rural area three and a half miles from Bodmin. The home is an adapted farmhouse set in three and a half acres of ground offering views of the surrounding countryside. Inside the home there is ample communal space with three lounges and a dining room. There is also a courtyard garden. The home has its own library facilities, including large-print books and arranges activities such as arts and crafts and skittles for the residents.

Clinton House Care Home

Manager: Patricia Nancarrow
Owner: Morleigh Ltd
Contact: 75 Truro Road,
St Austell, Cornwall, PL25 5JQ
☏ 01726 63663
@ clinton.house@btconnect.com

Clinton House is an extended period property situated around half a mile from St Austell town centre. The home is located near to important resources, such as a post office, library, and shopping centre. Residents may bring their own furniture and choose their room decoration. There is a lot of flexibility about meals. Residents can also bring their pets. Individual hobbies are catered for. The activities programme includes visiting entertainers and one-to-one sessions.

Registered places: 39
Guide weekly rate: £350–£550
Specialist care: Nursing, day care, respite
Medical services: Podiatry, physiotherapy
Qualified staff: Exceeds standard: 80% at NVQ level 2

Home details
Location: Residential area, 0.5 miles from St Austell
Communal areas: 2 lounges, 2 dining room, patio and garden
Accessibility: *Floors:* 2 • *Access:* Lift and stair lift
  Wheelchair access: Good
Smoking: ✗
Pets: ✓
Routines: Flexible

Room details
Single: 38
Shared: 1
En suite: Undisclosed
Facilities: TV point

Door lock: ✓
Lockable place: ✓

Services provided
Beauty services: Hairdressing
Mobile library: ✗
Religious services: ✗
Transport: ✗
Activities: *Coordinator:* ✓ • *Examples:* Themed evenings, visiting entertainers • *Outings:* ✗
Meetings: ✗

Clovelly House

Manager: June Hartigan
Owner: June Hartigan
Contact: St Michaels Road,
Newquay, Cornwall, TR7 1RA
☏ 01637 876 668
@ junehartigan@hotmail.com

A detached home set in its own grounds, Clovelly House combines sea views with close proximity to local amenities. The library and nearby bus stop are practically on its doorstep while the nearest shop is less than one minute's walk away, thus allowing residents much independence. Since opening in 1981, Clovelly House has been run by Mrs June Hartigan who doubles as the home's owner and manager. Clovelly House provides its residents with monthly outings while visits from Pets As Therapy provide residents with much enjoyment.

Registered places: 19
Guide weekly rate: £298–£340
Specialist care: Day care, respite
Medical services: Podiatry, dentist, optician, physiotherapy
Qualified staff: Exceeds standard: 68% at NVQ level 2

Home details
Location: Residential area, in Newquay
Communal areas: Lounge, dining room, smoking area, 2 conservatories, garden
Accessibility: *Floors:* 2 • *Access:* Lift • *Wheelchair access:* Good
Smoking: In designated area
Pets: At manager's discretion
Routines: Flexible

Room details
Single: 19
Shared: 0
En suite: 17
Facilities: TV point, telephone point

Door lock: ✓
Lockable place: ✓

Services provided
Beauty services: Hairdressing
Mobile library: ✗
Religious services: Weekly Anglican, Catholic and Methodist visits, monthly Communion service
Transport: ✗
Activities: *Coordinator:* ✗ • *Examples:* Bingo, visiting entertainers *Outings:* ✗
Meetings: ✗

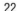

Registered places: 45
Guide weekly rate: £420–£600
Specialist care: Nursing, day care, physical disability, respite
Medical services: None
Qualified staff: Exceeds standard: 90% at NVQ level 2

Home details

Location: Rural area, 0.5 miles from Lostwithiel
Communal areas: 2 lounges, dining room, garden
Accessibility: *Floors:* 2 • *Access:* Lift • *Wheelchair access:* Good
Smoking: In designated area
Pets: At manager's discretion
Routines: Flexible

Room details

Single: 39
Shared: 3
En suite: 42
Facilities: TV point, telephone point

Door lock: ✓
Lockable place: ✓

Services provided

Beauty services: Hairdressing, aromatherapy
Mobile library: ✗
Religious services: Monthly Catholic Mass, monthly Anglican service
Transport: ✓
Activities: *Coordinator:* ✓ • *Examples:* Music therapy, Pets As Therapy
    Outings: ✓
Meetings: ✗

Collamere

Manager: Jane Eldridge
Owner: Pinerace
Contact: Grenville Road,
Lostwithiel, Cornwall, PL22 0RA
) 01208 872810
@ collamere@btconnect.com

Collamere is a traditional house that has been purposefully extended to better cater for the needs of residents. It has recently been redecorated. There is a garden with a patio area and gazebo. The home is situated in a rural area, half a mile from Lostwithiel. The home arranges a Catholic Mass once a month and an Anglican service once a month. The home also has its own transport, which is used when residents go on outings.

Registered places: 16
Guide weekly rate: £340–£375
Specialist care: Dementia, mental disorder, respite
Medical services: Podiatry, dentist, optician
Qualified staff: Exceeds standard: 80% at NVQ level 2

Home details

Location: Rural area, 1 mile from Liskeard
Communal areas: 2 lounges, dining room, garden
Accessibility: *Floors:* 2 • *Access:* Stair lift • *Wheelchair access:* Good
Smoking: ✗
Pets: ✓
Routines: Flexible

Room details

Single: 16
Shared: 0
En suite: Undisclosed
Facilities: None

Door lock: ✗
Lockable place: ✓

Services provided

Beauty services: Hairdressing
Mobile library: ✗
Religious services: ✗
Transport: ✗
Activities: *Coordinator:* ✓ • *Examples:* Equipment available
    Outings: ✗
Meetings: ✗

Coombe House

Manager: Ann Gray
Owner: Ann Gray
Contact: Coombe Lane,
Lamellion, Liskeard, Cornwall, PL14 4JU
) 01579 346819
@ anngray@clara.co.uk

Coombe House is located in a rural area, approximately one mile from Liskeard. The home is well maintained and the registered provider has invested in necessary equipment to aid the safety of residents. The home has no formal activities programme but has a variety of equipment available for residents' use. The home also has two lounges for residents to relax in.

Courtlands

Manager: Julie Hocking
Owner: Mark and Gillian Fairhurst
Contact: Rosudgeon,
Penzance, Cornwall, TR20 9PN
) 01736 710476

A large property that stands in its own grounds, Courtlands is about six miles from Penzance town centre. The home's owners are heavily involved with the day-to-day management and administration of the home. The home has a residents meeting once a month and provides a variety of services such as transportation and a fortnightly religious service.

Registered places: 35
Guide weekly rate: £293–£469
Specialist care: Day care, dementia, mental disorder, respite
Medical services: Podiatry, dentist, optician
Qualified staff: Meets standard

Home details
Location: Rural area, 6 miles from Penzance
Communal areas: 3 lounges, dining room, garden
Accessibility: *Floors:* 2 • *Access:* Lift • *Wheelchair access:* Good
Smoking: ✗
Pets: At manager's discretion
Routines: Flexible

Room details
Single: 29
Shared: 3
En suite: 16
Facilities: TV point, telephone point

Door lock: ✓
Lockable place: ✓

Services provided
Beauty services: Hairdressing
Mobile library: ✓
Religious services: Fortnightly nondenominational service
Transport: Cars
Activities: *Coordinator:* ✗ • *Examples:* Arts and crafts, reminiscence
  Outings: ✗
Meetings: ✓

Crantock Lodge

Manager: Carole Taylor
Owner: Carole Taylor
Contact: 34 Bonython Road,
Newquay, Cornwall, TR7 3AN
) 01637 872112
@ carendave@crantocklodge.
  wanadoo.co.uk

Permitting attractive sea views, Crantock Lodge is situated on level ground a few hundred yards from local facilities including small shops and a bank. The home is located in a residential area, one mile from Newquay. The home has its own library facilities and is also visited by a mobile library. There is a residents meeting twice a year to discuss any issues the residents may have. The home arranges outings for the residents as well as internal activities such as bingo.

Registered places: 10
Guide weekly rate: £400
Specialist care: Day care
Medical services: Podiatry, optician
Qualified staff: Meets standard

Home details
Location: Residential area, 1 mile from Newquay
Communal areas: Lounge, dining room, library, conservatory, garden
Accessibility: *Floors:* 2 • *Access:* Stair lift • *Wheelchair access:* Good
Smoking: ✗
Pets: ✗
Routines: Flexible

Room details
Single: 9
Shared: 1
En suite: 10
Facilities: TV point, telephone point

Door lock: ✓
Lockable place: ✓

Services provided
Beauty services: Hairdressing
Mobile library: ✓
Religious services: ✗
Transport: ✗
Activities: *Coordinator:* ✗ • *Examples:* Bingo • *Outings:* ✓
Meetings: ✓

Registered places: 12
Guide weekly rate: £340–£400
Specialist care: Day care, respite
Medical services: Podiatry, dentist, optician, physiotherapy
Qualified staff: Undisclosed

Home details
Location: Village location, in Tintagel
Communal areas: Lounge/dining room, garden
Accessibility: *Floors:* 1 • *Wheelchair access:* Good
Smoking: ✗
Pets: At manager's discretion
Routines: Flexible

Room details
Single: 8
Shared: 2
En suite: 0
Facilities: TV point

Door lock: ✓
Lockable place: ✓

Services provided
Beauty services: Hairdressing, massage
Mobile library: ✗
Religious services: Monthly nondenominational Communion service
Transport: ✗
Activities: *Coordinator:* ✓ • *Examples:* Bell ringing, bingo
  Outings: ✗
Meetings: ✓

Eirenikon Park Residential Home

Manager: Mrs Bennett
Owner: Mr and Mrs Bennett,
Mrs Van Zyl-Lamb
Contact: Bossiney Road,
Tintagel, Cornwall, PL34 0AE
☎ 01840 770252

A single-storey building situated in 'King Arthur's country', Tintagel, Eirenikon Park is within good reach of local amenities with the doctor's surgery, post office and shops within five minutes' walk. Permitting beautiful views of the nearby coast and countryside, Eirenikon is ideal for animal lovers, as the home currently has two small dogs and a cat.

Registered places: 18
Guide weekly rate: £320–£420
Specialist care: Day care, emergency admissions,
  mental disorder, respite
Medical services: Podiatry, dentist, optician, physiotherapy
Qualified staff: Undisclosed

Home details
Location: Rural area 6 miles from Liskeard
Communal areas: 2 lounges, dining room, garden
Accessibility: *Floors:* 3 • *Access:* Stair lift • *Wheelchair access:* Good
Smoking: In designated area
Pets: At manager's discretion
Routines: Flexible

Room details
Single: 14
Shared: 1
En suite: 2
Facilities: TV point, telephone point

Door lock: ✓
Lockable place: ✓

Services provided
Beauty services: Hairdressing, manicures
Mobile library: Library facilities
Religious services: Monthly Anglican service
Transport: ✗
Activities: *Coordinator:* ✗ • *Examples:* Bingo, painting, quizzes
  Outings: ✓
Meetings: ✓

Eldon House

Manager: Sharon Hancock
Owner: Sharob Care Homes Ltd
Contact: Downgate,
Upton Cross,
Liskeard, Cornwall, PL14 5AJ
☎ 01579 362686
@ care@eldonhouse.com
🖱 www.eldonhouse.com

A restored ex-mine captain's house – part of which is almost 200 years old – Eldon House is located in a rural area in the moorland hills and is set in five acres of ground. Home to two dogs and two horses who live in stables at the back of the gardens, Eldon House is a mile and a half from the nearest shop and a bus stop is located just outside the home with services to Launceston. Residents are free to explore the accessible grounds while the home holds summer fêtes and parties. A monthly newsletter is also sent out to relatives updating them on activities and events.

CORNWALL

The Elms Care Centre

Manager: Mrs Weaver
Owner: The Aldington Group Ltd
Contact: 108 Grenfell Avenue, Saltash, Cornwall, PL12 4JE

) 01752 846335
@ enquiries@elmscarecentre.co.uk
www.theelmscentre.co.uk

Situated in the thriving town of Saltash on the borders of Cornwall and Devon, The Elms Care Centre is within driving distance of the main shopping centre. Frequented by regular bus services, residents are able to make frequent visits out of the home and enjoy country living. With attractive flowerbeds in the garden and its own library facilities the home has ample resources for residents. As well as visits from Pets As Therapy, a cat belonging to a neighbour spends daytimes at the home. There is ample car parking at the home and a conservatory.

Registered places: 37
Guide weekly rate: £292–£626
Specialist care: Nursing, physical disability, respite
Medical services: Podiatry, dentist, optician
Qualified staff: Meets standard

Home details
Location: Residential area, 1 mile from Saltash
Communal areas: 3 lounges, dining room, conservatory, garden
Accessibility: *Floors:* 2 • *Access:* Lift • *Wheelchair access:* Good
Smoking: In designated area
Pets: At manager's discretion
Routines: Flexible

Room details
Single: 33
Shared: 2
En suite: 18
Facilities: TV point

Door lock: ✗
Lockable place: ✗

Services provided
Beauty services: Hairdressing
Mobile library: Library facilities
Religious services: Monthly Methodist and Anglican services
Transport: Car
Activities: *Coordinator:* ✗ • *Examples:* Arts and crafts, quizzes
    Outings: ✗
Meetings: ✗

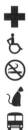

Eshcol House

Manager: Margaret Stobbart-Rowlands
Owner: Mark and Gillian Fairhurst
Contact: 12 Clifton Terrace, Portscatho, Truro, Cornwall, TR2 5HR

) 01872 580291

Set in its own grounds and located in the village of Portscatho in the Roseland Peninsula, the home has wonderful sea views. Eshcol House is located close to village facilities including a post office, a shop, a pub, churches and a doctor's surgery. The home is situated in a rural area, 16 miles from Truro. The home has its own transport for outings and arranges a monthly Communion service.

Registered places: 31
Guide weekly rate: £565–£725
Specialist care: Nursing, dementia, mental disorder, respite
Medical services: Podiatry, dentist, hygienist, optician, physiotherapy
Qualified staff: Exceeds standard: 90% at NVQ level 2

Home details
Location: Rural area, 16 miles from Truro
Communal areas: Lounge, dining room, TV room, garden
Accessibility: *Floors:* 3 • *Access:* Lift and stair lift
    Wheelchair access: Good
Smoking: ✗
Pets: ✓
Routines: Flexible

Room details
Single: 27
Shared: 2
En suite: Undisclosed
Facilities: TV point, telephone point

Door lock: ✓
Lockable place: ✓

Services provided
Beauty services: Hairdressing
Mobile Library: ✓
Religious services: Monthly Communion service
Transport: Car
Activities: *Coordinator:* ✓ • *Examples:* Art, cooking, music
    Outings: ✓
Meetings: ✗

Registered places: 30
Guide weekly rate: From £445
Specialist care: Day care, dementia, emergency admissions, respite
Medical services: Podiatry, dentist, optician, physiotherapy
Qualified staff: Exceeds standard: 75% at NVQ level 2

Home details
Location: Rural area, 3 miles from Bude
Communal areas: Lounge, dining room, hairdressing salon, garden
Accessibility: *Floors:* 1 • *Wheelchair access:* Good
Smoking: ✗
Pets: At manager's discretion
Routines: Flexible

Room details
Single: 26
Shared: 2   Door lock: ✓
En suite: 28   Lockable place: ✓
Facilities: TV point

Services provided
Beauty services: Hairdressing
Mobile library: ✓
Religious services: Fortnightly service
Transport: ✗
Activities: *Coordinator:* ✗ • *Examples:* Bingo, visiting karaoke
   Outings: ✓
Meetings: ✓

Fairfields Country Rest Home

Manager: Helen Goodgroves
Owner: Mr and Mrs Pantling
Contact: Launcells,
Nr Bude, Cornwall, EX23 9NH
☎ 01288 381241

Situated on a hill in five and a half acres of grounds this single-level house provides panoramic views across the open countryside and out towards the sea. With two acres of landscaped gardens which are regularly tended to, the home is a haven for gardeners, providing a well-stocked pond, flower and vegetable patch and greenhouse for residents to help with. There is also an internal Mediterranean-style garden with raised flowerbeds and ornamental pond. While local amenities are scarce, the home does provide outings to a variety of destinations and there is an in-house shopping trolley.

Registered places: 60
Guide weekly rate: £300–£550
Specialist care: Nursing, day care, physical disability, respite
Medical services: Podiatry
Qualified staff: Meets standard

Home details
Location: Residential area, 0.7 miles from Camborne
Communal areas: 3 lounges, dining room, conservatory, garden
Accessibility: *Floors:* 2 • *Access:* Lift • *Wheelchair access:* Good
Smoking: In designated area
Pets: ✓
Routines: Flexible

Room details
Single: 50
Shared: 5   Door lock: ✓
En suite: 14   Lockable place: ✓
Facilities: TV point, telephone point

Services provided
Beauty services: Hairdressing
Mobile library: ✗
Religious services: Weekly Catholic Mass, monthly Anglican
   Communion service
Transport: ✗
Activities: *Coordinator:* ✓ • *Examples:* Bingo, visiting entertainers
   Outings: ✗
Meetings: ✓

Fairholme

Manager: Douglas Hastings
Owner: Jaspal and Bhupender Mangat
Contact: Roskear, Camborne,
Cornwall, TR14 8DN
☎ 01209 714491
@ fairholmeuk@tiscali.co.uk

Formerly a children's home, Fairholme is located near Camborne town centre. It is approximately a 10-minute walk to the nearest supermarket and about 15 minutes to the centre of town. The home was recently refurbished and boasts a large garden with patio areas. The home also has three lounges for residents to relax in. There is a residents meeting which takes place every three months. The home arranges a Catholic Mass every week and an Anglican Communion service once a month.

Fernleigh House

Manager: Vacant
Owner: Alistair Tinto and Janet Cradick
Contact: Albaston, Gunnislake, Cornwall, PL18 9AJ

) 01822 832926
@ alistair.tinto@virgin.net

A small home set in a rural village location, Fernleigh House is 30 yards from village facilities that include a pub and post office. The home is approximately 18 miles from Plymouth. The home has a lounge and a conservatory for residents to socialise in and there are daily activities such as scrabble and reminiscence sessions. The home also arranges outings for the residents to enjoy.

Registered places: 11
Guide weekly rate: From £392
Specialist care: Day care, dementia, mental disorder
Medical services: Podiatry, optician
Qualified staff: Meets standard

Home details
Location: Village location, 1 mile from Gunnislake
Communal areas: Lounge, dining room, conservatory
Accessibility: *Floors:* 2 • *Access:* Stair lift • *Wheelchair access:* Limited
Smoking: In designated area
Pets: ✓
Routines: Flexible

Room details
Single: 9
Shared: 1
En suite: 10
Facilities: TV point, telephone point

Door lock: ✓
Lockable place: ✓

Services provided
Beauty services: Hairdressing, manicures
Mobile library: ✓
Religious services: Monthly Communion service
Transport: ✗
Activities: *Coordinator:* ✗ • *Examples:* Reminiscence, scrabble
   Outings: ✓
Meetings: ✗

Fistral House

Manager: Geoffrey Dowling
Owner: Geoffrey and Rita Dowling
Contact: 3 Esplanade Road, Pentire, Newquay, Cornwall, TR7 1PY

) 01637 878423

Fistral House is a care home for 13 individuals, situated in a residential area of Newquay, opposite Fistral Beach. The home enjoys sea views from its conservatory and some of its bed rooms. An activity is provided every day for residents to participate in if they wish. The home also arranges outings for the residents. The home also produces a regular newsletter for relatives.

Registered places: 13
Guide weekly rate: £300–£450
Specialist care: Respite
Medical services: Podiatry
Qualified staff: Exceeds standard: 70% at NVQ level 2

Home details
Location: Residential area, 1 mile from Newquay
Communal areas: Lounge, dining room, conservatory, garden
Accessibility: *Floors:* 2 • *Access:* Stair lift • *Wheelchair access:* Good
Smoking: ✗
Pets: ✓
Routine: Flexible

Room details
Single: 13
Shared: 0
En suite: 13
Facilities: Telephone point

Door lock: ✓
Lockable place: ✓

Services provided
Beauty services: Hairdressing
Mobile library: ✗
Religious services: ✗
Transport: ✗
Activities: *Coordinator:* ✗ • *Examples:* Bingo • *Outings:* ✓
Meetings: ✗

Registered places: 20
Guide weekly rate: £474–£625
Specialist care: Nursing, physical disability, respite
Medical services: Podiatry, hygienist, optician, physiotherapy
Qualified staff: Exceeds standard: 77% at NVQ level 2

Home details
Location: Village location, 3 miles from Hayle
Communal areas: 2 lounges, dining room, garden
Accessibility: *Floors:* 2 • *Access:* Lift • *Wheelchair access:* Good
Smoking: In designated area
Pets: At manager's discretion
Routines: Flexible

Room details
Single: 16
Shared: 2
En suite: 7
Facilities: TV point, telephone point

Door lock: ✓
Lockable place: ✓

Services provided
Beauty services: Hairdressing, manicures, massage
Mobile library: ✓
Religious services: Monthly Communion service
Transport: ✗
Activities: *Coordinator:* ✓ • *Examples:* Arts and craft, cookery
　　　Outings: ✓
Meetings: ✗

Glencoe Nursing Home

Manager: Tracey Brooking
Owner: Mrs Lunn
Contact: 23 Churchtown Road,
Gwithian, Hayle, Cornwall, TR27 5BX
☏ 01736 752216
@ info@glencoenursinghome.co.uk
🖰 www.glencoenursinghome.co.uk

Glencoe Nursing Home is set in the village of Gwithian with views over the surrounding countryside. The home is located approximately three miles from Hayle. The home is sheltered from the sea by sand dunes. Once a week there is a trolley shop, where residents can purchase small items such as toiletries and sweets. The home also has an activities coordinator who arranges events such as reminiscence sessions and cookey for the residents.

Registered places: 31
Guide weekly rate: Undisclosed
Specialist care: Day care, respite
Medical services: Podiatry, dentist, optician
Qualified staff: Meets standard

Home details
Location: Rural area, 1.8 miles from St Austell
Communal areas: 2 lounges, dining room, garden
Accessibility: *Floors:* 2 • *Access:* Lift • *Wheelchair access:* Good
Smoking: ✗
Pets: ✗
Routines: Flexible

Room details
Single: 15
Shared: 3
En suite: 18
Facilities: TV point, telephone point

Door lock: ✓
Lockable place: ✓

Services provided
Beauty services: Hairdressing
Mobile library: ✓
Religious services: Monthly Communion service
Transport: Minibus and car
Activities: *Coordinator:* ✓ • *Examples:* Games, poetry,
　　　Outings: ✓
Meetings: ✓

The Grove

Manager: Mr Stevens
Owner: Venetian Healthcare Ltd
Contact: 181 Charlestown Road,
St Austell, Cornwall, PL25 3NP
☏ 01726 76481

Standing in its own grounds on the approach to Charleston harbour, The Grove is situated about 1 mile from St Austell town centre and the train station. Some of the bedrooms in the home have sea views and the home also has a garden for residents to relax in. The home has a monthly Communion service and its own transport, having both a car and a minibus. There is a residents meeting every three months and the activities coordinator conducts one-to-one sessions with the residents as well as group activities.

Hansord

Manager: Heather Bunoomally
Owner: Chandruduth Bunoomally
Contact: Alexandra Road,
Penzance, Cornwall, TR18 4LZ
📞 01736 363311

Situated close to the promenade, Hansord is also very close to a park. The home is located in a residential area, half a mile from Penzance town centre. As well as a modestly sized garden, the home also has a courtyard that residents may access. The home arranges bingo in the home and also takes the residents on outings. The home also has visits from a mobile library.

Registered places: 10
Guide weekly rate: £293–£400
Specialist care: Day care, dementia, mental disorder
Medical services: Podiatry, hygienist, optician, physiotherapy
Qualified staff: Exceeds standard: 60% at NVQ level 2

Home details
Location: Residential area, 0.5 miles from Penzance
Communal areas: Lounge, dining room, garden
Accessibility: *Floors:* 4 • *Access:* Lift • *Wheelchair access:* Good
Smoking: ✗
Pets: ✗
Routines: Structured

Room details
Single: 10
Shared: 0
En suite: 0
Facilities: TV point, telephone point

Door lock: ✓
Lockable place: ✓

Services provided
Beauty services: Hairdressing
Mobile library: ✓
Religious services: ✗
Transport: ✗
Activities: *Coordinator:* ✗ • *Examples:* Bingo • *Outings:* ✓
Meetings: ✗

Highpoint Lodge

Manager: Mrs J Law
Owner: Mr and Mrs Law
Contact: 69 Molesworth Street,
Wadebridge, Cornwall, PL27 7DS
📞 01208 814525

Located on the main road leading towards Padstow, Highpoint Lodge is a large Victorian detached house situated close to the centre of Wadebridge and approximately two minutes' walk from both the shops and the banks of the Camel River. The entrance is up a graduated slope with a handrail. Residents reside on the ground and first floor while the registered providers use the second for their private accommodation. Residents with an interest in gardening are welcome to do so in the grounds.

Registered places: 11
Guide weekly rate: Undisclosed
Specialist care: Day care, mental disorder
Medical services: Podiatry, dentist, optician, physiotherapy
Qualified staff: Exceeds standard: 70% at NVQ level 2

Home details
Location: Residential area, in Wadebridge
Communal areas: Lounge, dining room, conservatory, garden
Accessibility: *Floors:* 2 • *Access:* Stair lift • *Wheelchair access:* Good
Smoking: ✗
Pets: ✗
Routines: Flexible

Room details
Single: 9
Shared: 1
En suite: 8
Facilities: TV, telephone point

Door lock: ✓
Lockable place: ✓

Services provided
Beauty services: Hairdressing
Mobile library: Library facilities
Religious services: Monthly Communion service
Transport: 7-seater vehicle
Activities: *Coordinator:* ✗ • *Examples:* Communication, exercise
   Outings: ✗
Meetings: ✗

Registered places: 88
Guide weekly rate: £453–£602
Specialist care: Nursing, dementia, mental disorder,
   physical disability, respite
Medical services: Podiatry, dentist, optician, physiotherapy
Qualified staff: Meets standard

Home details
Location: Residential area, 1.7 miles from Looe
Communal areas: Lounge, dining room, patio and garden
Accessibility: *Floors:* 2 • *Access:* Lift • *Wheelchair access:* Good
Smoking: ✗
Pets: At manager's discretion
Routines: Flexible

Room details
Single: 84
Shared: 2   Door lock: ✓
En suite: 86   Lockable place: ✓
Facilities: TV, telephone

Services provided
Beauty services: Hairdressing
Mobile library: ✓
Religious services: ✓
Transport: ✓
Activities: *Coordinator:* ✓ • *Examples:* Cinema night, singalongs
   Outings: ✓
Meetings: ✓

Hillcrest House

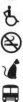

Manager: Sharon Keast
Owner: Hillcrest House Ltd
Contact: Barbican Road,
East Looe, Cornwall, PL13 1NN
☎ 01503 263489
@ care@hillcrestlooe.co.uk
🖱 www.hillcrestlooe.co.uk

A modern, purpose-built home, Hillcrest House is located in a scenic area in the outskirts of Looe, permitting views of the surrounding countryside and sea. The home has a lounge, a dining room and around two acres of ground. A monthly newsletter is produced which includes the activities programme for the residents. The activities coordinator arranges visiting entertainers and cinema nights for the residents as well as outings. There are two cats in the home and other pets would be allowed at the manager's discretion.

Registered places: 22
Guide weekly rate: £335–£373
Specialist care: Day care
Medical services: Podiatry, hygienist, optician, physiotherapy
Qualified staff: Exceeds standard: 70% at NVQ level 2

Home details
Location: Residential area, 1 mile from Callington
Communal areas: 2 lounges, 2 dining rooms, garden
Accessibility: *Floors:* 2 • *Access:* Stair lift • *Wheelchair access:* Good
Smoking: ✗
Pets: At manager's discretion
Routines: Flexible

Room details
Single: 18
Shared: 2   Door lock: ✓
En suite: 16   Lockable place: ✓
Facilities: TV point, telephone point

Services provided
Beauty services: Hairdressing
Mobile library: ✓
Religious service: Fortnightly
Transport: ✗
Activities: *Coordinator:* ✓ • *Examples:* Singalongs, quizzes, visiting
   entertainers • *Outings:* ✓
Meetings: ✓

Hillsborough

Manager: Marie Danvers
Owner: Marie Danvers
Contact: Southern Road,
Callington, Cornwall, PL17 7ER
☎ 01579 383138
@ hillsborough@tiscali.co.uk
🖱 www.hillsboroughresidentialhome.co.uk

Situated in its own gardens, Hillsborough is around 10 minutes' walk from Callington's local facilities. The home offers panoramic views of the surrounding countryside and is currently home to three cats. The home arranges a religious service every two weeks and also takes residents on outings in the local area. There is a residents meeting every six to eight months and the daily activities programme includes quizzes and visiting entertainers.

Hollybush

Manager: Neil and Nicola Brazier
Owner: Neil and Nicola Brazier
Contact: 45 Glamis Road,
Newquay, Cornwall, TR7 2RY
) 01637 874148

Hollybush resides in a residential area, one mile from the coast and a few hundred yards from local shops. The home is located over a mile from Newquay. The garden has recently been decked to improve wheelchair access and a water feature has been installed. The home also has a conservatory for residents to relax in. There is an Anglican Communion service once a month and the home arranges daily activities such as quizzes and exercise sessions.

Registered places: 14
Guide weekly rate: £325–£360
Specialist care: Dementia
Medical services: Podiatry, dentist, optician
Qualified staff: Fails standards

Home details
Location: Residential area, 1.2 miles from Newquay
Communal areas: Lounge/dining room, conservatory, garden
Accessibility: *Floors:* 2 • *Access:* Stair lift • *Wheelchair access:* Good
Smoking: ✗
Pets: ✓
Routines: Flexible

Room details
Single: 14
Shared: 0
En suite: 14
Facilities: TV point, telephone point

Door lock: ✓
Lockable place: ✓

Services provided
Beauty services: Hairdressing
Mobile library: ✓
Religious services: Monthly Anglican Communion service
Transport: ✗
Activities: *Coordinator:* ✗ • *Examples:* Cards, keep fit, quizzes
Outings: ✗
Meetings: ✗

Kenwyn

Manager: Amanda Trotter
Owner: Barchester Healthcare Ltd
Contact: Newmills Lane,
Kenwyn Hill, Truro, Cornwall, TR1 3EB
) 01872 223399
www.barchester.com

A purpose-built property in a semi-rural location on the outskirts of Truro, Kenwyn is split into four units providing care for 108 residents. With attractive gardens that have been the recipient of a number of awards, there are also numerous communal areas for residents. This includes several lounges and a separate dining room. The home has two activities coordinators who arrange activities such as a gardening club and bingo for the residents. There are also regular outings.

Registered places: 108
Guide weekly rate: £444–£1,523
Specialist care: Nursing, dementia, mental disorder, physical disability
Medical services: Podiatry, dentist, optician, physiotherapy
Qualified staff: Meets standard

Home details
Location: Rural area, 1.3 miles from Truro
Communal areas: Lounges, dining rooms, garden
Accessibility: *Floors:* 2 • *Access:* Lifts • *Wheelchair access:* Limited
Smoking: In designated area
Pets: Undisclosed
Routines: Flexible

Room details
Single: 100
Shared: 4
En suite: 104
Facilities: TV point, telephone point

Door lock: ✗
Lockable place: ✓

Services provided
Beauty services: Hairdressing
Mobile library: ✗
Religious services: ✗
Transport: ✗
Activities: *Coordinator:* ✓ • *Examples:* Bingo, gardening club, quizzes
Outings: ✓
Meetings: ✓

Registered places: 97
Guide weekly rate: £600–£2,000
Specialist care: Nursing, dementia, mental disorder,
    physical disability, respite
Medical services: Podiatry, dentist, dietician, optician, physiotherapy
Qualified staff: Undisclosed

Home details
Location: Rural area, in Launceston
Communal areas: 8 lounges, 4 dining rooms,
    hairdressing salon, garden
Accessibility: *Floors:* 2 • *Access:* Lift • *Wheelchair access:* Good
Smoking: In designated area
Pets: At manager's discretion
Routines: Flexible

Room details
Single: 85
Shared: 6 | Door lock: ✓
En suite: 91 | Lockable place: ✓
Facilities: TV point, telephone point

Services provided
Beauty services: Hairdressing, manicures, massage
Mobile library: ✓
Religious services: Nondenominational Communion service
    every 3 weeks
Transport: Minibus and car
Activities: *Coordinator:* ✓ • *Examples:* Film discussions, sewing group
    Outings: ✓
Meetings: ✓

Kernow House

Manager: Valerie Baggott
Owner: Barchester Healthcare Ltd
Contact: Landlake Road,
Launceston, Cornwall, PL15 9HP
☎ 01566 777841
@ kernow@barchester.com
🖰 www.barchester.com

A modern, purpose-built home on the outskirts of Launceston, Kernow House is in a semi-rural location close to the Cornish coast and nearby hospital, within 15 minutes' walk of a variety of local amenities. With landscaped gardens, the home also has a water feature at its main entrance and a sensory garden on its grounds. Offering a range of activities, outings are daily and can vary from trips into Truro to visits to the Eden project. Kernow House also has a specialist Huntington's disease unit at the attached Milaton Court, which accounts for the broad range in fees.

Registered places: 15
Guide weekly rate: £240–£342
Specialist care: Respite
Medical services: Podiatry, optician
Qualified staff: Undisclosed

Home details
Location: Residential area, 0.5 miles from Liskeard
Communal areas: Lounge, dining room, library, patio and garden
Accessibility: *Floors:* 2 • *Access:* Lift • *Wheelchair access:* Good
Smoking: In designated area
Pets: ✗
Routines: Flexible

Room details
Single: 13
Shared: 1 | Door lock: ✗
En suite: 3 | Lockable place: ✗
Facilities: TV point

Services provided
Beauty services: Hairdressing
Mobile library: ✓
Religious services: Anglican visits
Transport: ✗
Activities: *Coordinator:* ✗ • *Examples:* Bingo, skittles, games
    Outings: ✓
Meetings: ✓

Kilmar House

Manager: Stephen Corcoran
Owner: Stephen Corcoran
Contact: Higher Lux Street,
Liskeard, Cornwall, PL14 3JU
☎ 01579 343066

Kilmar House is situated near the centre of Liskeard and is within walking distance from the shops. Set on two floors, there is good wheelchair access throughout the home. A designated care worker organises daily activities such as board games and walks around the garden. A local vicar visits and other religious services can be arranged. There are two smoking rooms in the home. The home also has its own library facilities.

Little Trefawha Residential Care Home

Manager: Jacquelyn Elliott
Owner: Little Trefewha Ltd
Contact: Praze-an-Beeble,
Camborne, Cornwall, TR14 0JZ

☏ 01209 831566

@ j.elliott@trecaregroup.co.uk

This residential care home is located on the edge of the village of Praze-an-Beeble and nestled between the towns of Camborne and Heston. Little Trefewha is well suited for residents wanting easy access to the facilities and amenities the village has to offer. There is a greenhouse for those residents with an interest in gardening and residents are welcome to bring their own transport. It has an acre of grounds. The home arranges a monthly Communion service and takes the residents on outings in the local area.

Registered places: 20
Guide weekly rate: £375
Specialist care: Respite
Medical services: Podiatry, dentist, optician
Qualified staff: Exceeds standard: 79% at NVQ level 2

Home details
Location: Residential area, 2 miles from Camborne
Communal areas: 2 lounges, dining room, patio and garden
Accessibility: *Floors:* 2 • *Access:* Stair lift • *Wheelchair access:* Good
Smoking: ✗
Pets: At manager's discretion
Routines: Flexible

Room details
Single: 18
Shared: 1
En suite: 4
Facilities: TV point

Door lock: ✗
Lockable place: ✗

Services provided
Beauty services: Hairdressing
Mobile Library: ✓
Religious services: Monthly Communion service
Transport: ✗
Activities: *Coordinator:* ✗ • *Examples:* Poetry readings, quizzes
   Outings: ✓
Meetings: ✗

The Manse

Manager: Philippa Jewell
Owner: Underhill Care Ltd
Contact: Cargoll Road,
St Newlyn East,
Newquay, Cornwall, TR8 5LB

☏ 01872 510844

@ louise@themanse15.wanadoo.co.uk

The Manse is located a short walk from the nearest shops and around five miles from Newquay town centre. The home has a residents meeting every two months and arranges outings for the residents to take part in. There is a Communion service once a month and the home has its own transport. There are two lounges for residents to socialise in and a mobile library comes to the home.

Registered places: 23
Guide weekly rate: £347
Specialist care: Day care, dementia, respite
Medical services: Podiatry, dentist, optician, physiotherapy
Qualified staff: Meets standard

Home details
Location: Village location, 5 miles from Newquay
Communal areas: 2 lounges, dining room, garden
Accessibility: *Floors:* 3 • *Access:* Stair lift • *Wheelchair access:* Good
Smoking: ✗
Pets: At manager's discretion
Routines: Structured

Room details
Single: 19
Shared: 2
En suite: 21
Facilities: TV point, telephone point

Door lock: ✓
Lockable place: ✓

Services provided
Beauty services: Hairdressing
Mobile library: ✓
Religious services: Monthly Communion service
Transport: Car
Activities: *Coordinator:* ✗ • *Examples:* Exercises • *Outings:* ✓
Meetings: ✓

Registered places: 23
Guide weekly rate: £305–£350
Specialist care: Respite
Medical services: Podiatry, dentist, optician
Qualified staff: Meets standard

Home details

Location: Residential area, 0.2 miles from Saltash
Communal areas: Lounge/dining room, garden
Accessibility: *Floors:* 2 • *Access:* Stair lift • *Wheelchair access:* Good
Smoking: ✕
Pets: At manager's discretion
Routines: Flexible

Room details

Single: 19
Shared: 2 | Door lock: ✕
En suite: 0 | Lockable place: ✓
Facilities: TV point, telephone point

Services provided

Beauty services: Hairdressing
Mobile library: ✓
Religious services: Monthly Anglican Communion service
Transport: ✕
Activities: *Coordinator:* ✕ • *Examples:* Singers, games, exercises
     Outings: ✓
Meetings: ✓

Marray House

Manager: Enid Crofts
Owner: Enid and Peter Crofts
Contact: 12–14 Essa Road,
Saltash, Cornwall, PL12 4ED
☎ 01752 844488

Marray House is a detached house from which residents can easily access Saltash's community facilities, since the town centre is only half a mile away. The home is located a few hundred yards from the Tamar Bridge, the waterfront and the station. The home arranges an Anglican Communion service for the residents every month and also takes the residents on outings. The daily activities programme includes visiting singers and exercise sessions.

Registered places: 32
Guide weekly rate: £300–£525
Specialist care: Day care, dementia, mental disorder, respite
Medical services: Podiatry, hygienist, optician, physiotherapy
Qualified staff: Exceeds standard: 89% at NVQ level 2

Home details

Location: Rural area, 5 miles from Penzance
Communal areas: 3 lounges, dining room, hairdressing salon, garden
Accessibility: *Floors:* 3 • *Access:* Stair lift • *Wheelchair access:* Good
Smoking: In designated area
Pets: At manager's discretion
Routines: Flexible

Room details

Single: 30
Shared: 1 | Door lock: ✓
En suite: Undisclosed | Lockable place: ✓
Facilities: TV point, telephone point

Services provided

Beauty services: Hairdressing
Mobile library: ✓
Religious services: Weekly Communion service
Transport: Minibus
Activities: *Coordinator:* ✓ • *Examples:* Bingo, quizzes, reminiscence
     Outings: ✓
Meetings: ✕

Menwinnion Country House

Manager: Johanne Towson
Owner: Ablecare Ltd
Contact: Lamorna Valley,
Penzance, Cornwall, TR19 6BJ
☎ 01736 810233

Set in spacious grounds in a quiet rural area, Menwinnion Country Home is about five miles south of Penzance and around two miles from Mousehole. It is less than a mile to the coast. The home has visits from a mobile library and has its own hairdressing salon. There are three lounges and a garden for residents to socialise in and the home also arranges regular outings. The home has its own minibus for transportation and also organises a weekly Communion service for the residents.

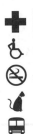

Millpond View Care Home

Manager: Maureen Tredinnick
Owner: Omar Thauoos and Joyceleen Lissenburg
Contact: 11 Millpond Avenue, Hayle, Cornwall, TR27 4HX
) 01736 752759
@ maureen2624@aol.com

Millpond View Care Home is an adapted Georgian house that overlooks the Millpond – a freshwater pond which is home to a variety of birds including ducks, swans and herons. It is five minutes' walk to Hayle's local amenities; there is also a vehicle suitable for wheelchairs provided free to residents with appointments in the community. Encouraging an active social life by means of a comprehensive activities programme, Millpond also welcomes visitors to stay, at no extra charge, for meals. The home will also provide residence for family if a relative is very ill and they are required to stay.

Registered places: 32
Guide weekly rate: £442–£513
Specialist care: Nursing, day care, emergency admissions, physical disability, respite
Medical services: Podiatry, dentist, optician, physiotherapy
Qualified staff: Undisclosed

Home details
Location: Residential area, in Hayle
Communal areas: 2 lounges, garden
Accessibility: *Floors:* 2 • *Access:* Lift • *Wheelchair access:* Good
Smoking: ✗
Pets: At manager's discretion
Routines: Flexible

Room details
Single: 28
Shared: 2   **Door lock:** ✗
En suite: 5   **Lockable place:** ✓
Facilities: TV point, telephone point

Services provided
Beauty services: Hairdressing
Mobile library: ✓
Religious services: Monthly Anglican Communion service
Transport: Car
Activities: *Coordinator:* ✓ • *Examples:* Arts and crafts, keep fit
Outings: ✓
Meetings: ✓

North Hill

Manager: Mandy Trask
Owner: David and Helen Smith
Contact: North Hill Park, St Austell, Cornwall, PL25 4BJ
) 01726 72647

North Hill is located in a quiet residential area of St Austell close to a train station. The home has a gazebo in the garden which residents enjoy during warmer weather. Although pets are not allowed in the home, north Hill has links to the Cinnamon Trust which provides new homes for pets. The home has an activities coordinator who arranges exercise sessions as well as quizzes. There are also regular outings for the residents.

Registered places: 24
Guide weekly rate: £444–£495
Specialist care: Nursing, physical disability
Medical services: Podiatry, dentist, occupational therapy, optician
Qualified staff: Meets standard

Home details
Location: Residential area, 0.5 miles from St Austell
Communal areas: 3 lounges, dining room, garden
Accessibility: *Floors:* 2 • *Access:* Lift • *Wheelchair access:* Good
Smoking: In designated area
Pets: ✗
Routines: Structured

Room details
Single: 20
Shared: 2   **Door lock:** ✓
En suite: 6   **Lockable place:** ✓
Facilities: TV point, telephone point

Services provided
Beauty services: Hairdressing, aromatherapy
Mobile library: ✓
Religious services: ✗
Transport: ✗
Activities: *Coordinator:* ✓ • *Examples:* Bingo, keep fit, quizzes
Outings: ✓
Meetings: ✓

Registered places: 14
Guide weekly rate: £300–£355
Specialist care: Day care, respite
Medical services: Podiatry, dentist, hygienist, optician, physiotherapy
Qualified staff: Exceeds standard: 90% at NVQ level 2

Home details
Location: Residential area, 0.3 miles from Penzance
Communal areas: 2 lounges, dining room, garden
Accessibility: *Floors:* 4 • *Access:* Lift • *Wheelchair access:* Good
Smoking: In designated area
Pets: At manager's discretion
Routines: Flexible

Room details
Single: 12
Shared: 1
En suite: 11
Facilities: TV point, telephone point

Door lock: ✓
Lockable place: ✓

Services provided
Beauty services: Hairdressing, aromatherapy, manicures
Mobile library: ✓
Religious services: ✗
Transport: Minibus
Activities: *Coordinator:* ✓ • *Examples:* Arts and crafts, games
    Outings: ✓
Meetings: ✗

The Old Manor House

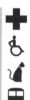

Manager: Kevin Edgar
Owner: Anson Care Services
Contact: 6 Regent Terrace,
Penzance, Cornwall, TR18 4DW
) 01736 363742

Boasting stunning sea views and situated a short walk from the town's amenities of the town, Old Manor House is set in beautiful surroundings next to the promonade in Penzance. Penlee botanical gardens are located in one direction while the port is in the other direction. The home has an activities coordinator who arranges activities in the home such as arts and crafts and games. The home also has its own minibus which is used in the outings organised by the home.

Registered places: 30
Guide weekly rate: Undisclosed
Specialist care: Nursing, respite, physical disability
Medical services: Podiatry, optician, physiotherapy
Qualified staff: Exceeds standard: 93% at NVQ level 2

Home details
Location: Village location, 0.6 miles from Par
Communal areas: 2 lounges, dining room, conservatory, garden
Accessibility: *Floors:* 2 • *Access:* Stair lift • *Wheelchair access:* Good
Smoking: In designated area
Pets: At manager's discretion
Routines: Flexible

Room details
Single: 24
Shared: 3
En suite: 6
Facilities: TV, telephone point

Door lock: ✗
Lockable place: ✓

Services provided
Beauty services: Hairdressing
Mobile library: ✓
Religious services: Weekly Communion service
Transport: Car
Activities: *Coordinator:* ✓ • *Examples:* Visiting entertainers
    Outings: ✗
Meetings: ✗

Old Roselyon Manor

Manager: Anthony Small
Owner: John and Marine Mobbs and Anthony Small
Contact: Old Roselyon,
Par, Cornwall, PL24 2DW
) 01726 814297

A converted 400-year-old Manor House, Old Roselyon Manor is set in two acres of its own land, home to a magnificent oak tree. The home is located in a village, half a mile from Par. There is a Communion service every week and the home has its own transportation in a car. The home also has an activities coordinator who arranges for visiting entertainers to come to the home.

The Old Vicarage

Manager: Anne Hetherington
Owner: Torcare Ltd
Contact: Antony,
Torpoint, Cornwall, PL11 3AQ
☎ 01752 812384
@ antony@torcare.co.uk
🖰 www.torcare.co.uk

An older building located in the village of Antony, residents at the Old Vicarage often make the five-minute minibus ride to the seaside. The home is in a residential area, three miles from Torpoint. The home prides itself on its food, offering classic dishes prepared with high-quality ingredients. Vegetables are always fresh and not cooked from frozen. The home provides a mobile library service and also arranges for choirs to come and perform at the home.

Registered places: 22
Guide weekly rate: £410–£420
Specialist care: Respite, dementia, mental disorder
Medical services: Podiatry, dentist, hygienist, optician, physiotherapy
Qualified staff: Exceeds standard: 88% at NVQ level 2

Home details
Location: Residential area, 3 miles from Torpoint
Communal areas: Lounge, dining room, TV room, garden
Accessibility: *Floors:* 3 • *Access:* Lift • *Wheelchair access:* Limited
Smoking: ✗
Pets: ✗
Routines: Structured

Room details
Single: 18
Shared: 2
En suite: 4
Facilities: TV point, telephone point

Door lock: ✓
Lockable place: ✓

Services provided
Beauty services: Hairdressing
Mobile Library: ✓
Religious services: Monthly Anglican Communion service
Transport: Minibus
Activities: *Coordinator:* ✗ • *Examples:* Choirs visit • *Outings:* ✓
Meetings: ✗

Parc Vro

Manager: Alison Stevenson
Owner: Alison Stevenson
Contact: Mawgan-in-Meneage,
Helston, Cornwall, TR12 6AY
☎ 01326 221275

Situated in a rural location, Parc Vro is close to a shop and a pub. The home is also close to a bus stop on a major route and it is a 15-minute journey to Helston. Showing a commitment to sustainable living, one resident has a vegetable patch in the gardens and provides staff with vegetables for meals while another is involved with the home's recycling policy. The home also arranges a weekly Anglican service and a monthly Methodist service for the residents. The home also has its own transportation.

Registered places: 15
Guide weekly rate: £301–£425
Specialist care: Day care, dementia, mental disorder, respite
Medical services: Podiatry
Qualified staff: Exceeds standard: 80% at NVQ level 2

Home details
Location: Rural area, 5 miles from Helston
Communal areas: Lounge, dining room, garden
Accessibility: *Floors:* 2 • *Access:* Lift • *Wheelchair access:* Good
Smoking: ✗
Pets: At manager's discretion
Routines: Flexible

Room details
Single: 13
Shared: 1
En suite: 0
Facilities: TV point, telephone point

Door lock: ✓
Lockable place: ✓

Services provided
Beauty services: Hairdressing
Mobile library: ✓
Religious services: Weekly Anglican Communion service, monthly Methodist service
Transport: Car
Activities: *Coordinator:* ✗ • *Examples:* Arts and crafts, keep fit
Outings: ✗
Meetings: ✗

Registered places: 18
Guide weekly rate: £330
Specialist care: Day care, respite
Medical services: Podiatry, dentist, optician
Qualified staff: Meets standard

Home details

Location: Rural area, 6 miles from Launceston
Communal areas: Lounge, dining room, patio and garden
Accessibility: *Floors: 2* • *Access:* Stair lift • *Wheelchair access:* Good
Smoking: ✗
Pets: At manager's discretion
Routines: Flexible

Room details

Single: 16
Shared: 1
En suite: 15
Facilities: TV point

Door lock: ✓
Lockable place: ✓

Services provided

Beauty services: Hairdressing
Mobile library: ✓
Religious services: Monthly church service
Transport: ✗
Activities: *Coordinator:* ✗ • *Examples:* Bingo, visiting entertainers
   Outings: ✗
Meetings: ✗

Pen Inney House

Manager: Elizabeth Ollerenshaw
Owner: Elizabeth Ollerenshaw
Contact: Lewannick,
Launceston, Cornwall, PL15 7QD
☎ 01566 782318
@ peninney@btopen.com

Situated in Lewannick, Pen Inney House is a 19th-century house that is set in over an acre of garden and easily accessed from the A30. Although access to local amenities is restricted, there is one village shop and one return bus journey each day to Launceston – where there are a number of shops and community facilities. A gardener is employed to ensure the gardens are well maintained, and the owner also lives on the site and doubles as the home's manager.

Registered places: 51
Guide weekly rate: £431–£553
Specialist care: Nursing, day care, respite
Medical services: Podiatry, dentist, optician
Qualified staff: Meets standard

Home details

Location: Residential area, 0.5 miles from Launceston
Communal areas: Lounge, dining room, conservatory,
   patio and garden
Accessibility: *Floors: 3* • *Access:* Lift • *Wheelchair access:* Good
Smoking: ✗
Pets: ✗
Routines: Flexible

Room details

Single: 51
Shared: 0
En suite: Undisclosed
Facilities: TV point, telephone point

Door lock: ✓
Lockable place: ✓

Services provided

Beauty services: Hairdressing, aromatherapy
Mobile library: ✓
Religious services: Monthly Communion service
Transport: ✓
Activities: *Coordinator:* ✓ • *Examples:* Arts and crafts, bingo,
   musical entertainment • *Outings:* ✓
Meetings: ✗

Pendruccombe House

Manager: Diane Kehoe and
Linda Winstone
Owner: AJ & Co Ltd
Contact: 23 Tazistock Road,
Launcestone, Cornwall, PL15 9HS
☎ 01566 776100
@ pendruccombe@btconnect.com
🖱 www.pendruccombe.co.uk

With communal rooms which permit views of the surrounding countryside, Pendruccombe House is situated five minutes from a nearby supermarket and the town of Launceston. Pendruccombe House is a family run home which was originally a school. The home offers both nursing and residential care, with 27 places for nursing and 24 for residential. There are two floors for nursing and three floors for residential care. Pets are allowed to visit but smoking is not permitted. There is an activities coordinator who arranges activities such as bingo and visiting entertainers as well as trips.

Penmeneth House

Manager: Felicity Richards
Owner: Philip and Felicity Richards
Contact: 16 Penpol Avenue,
Hayle, Cornwall, TR27 4NQ
☎ 01736 752359

A family-run home, Penmeneth is located near the station and Hayle town centre. The home has two lounges for residents to socialise in as well as a conservatory and a patio area for them to enjoy in the warmer months. The home holds a Methodist service every three months and has its own car to take residents on outings. The home also arranges for a mobile library to come to the home.

Registered places: 14
Guide weekly rate: £293–£340
Specialist care: Day care, dementia, respite
Medical services: Podiatry, dentist, optician
Qualified staff: Meets standard

Home details
Location: Residential area, 0.7 miles from Hayle
Communal areas: 2 lounges, dining room, conservatory, patio
Accessibility: *Floors:* 2 • *Access:* Stair lift
   Wheelchair access: Limited
Smoking: ✗
Pets: At manager's discretion
Routines: Flexible

Room details
Single: 12
Shared: 1 | **Door lock:** ✓
En suite: 4 | **Lockable place:** ✓
Facilities: TV point, telephone point

Services provided
Beauty services: Hairdressing
Mobile library: ✓
Religious services: Methodist service every 3 months
Transport: Car
Activities: *Coordinator:* ✗ • *Examples:* Bingo, visiting entertainers
   Outings: ✓
Meetings: ✗

Pine Trees

Manager: Tara Hughes
Owner: Guardian Care Homes Ltd
Contact: 15 Horsepool Road,
Connor Downs, Hayle,
Cornwall, TR27 5DZ
☎ 01736 753249
@ Pine_trees@btconnect.com

Set in its own grounds, Pine Trees is approximately four miles from Hayle town centre, and is on a local bus route. There are also some local shops nearby. The home prides itself on its homely atmosphere and offers a range of activities and takes residents on regular outings. Set on one floor, there is good wheelchair access around the home. The home also arranges a nondenominational religious service which takes place on a weekly basis.

Registered places: 24
Guide weekly rate: £293–£450
Specialist care: Day care, respite
Medical services: Podiatry, dentist, optician
Qualified staff: Exceeds standard: 75% at NVQ level 2

Home details
Location: Residential area, 4 miles from Hayle
Communal areas: Lounge, dining room, conservatory,
   patio and garden
Accessibility: *Floors:* 1 • *Wheelchair access:* Good
Smoking: ✗
Pets: ✗
Routines: Flexible

Room details
Single: 23
Shared: 1 | **Door lock:** ✗
En suite: 24 | **Lockable place:** ✓
Facilities: TV point, telephone point

Services provided
Beauty services: Hairdressing
Mobile library: ✓
Religious services: Weekly nondenominational service
Transport: ✗
Activities: *Coordinator:* ✓ • *Examples:* Arts and crafts, bingo,
   visiting entertainers • *Outings:* ✓
Meetings: ✗

Registered places: 63
Guide weekly rate: £450–£900
Specialist care: Nursing, day care, physical disability, respite
Medical services: Podiatry, dentist, optician
Qualified staff: Meets standard

Home details

Location: Rural area, 1 mile from Mullion
Communal areas: 2 lounges, dining room, conservatory, garden
Accessibility: *Floors:* 3 • *Access:* Lift • *Wheelchair access:* Good
Smoking: ✗
Pets: ✗
Routines: Flexible

Room details

Single: 45
Shared: 9
En suite: 40
Facilities: TV point, telephone point

Door lock: ✗
Lockable place: ✓

Services provided

Beauty services: Hairdressing
Mobile library: ✓
Religious services: Weekly nondenominational service
Transport: ✓
Activities: *Coordinator:* ✓ • *Examples:* Arts and crafts, bingo, music and movement • *Outings:* ✓
Meetings: ✗

The Poldhu Care Home

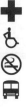

Manager: Tina Howard
Owner: Swallowcourt Ltd
Contact: Poldhu Cove,
Mullion, Helston, Cornwall, TR12 7JB
☎ 01326 240977
@ info@swallowcourt.com
🖰 www.swallowcourt.com

Situated in nearly 10 acres of landscaped grounds and overlooking spectacular views of Poldhu Cove on the Lizard Peninsula, The Poldhu began life as a luxury hotel. With tall ceilings and large double-glazed windows, The Poldhu has the sensation of being spacious and bright. Although not within easy walking distance of amenities, the home is positioned a short drive away from Helston and Mullion and residents are offered free transport to the supermarkets or activity centres nearby. There is also a coastal footpath that may tempt more active.

Registered places: 13
Guide weekly rate: £425–£475
Specialist care: Dementia, mental disorder
Medical services: Podiatry
Qualified staff: Exceeds standard: 90% at NVQ level 2

Home details

Location: Residential area, 0.5 miles from Redruth
Communal areas: Lounge, dining room, conservatory, garden
Accessibility: *Floors:* 2 • *Access:* Stair lift • *Wheelchair access:* Good
Smoking: In designated area
Pets: Undisclosed
Routines: Flexible

Room details

Single: 11
Shared: 1
En suite: 5
Facilities: None

Door lock: ✗
Lockable place: ✗

Services provided

Beauty services: Hairdressing
Mobile library: ✗
Religious services: ✓
Transport: ✗
Activities: *Coordinator:* ✗ • *Examples:* Undisclosed
    Outings: Undisclosed
Meetings: Undisclosed

Polsloe House

Manager: Mary Butland
Owner: Polsloe House Ltd
Contact: 22 Park Road,
Redruth, Cornwall, TR15 2JG
☎ 01209 215337

Polsloe House is a detached building set in its own grounds and approximately half a mile from Redruth. The home is close to local GP surgeries with Camborne and Redruth Hospital one and a half miles away. There are nice views of the front garden from the lounge and conservatory and a separate dining room. Activities are displayed on the white board in the main lounge. The home also arranges religious services for the residents.

Polventon Residential Home

Manager: Christine Stewart
Owner: Melita Care Homes Ltd
Contact: High Street, St Keverne, Helston, Cornwall, TR12 6NS

☎ 01326 280734

Polventon Residential Home is a detached country house that is set in one acre of land, permitting wonderful views of the surrounding countryside while remaining a short walk to nearby amenities. These include shops, a post office and a pub. New providers took over the home in 2006, and Polventon has undertaken a modern extension. With one of the lounges dedicated as a quiet lounge, the home has attractive gardens surrounding the building and there is also a putting green in the grounds for those with an interest in golf.

Registered places: 19
Guide weekly rate: £385–£480
Specialist care: Day care, dementia, mental disorder, physical disability, respite
Medical services: Podiatry, dentist, optician
Qualified staff: Exceeds standard: 69% at NVQ level 2

Home details
Location: Village location, 12 miles from Helston
Communal areas: 2 lounges, dining room, garden
Accessibility: *Floors:* 2 • *Access:* Lift • *Wheelchair access:* Good
Smoking: In designated area
Pets: ✗
Routines: Flexible

Room details
Single: 19
Shared: 0
En suite: 0
Facilities: TV point, telephone point

Door lock: ✓
Lockable place: ✓

Services provided
Beauty services: Hairdressing
Mobile library: ✓
Religious services: Monthly Anglican Communion service, monthly Methodist Communion service
Transport: ✗
Activities: *Coordinator:* ✗ • *Examples:* Bingo, quizzes *Outings:* ✓
Meetings: ✗

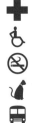

Ponsandane

Manager: Penelope Hicks
Owner: Swallowcourt Ltd
Contact: Chy-an-dour, Penzance, Cornwall, TR18 3LT

☎ 01736 330063
@ ponsandane@swallowcourt.com
🖱 www.swallowcourt.com

Close to both bus routes and Penzance railway station, Ponsandane is a Georgian building set in its own grounds. The building was once the home of the Bolitho family who were major landowners in the area. The home has large drawing rooms with fireplaces and ornate ceilings, which have been converted into lounges for residents. In keeping with this setting, the activities coordinator arranges candlelight dinners for the residents and their families. The home offers views across Mounts Bay towards St Michael's Mount.

Registered places: 58
Guide weekly rate: £293–£750
Specialist care: Nursing, dementia, learning disability, physical disability, respite
Medical services: Podiatry, optician
Qualified staff: Meets standard

Home details
Location: Residential area, 0.7 miles from Penzance
Communal areas: 3 lounges, dining room, garden
Accessibility: *Floors:* 3 • *Access:* Lift and stair lift *Wheelchair access:* Good
Smoking: ✗
Pets: At manager's discretion
Routines: Flexible

Room details
Single: 34
Shared: 12
En suite: 0
Facilities: TV point, telephone point

Door lock: ✓
Lockable place: ✓

Services provided
Beauty services: Hairdressing
Mobile library: ✓
Religious services: Fortnightly service
Transport: Minibus
Activities: *Coordinator:* ✓ • *Examples:* Candlelight dinners *Outings:* ✓
Meetings: ✓

Registered places: 30
Guide weekly rate: £350–£385
Specialist care: Day care
Medical services: None
Qualified staff: Meets standard

Home details

Location: Residential area, 0.8 miles from Bude
Communal areas: 2 lounges, dining room, conservatory,
    patio and garden
Accessibility: *Floors:* 2 • *Access:* Lift • *Wheelchair access:* Good
Smoking: In designated area
Pets: ✓
Routines: Flexible

Room details

Single: 26
Shared: 2
En suite: 19
Facilities: TV point, telephone point

Door lock: ✓
Lockable place: ✓

Services provided

Beauty services: Hairdressing
Mobile Library: ✓
Religious services: Monthly Anglican service
Transport: ✗
Activities: *Coordinator:* ✗ • *Examples:* Bingo, exercise, singing
    Outings: ✗
Meetings: ✗

Red Gables

Manager: Andrew Renshaw
Owner: George Kneebone
Contact: 59 Killerton Road,
Bude, Cornwall, EX23 8EW
✆ 01288 355250

Red Gables is a red brick stately home set in its own grounds. It has been converted to meet the needs of its residents. The management are currently looking into purchasing a minibus which would allow the residents to take trips to the nearby beaches. Musical entertainment is prov-ided at Christmas and Easter by the choirs of local schools, and throughout the year volunteers often perform recitals. The home also organises an Anglican service once a month.

Registered places: 36
Guide weekly rate: £370
Specialist care: Day care, dementia, mental disorder, respite
Medical services: Podiatry, dentist, optician, physiotherapy
Qualified staff: Meets standard

Home details

Location: Residential area, 5 miles from Looe
Communal areas: 4 lounges, dining room, patio and garden
Accessibility: *Floors:* 3 • *Access:* Lift and 2 stair lifts
    Wheelchair access: Good
Smoking: ✗
Pets: ✓
Routines: Flexible

Room details

Single: 32
Shared: 2
En suite: 31
Facilities: TV, telephone system
Offer

Door lock: ✓
Lockable place: ✓

Services provided

Beauty services: Hairdressing, manicures
Mobile library: ✓
Religious services: ✓
Transport: ✓
Activities: *Coordinator:* ✓ • *Examples:* Exercises, visiting entertainers
    Outings: ✓
Meetings: ✗

Restgarth Care Home

Manager: Helen Taylor
Owner: Restgarth Care Ltd
Contact: Langreek Lane,
Polperro, Cornwall, PL13 2PW
✆ 01503 272016
@ lesliefoggy@hotmail.com

A modern house set in its own grounds half a mile from the village of Polperrow and its local amenities, Restgarth Care Home is a family-run home with 36 places. The home is five miles from the town of Looe and there is a bus service. The home has a self-contained flat for residents to prepare to return home. The home has its own books and also arranges for mobile library visits. Small pets are allowed if the resident can care for the animal themselves.

Roscarrack House

Manager: Malcolm Gibbs
Owner: David and Maureen Edwards
Contact: Bickland Water Road,
Budock, Falmouth, Cornwall, TR11 5BP
☎ 01326 312498
@ roscarrack@aol.com

A Victorian family home set in five and a half acres of ground, Roscarrack House is situated on the outskirts of Falmouth in an elevated position. Permitting wonderful views of the valley, some of the home's bedrooms also look out towards the sea. Approximately one mile from the beach, the home has attractive gardens which have three ponds and a vegetable patch. Roscarrack also offers weekly outings in addition to the daily activities programme which includes flower arranging. The home has two resident cats.

Registered places: 19
Guide weekly rate: From £370
Specialist care: Emergency admissions
Medical services: Podiatry, dentist, optician
Qualified staff: Exceeds standard: 75% at NVQ level 2

Home details
Location: Residential area, 2 miles from Falmouth
Communal areas: Lounge, dining room, library facilities, garden
Accessibility: *Floors:* 2 • *Access:* Stair lift • *Wheelchair access:* Good
Smoking: ✗
Pets: At manager's discretion
Routines: Flexible

Room details
Single: 19
Shared: 0
En suite: 17
Facilities: TV point, telephone point

Door lock: ✓
Lockable place: ✓

Services provided
Beauty services: Hairdressing
Mobile library: ✗
Religious services: Monthly Anglican church service
Transport: Minibus
Activities: *Coordinator:* ✓ • *Examples:* Discussions, flower arranging
 Outings: ✓
Meetings: ✗

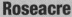

Roseacre

Manager: Pauline Knight
Owner: Anthony Knight
Contact: St Winnolls, Polbathick,
Torpoint, Cornwall, PL11 3DX
☎ 01503 230256
@ Roseacre333@aol.com
🖱 www.roseacrecare.co.uk

A family-run home in a rural location, Roseacre permits spectacular views across farmland to Rame Head and Whitsand Bay. The building itself is a converted 16th-century farmhouse, which, despite being modernised, retains its 'old-world charm'. Although the home has a stair lift to assist residents in accessing the upper floor, a degree of mobility is still required. The home arranges an activities schedule for the residents, which includes arts and crafts and music sessions.

Registered places: 22
Guide weekly rate: £293–£370
Specialist care: Day care, learning disability, mental disorder, respite
Medical services: Podiatry, dentist
Qualified staff: Meets standard

Home details
Location: Rural area, 7 miles from Torpoint
Communal areas: 2 lounges, dining room, conservatory, garden
Accessibility: *Floors:* 2 • *Access:* Stair lift • *Wheelchair access:* Good
Smoking: ✗
Pets: ✓
Routines: Flexible

Room details
Single: 20
Shared: 1
En suite: Undisclosed
Facilities: TV point, telephone point

Door lock: ✗
Lockable place: ✓

Services provided
Beauty services: Hairdressing
Mobile library: ✓
Religious services: ✗
Transport: ✗
Activities: *Coordinator:* ✗ • *Examples:* Arts and crafts, bingo
 Outings: ✓
Meetings: ✗

Registered places: 20
Guide weekly rate: £300–£380
Specialist care: Day care
Medical services: Podiatry, optician
Qualified staff: Exceeds standard: 80% at NVQ level 2

Home details
Location: Residential area, in Truro
Communal areas: Lounge, dining room, garden
Accessibility: *Floors:* 2 • *Access:* Lift • *Wheelchair access:* Good
Smoking: ✗
Pets: ✗
Routines: Flexible

Room details
Single: 18
Shared: 1
En suite: 0
Facilities: TV point, telephone point

Door lock: ✓
Lockable place: ✓

Services provided
Beauty services: Hairdressing
Mobile library: ✗
Religious services: Monthly Anglican Communion service
Transport: ✗
Activities: *Coordinator:* ✗ • *Examples:* Bingo, games • *Outings:* ✓
Meetings: ✗

Wyn House

Manager: Jennifer Spargo
Owner: William Dawes and
Gregory Murrell
Contact: Alverton Terrace,
Truro, Cornwall, TR1 1JE
☎ 01872 279107
@ rosewynhouse@gmail.com

Rosewyn lies in the centre of Truro, close to shops and the train station. The home is next door to a block of supported living flats which are managed by the home's providers. As a result, there is frequent cause for interaction between both sets of residents. The home provides residents with regular minibus trips that include a drive out to the Roseland Peninsula. The home also organises a monthly Anglican Communion service.

Registered places: 9
Guide weekly rate: £300–£370
Specialist care: None
Medical services: Podiatry, optician, physiotherapy
Qualified staff: Exceeds standard: 71% at NVQ level 2

Home details
Location: Residential area, 1.7 miles from St Agnes
Communal areas: Lounge, dining room, garden
Accessibility: *Floors:* 2 • *Access:* Stair lift • *Wheelchair access:* Limited
Smoking: ✗
Pets: ✓
Routines: Flexible

Room details
Single: 9
Shared: 0
En suite: 2
Facilities: TV point, telephone point

Door lock: ✓
Lockable place: ✓

Services provided
Beauty services: Hairdressing
Mobile library: ✓
Religious services: ✗
Transport: Car
Activities: *Coordinator:* ✗ • *Examples:* Aerobics, arts and crafts
   Outings: ✗
Meetings: ✗

The Rowans

Manager: Ian Hirsch
Owner: Ian and Rosemary Hirsch
Contact: 31 Goonown,
St Agnes, Cornwall, TR5 0UY
☎ 01872 552147
@ rowian@aol.com

A large Victorian property set in its own secluded gardens, The Rowans is a family-run care home where the owners live next door. The home is located in a residential area, almost two miles from St Agnes. Activities are available as and when they are requested. These can include arts and crafts sessions and aerobics. The home also has its own transport and arranges for a mobile library to come to the home.

Springfield House

Manager: Vacant
Owner: Eugene and Jennifer Huntley
Contact: North Hill,
Launceston, Cornwall, PL15 7PQ

📞 01566 782361
@ info@springfieldhouse.com
🖰 www.springfieldhouse.com

Situated in a small village seven miles from the town centre, Springfield House is a small home which specialises in the care of the confused elderly. The home is situated across the road from the Anglican church. The staff are highly trained with qualifications in fire safety and first aid. The home has an activities programme which includes visiting entertainers and there are numerous seating areas throughout the home. The home has its own cats. The home is setting up a Friends of Springfield House association which will allow relatives and residents to express their views.

Registered places: 23
Guide weekly rate: From £372
Specialist care: Dementia, mental disorder
Medical services: Podiatry, dentist, optician, physiotherapy
Qualified staff: Exceeds standard: 100% at NVQ level 2

Home details
Location: Residential area, 7 miles from Launceston
Communal areas: Lounge, dining room, seating areas, patio and garden
Accessibility: *Floors:* 2 • *Access:* Stair lift • *Wheelchair access:* Good
Smoking: ✗
Pets: ✗
Routines: Flexible

Room details
Single: 23
Shared: 0
En suite: 7
Facilities: TV point

Door lock: ✓
Lockable place: ✓

Services provided
Beauty services: Hairdressing
Mobile library: ✓
Religious services: ✗
Transport: Minibus
Activities: *Coordinator:* ✓ • *Examples:* Bingo, visiting entertainers *Outings:* ✓
Meetings: ✓

St Anne's

Manager: Dawn Parnell
Owner: Helen and Herbert Medland
Contact: Whitstone,
Holsworthy, Cornwall, EX22 6UA

📞 01288 341355

St Anne's is located in a small village 10 miles from Holsworthy. The communal areas are large, as are the bedrooms. The home also has a conservatory and a garden for residents to enjoy. The home has an activities coordinator who arranges bingo and quizzes for the residents, as well as performances from visiting entertainers.

Registered places: 28
Guide weekly rate: £280–£360
Specialist care: Respite
Medical services: Podiatry, physiotherapy, optician
Qualified staff: Meets standard

Home details
Location: Village location, 10 miles from Holsworthy
Communal areas: Lounge, dining room, conservatory, garden
Accessibility: *Floors:* 2 • *Access:* Lift • *Wheelchair Access:* Good
Smoking: ✗
Pets: ✗
Routines: Flexible

Room details
Single: 27
Shared: 0
En suite: 27
Facilities: None

Door lock: ✓
Lockable place: ✓

Services provided
Beauty services: Hairdressing
Mobile library: ✗
Religious services: ✗
Transport: ✗
Activities: *Coordinator:* ✓ • *Examples:* Bingo, quizzes, visiting entertainers • *Outings:* ✓
Meetings: ✗

Registered places: 16
Guide weekly rate: Undisclosed
Specialist care: Dementia, day care, respite
Medical services: Podiatry, dentist, optician
Qualified staff: Meets standard

Home details

Location: Rural area, 0.5 miles from Liskeard
Communal areas: Lounge, dining room, garden
Accessibility: *Floors:* 2 • *Access:* Stair lift • *Wheelchair access:* Good
Smoking: ✗
Pets: ✗
Routines: Undisclosed

Room details

Single: 16
Shared: 0
En suite: 9
Door lock: ✗
Lockable place: ✗
Facilities: TV point, telephone point

Services provided

Beauty services: Hairdressing
Mobile library: ✓
Religious services: ✓
Transport: ✗
Activities: *Coordinator:* ✓ • *Examples:* Bingo, games • *Outings:* ✗
Meetings: Undisclosed

St Anthonys Care Home

Manager: Judith Lingham
Owner: St Anthonys Ltd
Contact: Station Road,
Liskeard, Cornwall, PL14 4BY
☎ 01579 342308

St Anthony's is situated 100 yards from the town's local amenities, which include shops, a health centre and a railway station. The home has places for 16 residents, with five of those places for dementia patients. The home also offers respite and day care if there is availability. The home has a lounge and a dining room and work is currently being done on the garden. The home has its own activities coordinator. Smoking and pets are not allowed in the home.

Registered places: 18
Guide weekly rate: £460
Specialist care: Respite, day care
Medical services: Podiatry, dentist, optician
Qualified staff: Exceeds standard: 100% at NVQ level 2

Home details

Location: Residential area, 0.2 miles from Camborne
Communal areas: Lounges, dinning room, conservatory,
    patio and garden
Accessibility: *Floors:* 2 • *Access:* Lift • *Wheelchair access:* Good
Smoking: ✗
Pets: ✓
Routines: Flexible

Room details

Single: 14
Shared: 2
En suite: Undisclosed
Door lock: ✓
Lockable place: ✓
Facilities: TV, telephone

Services provided

Beauty services: Hairdressing, manicures
Mobile library: ✗
Religious services: ✓
Transport: ✓
Activities: *Coordinator:* ✗ • *Examples:* Arts and crafts, bingo, games
    Outings: ✓
Meetings: ✓

St Clair House Care Home

Manager: David Maund
Owner: St Clair Care Ltd
Contact: 32 Basset Road,
Camborne, Cornwall, TR14 8SL
☎ 01209 713273
@ stclaircare@btconnect.com

A Georgian building that has been extended, St Clair House is a home where residents take their tea in comfortable surroundings using china cups. The home has several lounges, as well as a dining room, a garden with a patio area and a conservatory. The home has a varied activities programme including keep fit, bingo, arts and crafts and visiting entertainers. There are also outings in the home's own transport to the theatre. There are weekly residents meetings. The home offers a buffet for breakfast and a relaxed evening meal.

St Margaret's

Manager: Christopher Lydon
Owner: Blakeshields Ltd
Contact: Mylord Road,
Fraddon, St Columb, Cornwall, TR9 6LX
) 01726 861497
@ clydon@btinternet.com

Located on the main road leading into Fraddon, St Margaret's is half a mile from the local village and on the main bus route to Newquay. The nurses in the home are trained to deal with a variety of conditions. The home has an activities coordinator who arranges visiting entertainment, weekly craft sessions and bingo. There are also two outings a month. Pets are allowed in the home and smoking is permitted in a designated area. There are residents meetings once a week to discuss any issues the residents may have.

Registered places: 29
Guide weekly rate: £450–£600
Specialist care: Nursing, day care, respite, physical disability
Medical services: Podiatry, dentist, optician, physiotherapy
Qualified staff: Exceeds standard: 60% at NVQ level 2

Home details
Location: Village location, 0.5 miles from Fraddon
Communal areas: 2 lounges, dining room, patio and garden
Accessibility: *Floors:* 2 • *Access:* Lift • *Wheelchair access:* Good
Smoking: In designated area
Pets: ✓
Routines: Flexible

Room details
Single: 27
Shared: 1
En suite: 20
Facilities: TV

Door lock: ✓
Lockable place: ✓

Services provided
Beauty services: Hairdressing, aromatherapy, manicures
Mobile library: ✓
Religious services: ✓
Transport: ✗
Activities: *Coordinator:* ✓ • *Examples:* Arts and crafts, bingo, visiting entertainers • *Outings:* ✓
Meetings: ✓

St Petrocs Care Home

Manager: Fiona Searle
Owner: Stonehaven Healthcare Ltd
Contact: St Nicholas Street,
Bodmin, Cornwall, PL31 1AG
) 01208 76152
@ stpetrocs@stone-haven.co.uk
⌂ www.stone-haven.co.uk

Located in its own grounds and set back from the main road, St Petrocs lies close to local amenities and public transport links. The home is situated in a residential area, half a mile from Bodmin. The staff have good working relationships with healthcare professionals and the professionals make regular visits to the people in the home to ensure that their healthcare needs are being met. The home has an activities coordinator who arranges exercises and pampering sessions for the residents.

Registered places: 30
Guide weekly rate: £293–£400
Specialist care: Dementia, mental disorder
Medical services: Podiatry
Qualified staff: Exceeds standard: 60% at NVQ level 2

Home details
Location: Residential area, 0.3 miles from Bodmin
Communal areas: Lounge, dining room, conservatory
Accessibility: *Floors:* 2 • *Access:* Lift and stair lift
Wheelchair access: ✗
Smoking: In designated area
Pets: At manager's discretion
Routines: Flexible

Room details
Single: 27
Shared: 3
En suite: 8
Facilities: TV

Door lock: ✓
Lockable place: ✗

Services provided
Beauty services: Hairdressing
Mobile library: ✗
Religious services: ✗
Transport: ✗
Activities: *Coordinator:* ✓ • *Examples:* Exercise, entertainment, *Outings:* ✗
Meetings: ✗

Registered places: 45
Guide weekly rate: Undisclosed
Specialist care: Nursing, physical disability, respite
Medical services: Podiatry, dentist, optician
Qualified staff: Meets standard

Home details

Location: Residential area, 0.5 miles from Callington
Communal areas: 3 lounges, dining room, garden
Accessibility: *Floors:* 1 • *Wheelchair access:* Good
Smoking: ✗
Pets: At manager's discretion
Routines: Flexible

Room details

Single: 41
Shared: 2
En suite: 17
Facilities: TV point

Door lock: ✗
Lockable place: ✗

Services provided

Beauty services: Hairdressing
Mobile library: Library facilities
Religious services: ✓
Transport: ✗
Activities: *Coordinator:* ✓ • *Examples:* Exercises, games
        Outings: ✓
Meetings: ✗

St Theresa's Care Centre

Manager: Vivienne Milden
Owner: The Aldington Group Ltd
Contact: St Therese Close,
Callington, Cornwall, PL17 7QF
☎ 01579 383488

St Theresa's Care Home is situated on the outskirts of Callington, approximately half a mile from the town centre. There are three lounges, a dining room and a garden for residents to enjoy. The home has its own library facilities and organises religious services for the residents. There is an activities coordinator and the home also arranges outings. Pets would be allowed only at the manager's discretion and smoking is not permitted in the home. The home is spread across one level, providing good wheelchair access.

Registered places: 21
Guide weekly rate: £293–£495
Specialist care: Nursing, dementia, mental disorder,
        physical disability, respite
Medical services: Podiatry, optician
Qualified staff: Meets standard

Home details

Location: Residential area, 0.7 miles from Saltash
Communal areas: Lounge, dining room, garden
Accessibility: *Floors:* 2 • *Access:* Lift • *Wheelchair access:* Good
Smoking: In designated area
Pets: At manager's discretion
Routines: Flexible

Room details

Single: 14
Shared: 3
En suite: 0
Facilities: TV point, telephone point

Door lock: ✓
Lockable place: ✓

Services provided

Beauty services: Hairdressing
Mobile library: ✗
Religious services: ✗
Transport: ✗
Activities: *Coordinator:* ✗ • *Examples:* Singalongs
        Outings: ✗
Meetings: ✗

Tamar House

Manager: Paula Hannon
Owner: Mary Beaumont
Contact: 175 Old Ferry Road,
Saltash, Cornwall, PL12 6BN
☎ 01752 843579

Tamar House is located three miles from Plymouth. It is a manageable walk from the nearest shops, the Tamar Bridge and the waterfront of the river Tamar. The home allows smoking in a designated area and pets would be allowed at the manager's discretion. The home organises singalongs for the residents to participate in and also offers a hairdressing service.

Torpoint Nursing Centre

Manager: Elizabeth Fourniss
Owner: Torcare Ltd
Contact: Vicarage Road,
Torpoint, Cornwall, PL11 2BW
) 01752 813677
@ torpoint@torcare.co.uk
⌐ www.torcare.co.uk

Torpoint Nursing Centre is a purpose-built home a few hundred yards, level walk from Torpoint. It is located across the river Tamar from Plymouth. The home has its own supply of books and a mobile shop. There is a minibus at the home to take residents on outings and in the home itself the activities coordinator arranges arts and crafts and performances by visiting entertainers.

Registered places: 57
Guide weekly rate: £444–£600
Specialist care: Nursing, day care, dementia, mental disorder, physical disability, respite
Medical services: Podiatry, dentist, occupational therapy
Qualified staff: Meets standard

Home details
Location: Residential area, 0.5 miles from Torpoint
Communal areas: 2 lounges, 3 dining rooms, 2 conservatories, library, garden
Accessibility: *Floors:* 2 • *Access:* Lift • *Wheelchair access:* Good
Smoking: In designated area
Pets: ✗
Routines: Flexible

Room details
Single: 49
Shared: 4
En suite: 53
Facilities: TV point

Door lock: ✓
Lockable place: ✓

Services provided
Beauty services: Hairdressing
Mobile library: Library facilities
Religious services: ✗
Transport: Minibus
Activities: *Coordinator:* ✓ • *Examples:* Arts and crafts, visiting entertainers • *Outings:* ✓
Meetings: ✗

Trefula House

Manager: Pamela Davey
Owner: Issuemarket Ltd
Contact: St Day,
Redruth, Cornwall, TR16 5ET
) 01209 820215

Trefula Nursing Home is located in a quiet, secluded area with attractive views of the surrounding countryside. The home is situated in a village, approximately one mile from Redruth. The home arranges a variety of activities for the residents including performances by visiting entertainers and one-to-one sessions. There are also outings in the local area.

Registered places: 34
Guide weekly rate: £470–£700
Specialist care: Nursing, dementia, mental disorder, physical disability
Medical services: None
Qualified staff: Exceeds standard: 60% at NVQ level 2

Home details
Location: Village location, 1 mile from Redruth
Communal areas: Lounge, dining room, conservatory, garden
Accessibility: *Floors:* 2 • *Access:* Lift • *Wheelchair access:* Good
Smoking: ✗
Pets: ✗
Routines: Flexible

Room details
Single: 32
Shared: 2
En suite: 3
Facilities: TV point, telephone point

Door lock: ✗
Lockable place: ✗

Services provided
Beauty services: Hairdressing
Mobile library: ✗
Religious services: ✗
Transport: ✗
Activities: *Coordinator:* ✗ • *Examples:* One-to-one sessions, visiting entertainers • *Outings:* ✓
Meetings: ✗

Registered places: 25
Guide weekly rate: £550–£850
Specialist care: Respite
Medical services: Podiatry, hygienist, optician, physiotherapy
Qualified staff: Exceeds standard: 82% at NVQ level 2

Home details

Location: Residential area, 0.5 miles from Truro
Communal areas: 2 lounges, dining room, garden
Accessibility: *Floors:* 3 • *Access:* Lift • *Wheelchair access:* Good
Smoking: ✗
Pets: At manger's discretion
Routines: Flexible

Room details

Single: 22
Shared: 2
En suite: 22
Facilities: TV point, telephone point

Door lock: ✓
Lockable place: ✓

Services provided

Beauty services: Hairdressing
Mobile library: ✗
Religious services: Monthly Anglican Communion service
Transport: Minibus and car
Activities: *Coordinator:* ✓ • *Examples:* Bingo, quizzes • *Outings:* ✓
Meetings: ✗

Tregolls Manor

Manager: Rosemary Evans
Owner: Tregolls Manor Homes Ltd
Contact: Tregolls Road,
Truro, Cornwall, TR1 1XQ
) 01872 223330
@ tregolls.manor@btconnect.com

In an elevated position just off one of the main routes leading from Truro, Tregolls Manor occupies a fairly central location in the town. Residents enjoy trips all over the county of Cornwall including trips to the seaside and even trips on the Scillonian over to the Scilly Isles. The home has its own transport for these trips, in both a car and a minibus. The home also arranges an Anglican Communion service once a month as well as daily activities such as bingo and quizzes.

Registered places: 50
Guide weekly rate: £350–£750
Specialist care: Nursing, dementia, emergency admissions, physical disability, respite
Medical services: Podiatry, dentist, optician
Qualified staff: Meets standard

Home details

Location: Rural area, 1.5 miles from Bude
Communal areas: 4 lounges, dining room, activity/therapy room, hairdressing salon, library, patio and garden
Accessibility: *Floors:* 2 • *Access:* Lift • *Wheelchair access:* Good
Smoking: ✗
Pets: At manager's discretion
Routines: Flexible

Room details

Single: 44
Shared: 3
En suite: 46
Facilities: TV, telephone point

Door lock: ✓
Lockable place: ✓

Services provided

Beauty services: Hairdressing, reflexology
Mobile library: Library facilities
Religious services: Weekly nondenominational service
Transport: ✗
Activities: *Coordinator:* ✗ • *Examples:* Arts and crafts, chairobics
Outings: ✗
Meetings: ✓

Trelana Nursing Home

Manager: Jacqueline Welch
Owner: European Care Ltd
Contact: Poughill,
Bude, Cornwall, EX23 9EL
) 01288 354613
@ trelanacare@aol.com

A 19th-century home that is set in its own gardens on a hill, Trelana Nursing Home is approximately 10 minutes' walk from village facilities which include shops, a post office, church and pub. The home also permits wonderful views of both the surrounding countryside and the ocean. As well as extensive gardens, Trelana also benefits from the way the communal areas have been divided up. As well as a room with satellite TV dubbed the 'viewing zone', there are also quiet areas for reading or chatting. The home has a residents meeting once a month.

Trelawney House

Manager: Vacant
Owner: Christine and Rigas Gatzianidis
Contact: Polladras, Carleen,
Helston, Cornwall, TR13 9NT
) 01736 763334

Situated in a rural area with views of the surrounding countryside, Trelawney House sits in its own grounds. The gardens are accessible, with seating areas and a pond. The home is pet friendly, and currently cats and dogs are living at the home. Trelawney also provide a 'meals on wheels' facility supplying a small number of homes in the surrounding area. The home has its own transport and arranges a Communion service every two weeks.

Registered places: 11
Guide weekly rate: £365–£500
Specialist care: Day care, respite
Medical services: Podiatry, dentist, optician
Qualified staff: Meets standard

Home details
Location: Rural area, 4 miles from Helston
Communal areas: 2 lounges, dining room, garden
Accessibility: *Floors:* 2 • *Access:* Lift • *Wheelchair access:* Good
Smoking: ✗
Pets: At manager's discretion
Routines: Flexible

Room details
Single: 9
Shared: 1
En suite: 9
Facilities: TV point, telephone point

Door lock: ✗
Lockable place: ✓

Services provided
Beauty services: Hairdressing
Mobile library: ✗
Religious services: Fortnightly Communion service
Transport: Car
Activities: *Coordinator:* ✗ • *Examples:* Barbecues, bingo, quizzes
  Outings: ✗
Meetings: ✓

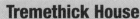

Tremethick House

Manager: Denise Ball
Owner: Mary and John Anson
Contact: Meadowside,
Redruth, Cornwall, TR15 3AL
) 01209 215713
@ info@anson-care-services.co.uk

Situated on the edge of Redruth town, Tremethick House allows residents easy access to the town's leisure and health facilities and is a bus ride from the nearest shop. There has recently been a new wing added to the home. Residents have their own choice in activities, and the activities coordinator will try to be flexible to their preferences. There is a mobile library which visits the home and there are regular visits from clergy of varying denominations.

Registered places: 42
Guide weekly rate: £335–£410
Specialist care: Dementia
Medical services: Podiatry, hygienist, optician, physiotherapy
Qualified staff: Exceeds standard: 80% at NVQ level 2

Home details
Location: Residential area, 1.2 miles from Redruth
Communal areas: 3 Lounges, dining room, patio and garden
Accessibility: *Floors:* 2 • *Access:* 2 lifts • *Wheelchair access:* Good
Smoking: ✗
Pets: At manager's discretion
Routines: Flexible

Room details
Single: 38
Shared: 2
En suite: 32
Facilities: TV point, telephone point

Door lock: ✓
Lockable place: ✓

Services provided
Beauty services: Hairdressing
Mobile Library: ✓
Religious services: Regular visits
Transport: ✓
Activities: *Coordinator:* ✓ • *Examples:* Games • *Outings:* ✓
Meetings: ✗

Registered places: 73
Guide weekly rate: £562–£650
Specialist care: Nursing, dementia, mental disorder,
 physical disability
Medical services: Podiatry, dentist, optician
Qualified staff: Meets standard

Home details

Location: Residential area, 2 miles from Penzance
Communal areas: Lounge, dining room, garden
Accessibility: *Floors:* 2 • *Access:* Undisclosed
 Wheelchair access: Undisclosed
Smoking: ✗
Pets: ✓
Routines: Flexible

Room details

Single: 73
Shared: 0
En suite: Undisclosed
Facilities: None

Door lock: ✓
Lockable place: ✓

Services provided

Beauty services: Hairdressing
Mobile library: ✗
Religious services: ✗
Transport: Minibus
Activities: *Coordinator:* ✓ • *Examples:* Games • *Outings:* ✓
Meetings: ✓

Trevaylor Manor

Manager: Janet Prela
Owner: Swallowcourt Ltd
Contact: Newmill Road,
Gulval, Penzance, Cornwall, TR20 8UR
☎ 01736 350856
@ trevaylor@swallowcourt.com

Trevaylor Manor is a detached manor house set in spacious grounds, approximately two miles from Penzance. The home has a designated dementia wing and organises daily outings for residents. The home supports a group where residents have regular meetings. There is a wide variety of activities on offer and throughout the home and the home has its own minibus for outings.

Registered places: 10
Guide weekly rate: £310
Specialist care: Day care, respite, mental disorder
Medical services: Podiatry
Qualified staff: Fails standards

Home details

Location: Residential area, 1 mile from St Columb Major
Communal areas: Lounge, dining room, garden
Accessibility: *Floors:* 2 • *Access:* None • *Wheelchair access:* Limited
Smoking: ✗
Pets: ✓
Routines: Flexible

Room details

Single: 8
Shared: 1
En suite: 5
Facilities: TV point, telephone point

Door lock: ✓
Lockable place: ✓

Services provided

Beauty services: Hairdressing
Mobile library: Library facilities
Religious services: ✗
Transport: ✗
Activities: *Coordinator:* ✗ • *Examples:* Board games, films, reading
 Outings: ✗
Meetings: ✗

Tropicana

Manager: Vacant
Owner: Ernest and Marina Westbrook
Contact: Newquay Road,
St Columb Major, Cornwall, TR9 6TJ
☎ 01637 880779
@ info@trop.ssnet.co.uk

A family-run home where the owners live on site, Tropicana is a Victorian property situated six miles from the sea and around one mile from St Columb Major. The home is a short walk from the town. Tropicana has a pond in the garden and the home has a large library of books and films on DVD. The home arranges activities such as board games and film showing for the residents.

The White House Care Home

Manager: Eves Carkeek
Owner: Platinum Care Ltd
Contact: 40 Castle Street, Bodmin, Cornwall, PL31 2DU

☎ 01208 72310
@ thewhitehouse@surf3.co.uk
🖱 www.whitehousecarehome.co.uk

The White House is a modernised Victorian house located on a hill overlooking Bodmin and the surrounding Cornish countryside. In easy walking distance of local amenities, the home also has an hourly bus service running from the back gate, thus enabling residents to maintain a degree of independence outside of the home. With an extensive and varied activities programme on offer, residents with an interest in gardening are also encouraged to pursue their hobby. As well as twice-monthly residents meetings, the home publishes a newsletter with news on activities, useful addresses, birthday messages and tips.

Registered places: 34
Guide weekly rate: From £330
Specialist care: Day care, dementia, emergency admissions, mental disorder, physical disability, respite
Medical services: Podiatry, dentist, optician, physiotherapy
Qualified staff: Meets standard

Home details
Location: Residential area, 0.2 miles from Bodmin
Communal areas: 2 lounges, 2 dining rooms, garden
Accessibility: *Floors:* 3 • *Access:* Lift and stair Lift *Wheelchair Access:* Good
Smoking: In designated area
Pets: At manager's discretion
Routines: Flexible

Room details
Single: 34	
Shared: 0	Door lock: ✓
En suite: 19	Lockable place: ✓
Facilities: TV point	

Services provided
Beauty services: Hairdressing, manicures
Mobile library: ✓
Religious services: Weekly Catholic Communion service, monthly Methodist Communion service, monthly Anglican visits
Transport: ✗
Activities: *Coordinator:* ✗ • *Examples:* Bingo, visiting entertainers *Outings:* ✓
Meetings: ✓

Windmill Court

Manager: Fiona Khouri
Owner: Thomas Henry Mallaband Ltd
Contact: St Minver, Wadebridge, Cornwall, PL27 6RD

☎ 01208 863831

Set in its own grounds and permitting attractive views of the surrounding area, Windmill Court is located in a rural area, approximately five miles from Wadebridge. The home has a conservatory and a garden for residents to enjoy in the warmer months and two activities coordinators who arrange a varied program. This includes armchair yoga and one-to-one sessions. The home also arranges a Communion service which takes place every two weeks.

Registered places: 34
Guide weekly rate: £675–£795
Specialist care: Nursing, physical disability, sensory impairment
Medical services: Podiatry, dentist, optician
Qualified staff: Exceeds standard: 82% at NVQ level 2

Home details
Location: Rural area, 5 miles from Wadebridge
Communal areas: Lounge, dining room, hairdressing salon, conservatory, garden
Accessibility: *Floors:* 2 • *Access:* Lift • *Wheelchair access:* Good
Smoking: ✗
Pets: ✓
Routines: Flexible

Room details
Single: 34	
Shared: 0	Door lock: ✓
En suite: 34	Lockable place: ✓
Facilities: TV point	

Services provided
Beauty services: Hairdressing
Mobile library: ✓
Religious services: Fortnightly Communion service
Transport: ✗
Activities: *Coordinator:* ✓ • *Examples:* Armchair yoga, one-to-one sessions • *Outings:* ✗
Meetings: ✗

Registered places: 32
Guide weekly rate: Undisclosed
Specialist care: Nursing, dementia
Medical services: Podiatry, hygienist, optician, physiotherapy
Qualified staff: Undisclosed

Home details

Location: Residential area, 1 mile from Okehampton
Communal areas: 2 lounges, dining room, activity room, conservatory, garden
Accessibility: *Floors:* 3 • *Access:* Lift • *Wheelchair Access:* Good
Smoking: In designated area
Pets: At manager's discretion
Routines: Structured

Room details

Single: 32
Shared: 0
En suite: 32
Facilities: TV point, telephone point

Door lock: ✓
Lockable place: ✓

Services provided

Beauty services: Hairdressing
Mobile library: ✗
Religious services: ✗
Transport: ✗
Activities: *Coordinator:* ✓ • *Examples:* Painting, gardening
    Outings: ✗
Meetings: ✗

Aalen House

Manager: Jan Hazell
Owner: PSP Group Ltd
Contact: 12 Parklands, Okehampton, Devon, EX20 1EG
) 01837 52039
@ Manager@aalenhouse.com
⌂ www.aalenhouse.com

Aalen House is an extended property in a rural location. It is approximately one mile from the Okehampton. The facilities there include a post office, hotel, pub and health centre. A conservatory is being built at the home. The home also has two lounges and an activity room. The home has a dedicated activities coordinator who organises painting and gardening for the residents.

Registered places: 9
Guide weekly rate: From £350
Specialist care: Day care, respite
Medical services: Podiatry, dentist, optician
Qualified staff: Meets standard

Home details

Location: Residential area, 1 mile from Torquay
Communal areas: Lounge, dining room, patio
Accessibility: *Floors:* 3 • *Access: Stair lift* • *Wheelchair access:* Good
Smoking: ✗
Pets: ✓
Routines: Flexible

Room details

Single: 7
Shared: 1
En suite: 7
Facilities: TV point, telephone point

Door lock: ✓
Lockable place: ✓

Services provided

Beauty services: Hairdressing
Mobile library: ✓
Religious services: Communion
Transport: People carrier
Activities: *Coordinator:* ✓ • *Examples:* Bingo, visiting entertainers
    Outings: ✓
Meetings: ✓

Abbott's Residential Care Home

Manager: Alison Goodrich
Owner: David Trulock
Contact: 74 Windsor Road, Babbacombe, Torquay, Devon, TQ1 1SX
) 01803 327574
@ enquiries@abbottresidential.co.uk
⌂ www.abbottresidential.co.uk

Abbott's Residential Care Home is a large semi-detached Victorian property situated one mile from Torquay. The home has a lounge and a dining room as well as a patio area for residents to enjoy in the warmer weather. There are daily activities such as bingo and one-to-one sessions and the home also arranges performances by visiting entertainers. There are arranged outings, for example to the nearby butterfly farm, and there are photographs on display from parties held in the home.

Adelaide Lodge Retirement Home

Manager: Melissa Salter
Owner: Adelaide Lodge Care Home Ltd
Contact: 27 Kings Road,
Honiton, Devon, EX14 1HW
☏ 01404 42921
🖥 www.adelaidelodge.co.uk

Occupying a one-acre site, Adelaide Lodge is a detached property situated on the edge of the attractive market town of Honiton, approximately 10 minutes' walk from the centre. This is a fast-growing area with great shopping links and well known for its antique shops, ideal for active retirees. The vegetable gardens and sensory garden with water feature at the home offer a place for relaxation. The home is a few minutes' drive from Honiton Hospital and near a train station.

Registered places: 37
Guide weekly rate: £400–£450
Specialist care: Day care, dementia, physical disability, respite
Medical services: Podiatry, dentist, optician, physiotherapy
Qualified staff: Undisclosed

Home details
Location: Residential area, 0.5 miles from Honiton centre
Communal areas: 2 lounges, dining room, patio and garden
Accessibility: *Floors:* 3 • *Access:* Lift and stair Lift
   Wheelchair access: Good
Smoking: ✗
Pets: ✗
Routines: Flexible

Room details
Single: 31
Shared: 3
En suite: 15
Facilities: TV point, telephone point

Door lock: ✓
Lockable place: ✗

Services provided
Beauty services: Hairdressing
Mobile library: ✗
Religious services: Monthly Communion service
Transport: Minibus
Activities: *Coordinator:* ✓ • *Examples:* Arts and crafts, bingo, exercise
   Outings: ✓
Meetings: ✓

Alban House

Manager: Frances Svenson
Owner: David and Frances Svenson
Contact: 8–10 Apsley Terrace,
Highfield Road, Ilfracombe,
Devon, EX34 9JU
☏ 01271 863217
@ fran@albanhouse.co.uk
🖥 www.albanhouse.co.uk

Alban House in an older property which incorporates what used to be three separate buildings. The home is located close to Ilfracombe's high street and the local facilities. It is also a few hundred yards from the coast. The home has its own car for transport and takes the residents on outings in the local area.

Registered places: 22
Guide weekly rate: £270–£400
Specialist care: Day care, dementia, mental disorder
Medical services: Podiatry, optician, physiotherapy
Qualified staff: Undisclosed

Home details
Location: Residential area, in Ilfracombe
Communal areas: Lounge, dining room, 3 conservatories, garden
Accessibility: *Floors:* 4 • *Access:* Lift • *Wheelchair access:* Good
Smoking: In designated area
Pets: At manager's discretion
Routines: Flexible

Room details
Single: 22
Shared: 0
En suite: Undisclosed
Facilities: TV point

Door lock: ✓
Lockable place: ✓

Services provided
Beauty services: Hairdressing
Mobile library: ✗
Religious services: ✗
Transport: Car
Activities: *Coordinator:* ✗ • *Examples:* Exercises, games
   Outings: ✓
Meetings: ✓

Registered places: 28
Guide weekly rate: £400–£450
Specialist care: Undisclosed
Medical services: Podiatry, hygienist, optician
Qualified staff: Fails standards

Home details

Location: Residential area, 2 miles from Exeter centre
Communal areas: 3 lounges, garden
Accessibility: *Floors:* 3 • *Access:* Lift • *Wheelchair access:* Good
Smoking: ✗
Pets: ✗
Routines: Flexible

Room details

Single: 28
Shared: 0
En suite: 14
Facilities: TV point, telephone point

Door lock: ✓
Lockable place: ✓

Services provided

Beauty services: Hairdressing
Mobile library: ✓
Religious services: Weekly Catholic Mass,
    fortnightly Anglican Communion service
Transport: ✗
Activities: *Coordinator:* ✓ • *Examples:* Bingo, flower arranging
    Outings: ✓
Meetings: Undisclosed

Alphington Lodge Residential Home

Manager: Susan Reynolds
Owner: Nicola and Anna Hitchcott
Contact: 1 St Michaels Close,
Alphington, Exeter, Devon, EX2 8XH

☎ 01392 216352
@ jan@alphingtonlodge.co.uk
🖰 www.alphingtonlodge.co.uk

Alphington Lodge is a Grade II listed period property in the centre of Alphington. It is located near to local amenities, including shops, pubs and a health centre. Alphington Lodge is currently home to a cat, and there is a fishpond in the garden. The home arranges a range of religious services and also takes residents on outings in the local area.

Registered places: 39
Guide weekly rate: Undisclosed
Specialist care: Day care, dementia, mental disorder,
    physical disability, respite
Medical services: Podiatry, optician
Qualified staff: Undisclosed

Home details

Location: Residential area, in Plympton
Communal areas: 4 lounges, 3 dining rooms, garden
Accessibility: *Floors:* 3 • *Access:* Lift and stair lifts
    Wheelchair access: Good
Smoking: ✗
Pets: At manager's discretion
Routines: Structured

Room details

Single: 39
Shared: 0
En suite: 37
Facilities: TV point, telephone point

Door lock: ✓
Lockable place: ✓

Services provided

Beauty services: Hairdressing
Mobile library: ✓
Transport: Minibus and car
Religious services: Monthly Anglican Communion service,
    weekly Catholic Mass
Activities: *Coordinator:* ✓ • *Examples:* Bingo, visiting entertainers
    Outings: ✗
Meetings: ✓

Amberley House

Manager: Lisa Webb
Owner: A & L Care Homes Ltd
Contact: 171–175 Ridgeway,
Plympton, Plymouth, Devon, PL7 2HJ

☎ 01752 336960
@ amberleyhouse@plympton51.fsnet.co.uk

Located in central Plymouth, Amberley House offers easy access to local amenities. It is a few hundred yards walk to local shops, including a supermarket and chemist. The home has its own transport and arranges both Anglican and Catholic services for the residents. The activities coordinator arranges bingo for the residents and performances by visiting entertainers.

DEVON

Amelia House

Manager: Nuala Baxendale
Owner: Nuala and Alan Baxendale
Contact: Pocombe Bridge,
Exeter, Devon, EX2 9SX
☎ 01392 213631
@ AmeliaHouseRes@aol.com

Situated in a rural location with attractive views, Amelia House is an old building which retains much of its character. The home boasts a large garden with a greenhouse. The owners live in adjoining premises and so are always close at hand. The home has an Anglican Communion service once a month and arranges other activities such as exercise sessions and musical entertainment.

Registered places: 18
Guide weekly rate: £390–£420
Specialist care: Dementia, respite
Medical services: Podiatry, dentist, optician
Qualified staff: Undisclosed

Home details
Location: Residential area, 2 miles from Exeter centre
Communal areas: 2 lounges, 2 dining rooms, conservatory, garden
Accessibility: *Floors:* 2 • *Access:* Stair Lift • *Wheelchair access:* Limited
Smoking: In designated area
Pets: At manager's discretion
Routines: Flexible

Room details
Single: 18
Shared: 0
En suite: 10
Facilities: TV point, telephone point

Lockable place: ✓
Door lock: ✓

Services provided
Beauty services: Hairdressing
Mobile library: ✗
Religious services: Monthly Anglican Communion service
Transport: ✗
Activities: *Coordinator:* ✗ • *Examples:* Exercise sessions, quizzes
　　　　Outings: ✗
Meetings: ✗

Amersham Care Home

Manager: Richard Conway
Owner: Amersham House Care Ltd
Contact: 454 Babbacombe Road,
Torquay, Devon, TQ1 1HW
☎ 01803 292762

Amersham Care Home is a converted, period property. The home's garden is partly accessible to residents. The home is located in a residential area, half a mile from Torquay harbour. The home has its own minibus and often takes residents on outings. The home also has its own activities coordinator.

Registered places: 15
Guide weekly rate: £360
Medical services: Podiatry, dentist, optician
Specialist care: Dementia, physical disability
Qualified staff: Undisclosed

Home details
Location: Residential area, 0.5 miles from Torquay harbour
Communal areas: Lounge, conservatory, dining room
Accessibility: *Floors:* 2 • *Access:* Stair lift • *Wheelchair access:* Good
Smoking: ✗
Pets: ✓
Routines: Flexible

Room details
Single: 11
Shared: 2
En suite: 13
Facilities: TV

Door lock: ✓
Lockable place: ✓

Services provided
Beauty services: None
Mobile library: ✗
Religious services: ✗
Transport: Minibus
Activities: *Coordinator:* ✓ • *Examples:* Bingo • *Outings:* ✓
Meetings: ✗

Registered places: 37
Guide weekly rate: £350–£500
Specialist care: Respite, dementia, physical disability
Medical services: Podiatry, optician
Qualified staff: Meets standard

Home details
Location: Rural area, 0.5 miles from Tipton St John
Communal areas: Lounge, dining room, hairdressing salon, garden
Accessibility: *Floors:* 2 • *Access:* Lift • *Wheelchair access:* Good
Smoking: In designated area
Pets: ✓
Routines: Flexible

Room details
Single: 37
Shared: 0
En suite: 14
Facilities: TV point

Door lock: ✓
Lockable place: ✓

Services provided
Beauty services: Hairdressing
Mobile library: ✗
Religious services: ✗
Transport: ✗
Activities: *Coordinator:* ✓ • *Examples:* Visiting entertainers
   Outings: ✓
Meetings: ✗

Angela Court

Manager: Mary Bavidge
Owner: Pliahurst Ltd
Contact: Tipton St John,
Sidmouth, Devon, EX10 0AG
☎ 01404 812495

Angela Court is situated next to the church in the village of Tipton St John. The home currently owns two budgies and is considering having a cat within the home as well. Angela Court possesses its own hairdressing salon, where hairdressers come in two or three times a week. The home also has an activities coordinator who arranges performances by visiting entertainers as well as outings in the local area.

Registered places: 28
Guide weekly rate: Undisclosed
Specialist care: Day care, dementia, physical disability
Medical services: Podiatry, hygienist, optician
Qualified staff: Meets standard

Home details
Location: Residential area, 1.3 miles from Torquay
Communal areas: Lounge, dining room, visiting room, garden
Accessibility: *Floors:* 3 • *Access:* Stair Lift • *Wheelchair access:* Limited
Smoking: ✗
Pets: At manager's discretion
Routines: Flexible

Room details
Single: 28
Shared: 0
En suite: Undisclosed
Facilities: TV point, telephone point

Door lock: ✗
Lockable place: ✓

Services provided
Beauty services: Hairdressing
Mobile library: ✗
Religious services: ✗
Transport: Minibus
Activities: *Coordinator:* ✗ • *Examples:* Exercises, games
   Outings: ✓
Meetings: ✗

Ashbourne House

Manager: Sandra Brown
Owner: Robert and Diana Williamson
Contact: 213 St Marychurch Road,
Torquay, Devon, TQ1 3JT
☎ 01803 327041

Situated in a residential area close to the St Marychurch precinct, Ashbourne House provides a varied programme of activities including trips in the home's minibus. The home has a lounge and a garden for residents to relax in, as well as a visiting room to enjoy some privacy with their guests.

Ashdowne Care Centre

Manager: Kate Ley
Owner: Ashdown Care Ltd
Contact: Orkney Mews, Pinnex Moor Road, Tiverton, Devon, EX16 6SJ
) 01884 252527
@ ashdownecare@onetel.com

Ashdowne is a purpose-built property and is split into two sections: Ashdowne and Pinnex (which cares for those with mental disorders). The two are connected by a covered walkway. There are garden areas adjoining the properties. The home is situated a 20-minute walk from the town centre and there is a bus service into town. The home has deliveries of books from the local library. The home also offers regular religious services including Communion.

Registered places: 60
Guide weekly rate: Undisclosed
Specialist care: Nursing, dementia, mental disorder
Medical services: Podiatry, dentist, optician
Qualified staff: Fails standards

Home details
Location: Residential area, 1.6 miles from Tiverton
Communal areas: Lounges, dining area, garden
Accessibility: *Floors:* Undisclosed • *Access:* Undisclosed
    Wheelchair access: Undisclosed
Smoking: In designated area
Pets: At manager's discretion
Routines: Flexible

Room details
Single: 60
Shared: 0
En suite: 0
Facilities: TV, telephone

Door lock: ✓
Lockable place: ✓

Services provided
Beauty services: Hairdressing
Mobile library: Library facilities
Religious services: ✓
Transport: ✗
Activities: *Coordinator:* ✓ • *Examples:* Pets As Therapy
    Outings: ✓
Meetings: ✓

Ashleigh Manor

Manager: Maureen Lawley
Owner: Maureen and Loretta Maher-Lawley
Contact: 1–3 Vicarage Road, Plympton, Plymouth, Devon, PL7 4JU
) 01752 346662

A detached house set in its own grounds, Ashleigh Manor is located in a residential area close to local amenities and on a bus route to Plympton. The home is a 15-minute walk from The Ridgeway shopping centre. Permitting attractive views of the surrounding countryside it also has a large garden, which is currently home to Ashleigh Manor's two cats. The home publishes a quarterly newsletter with details of activities and outings.

Registered places: 38
Guide weekly rate: £333–£406
Specialist care: Dementia, physical disability
Medical services: Podiatry, hygienist, optician
Qualified staff: Exceeds standard: 70% at NVQ level 2

Home details
Location: Residential area, 0.2 miles from Plympton
Communal areas: 4 lounges, 4 dining rooms, library conservatory, garden
Accessibility: *Floors:* 2 • *Access:* Lift and stair Lift
    Wheelchair access: Good
Smoking: ✗
Pets: ✓
Routines: Flexible

Room details
Single: 37
Shared: 1
En suite: 30
Facilities: TV point, telephone point

Door lock: ✓
Lockable place: ✓

Services provided
Beauty services: Hairdressing, aromatherapy, massage
Mobile library: ✓
Religious services: ✗
Transport: ✗
Activities: *Coordinator:* ✓ • *Examples:* Musical entertainment
    Outings: ✓
Meetings: ✓

Registered places: 33
Guide weekly rate: £350–£540
Specialist care: Nursing, physical disability
Medical services: Podiatry, physiotherapy
Qualified staff: Fails standards

Home details
Location: Residential area, 1 mile from Torquay
Communal areas: 2 lounges, dining room, hairdressing salon, garden
Accessibility: *Floors:* Undisclosed • *Access:* Lift
    Wheelchair access: Undisclosed
Smoking: ✗
Pets: ✓
Routines: Flexible

Room details
Single: 31
Shared: 2
En suite: Undisclosed
Facilities: TV

Door lock: ✗
Lockable place: ✗

Services provided
Beauty services: Hairdressing
Mobile library: ✗
Religious services: ✗
Transport: ✗
Activities: • *Coordinator:* ✗ • *Examples:* Visiting musicians, quizzes
    Outings: ✗
Meetings: ✗

Aspreys Nursing Home

Manager: Sandra Todd
Owner: Friendly Care Homes Ltd
Contact: 1 Kents Road,
Torquay, Devon, TQ1 2NL
☎ 01803 201500
@ matron@aspreys.co.uk

Aspreys Nursing Home is found in Wellswood, one mile from Torquay town centre. The local shops, a pub and restaurants are around 100 yards from the home. The local church is less than 200 yards. Weekly activities are organised for residents such as quizzes and musical entertainment. The home has two lounges and a garden for residents to enjoy as well as a dedicated hairdressing salon.

Registered places: 30
Guide weekly rate: £370–£450
Specialist care: Day care, dementia, mental disorder,
    physical disability
Medical services: Undisclosed
Qualified staff: Fails standard: 33% at NVQ level 2

Home details
Location: Residential area, 1.3 miles from Torquay
Communal areas: Lounge, dining room, garden
Accessibility: *Floors:* 2 • *Access:* Lift and stair Lift
    Wheelchair access: Good
Smoking: ✗
Pets: Undisclosed
Routines: Flexible

Room details
Single: 22
Shared: 4
En suite: Undisclosed
Facilities: None

Door lock: ✗
Lockable place: ✗

Services provided
Beauty services: None
Mobile library: ✗
Religious services: ✗
Transport: Minibus
Activities: *Coordinator:* ✗ • *Examples:* Flower arranging, music
    Outings: ✓
Meetings: Undisclosed

Aveland Court

Manager: Gina Coplestone
Owner: Christina Walton
Contact: Aveland Road,
Torquay, Devon, TQ1 3PT
☎ 01803 326259

Aveland Court is detached and set in quiet level gardens to the front and back. The shops, parks and other local amenities at Babbacombe are within level walking distance. A minibus is provided, for trips out and healthcare appointments.
Although the home is registered for 30 places, there are normally no more than 26 residents. Most bedrooms have an en suite toilet, and some have patio doors. Recent outings include picnics to both Dartmouth and Dartmoor, cream teas at Lustleigh and ice creams on the beach at Goodrington.

Barton House

Manager: Sally Child
Owner: Mr and Mrs Child
Contact: 1 Barton Terrace,
Dawlish, Devon, EX7 9QH
☏ 01626 864474

Barton House is a Grade II listed building situated in a prominent position close to the centre of Barton Terrace. A five-minute walk from shops in the town centre, the home is also a few minutes' walk from the hospital and nearby Manor Gardens. Residents may also wander up to the large public lawn that is home to Dawlish's famous black swans. Residents are encouraged to live as 'full and normal life as possible' and many enjoy spending time in the home's gardens with its plants, flowers, rockery and pond.

Registered places: 11
Guide weekly rate: £297–£465
Specialist care: Day care, dementia, mental disorder, physical disability, respite
Medical services: Podiatry, dentist, optician, physiotherapy
Qualified staff: Fails standards

Home details
Location: Residential area, in Dawlish
Communal areas: 2 lounge/dining rooms, patio and garden
Accessibility: *Floors:* 2 • *Access:* Lift • *Wheelchair access:* ✗
Smoking: In designated area
Pets: ✗
Routines: Flexible

Room details
Single: 11
Shared: 0
En suite: 2
Facilities: TV point

Door lock: ✓
Lockable place: ✓

Services provided
Beauty services: Hairdressing
Mobile library: ✗
Religious services: Monthly Anglican and Methodist visits, monthly Communion service
Transport: ✗
Activities: *Coordinator:* ✓ • *Examples:* Bingo, exercise class
Outings: ✗
Meetings: ✓

Barton Lodge

Manager: Sally and Glen Child
Owner: Sally and Glen Child
Contact: 12 Longlands, Dawlish, Devon,
EX7 9NF
☏ 01626 866724
@ bartoncare@supernet.com

Barton Lodge is located in a residential area, half a mile from the town of Dawlish. There is a lounge and a dining room in the home as well as a conservatory and a garden. The home arranges walks in the local area for the residents in addition to activities in the home such as bingo and music sessions. There are also outings to the local theatre. The home arranges a Communion service to take place on a monthly basis and there are visits from a mobile library.

Registered places: 11
Guide weekly rate: £294–£430
Specialist care: Dementia, respite
Medical services: Podiatry, dentist, optician
Qualified staff: Meets standard

Home details
Location: Residential area, 0.5 miles from Dawlish
Communal areas: Lounge, dining room, conservatory, garden
Accessibility: *Floors:* 2 • *Access:* Stair lift • *Wheelchair access:* Good
Smoking: ✗
Pets: At manager's discretion
Routines: Flexible

Room details
Single: 7
Shared: 2
En suite: 9
Facilities: TV, telephone

Door lock: ✓
Lockable place: ✓

Services provided
Beauty services: Hairdressing
Mobile library: ✓
Religious services: Monthly Communion
Transport: ✗
Activities: *Coordinator:* ✗ • *Examples:* Bingo, music, reminiscence sessions • *Outings:* ✓
Meetings: ✓

Registered places: 30
Guide weekly rate: £650–£750
Specialist care: Nursing, dementia, mental disorder
Medical services: Podiatry, hygienist, optician, physiotherapy
Qualified staff: Exceeds standard: 80% at NVQ level 2

Home details
Location: Residential area, 2 mile from Exeter
Communal areas: 3 lounges, library, garden
Accessibility: *Floors:* 3 • *Access:* Lift • *Wheelchair access:* Good
Smoking: ✗
Pets: At manager's discretion
Routines: Structured

Room details
Single: 20
Shared: 5 | Door lock: ✓
En suite: 15 | Lockable place: ✗
Facilities: None

Services provided
Beauty services: Hairdressing
Mobile library: Library facilities
Religious services: Monthly
Transport: ✗
Activities: *Coordinator:* ✓ • *Examples:* Arts and crafts
  Outings: ✗
Meetings: ✗

Barton Place Independent Care Hotel

Manager: Michaela Harris
Owner: Barton Place Ltd
Contact: Wrefords Link,
Cowley Bridge, Exeter, Devon, EX4 5AX
☎ 01392 211099
@ kh.barton-place@btconnect.com

A grand Georgian house with several acres of established gardens, Barton Place is located close to Cowley Hill and the river Exe. The home recently received funding to install a new sensory garden. The home also has three lounges for residents to relax in and its own library facilities. There are monthly religious services in the home and the activities coordinator arranges both group and on-to-one sessions.

Registered places: 31
Guide weekly rate: From £395
Specialist care: Day care, physical disability, respite
Medical services: Podiatry, dentist, optician, physiotherapy
Qualified staff: Exceeds standard: 90% at NVQ level 2

Home details
Location: Residential area, 4.5 miles from Torbay
Communal areas: 2 lounges, dining room, patio and garden
Accessibility: *Floors:* 3 • *Access:* Lift • *Wheelchair access:* Good
Smoking: ✗
Pets: ✓
Routines: Flexible

Room details
Single: 23
Shared: 4 | Door lock: ✓
En suite: 31 | Lockable place: ✓
Facilities: TV point, telephone point

Services provided
Beauty services: Hairdressing, manicures
Mobile library: ✓
Religious services: Monthly Anglican service
Transport: ✓
Activities: *Coordinator:* ✗ • *Examples:* Bingo, piano playing
  Outings: ✓
Meetings: ✓

Bascombe Court

Manager: Jill Wakeham
Owner: The Manor Collection
Contact: Bascombe Road,
Churston Ferrers, Brixham,
Devon, TQ5 0JS
☎ 01803 842360
@ info@thecourtgroup.co.uk
🖰 www.thecourtgroup.co.uk

Standing in two acres of landscaped gardens, with features which include a water garden and terraced walkways, Bacombe Court offers care for 31 residents. From the patios and terraces around the house there are wonderful views across to the coastal charms of Broadsands and Elbury Cove. All bedrooms offer en suite facilities and some rooms can provide the added luxury of their own sitting rooms. The home also benefits from having a minibus service which takes residents on frequent trips out.

Bay Court Nursing and Residential Home

Manager: Susan Stevens
Owner: Court Healthcare Ltd
Contact: 16–18 West Hill,
Budleigh Salterton, Devon, EX9 6BS
✆ 01395 442637
@ matron@baycourt.net
🖰 www.baycourt.net

Bay Court is located in the centre of Budleigh Salterton, a town on the Devon coast. It is less then 200 yards level walk to the centre of town, and approximately the same distance to the seafront. The home has visits from a mobile library and there is an Anglican Communion service once a month. The activities programme at the home includes poetry readings and board games.

Registered places: 29
Guide weekly rate: £496–£650
Specialist care: Nursing, respite
Medical services: Podiatry, optician, physiotherapy
Qualified staff: Exceeds standard: 64% at NVQ level 2

Home details
Location: Residential area, 0.2 miles from Budleigh Salterton
Communal areas: 3 lounges, dining room, garden
Accessibility: *Floors:* 4 • *Access:* Lift • *Wheelchair access:* Good
Smoking: In designated area
Pets: ✗
Routines: Flexible

Room details
Single: 24
Shared: 5
En suite: Undisclosed
Facilities: TV point, telephone point

Door lock: ✓
Lockable place: ✓

Services provided
Beauty services: Hairdressing, massage
Mobile library: ✓
Religious services: Monthly Anglican Communion service
Transport: ✗
Activities: *Coordinator:* ✗ • *Examples:* Poetry reading, board games
　　　Outings: ✗
Meetings: ✗

Beacon Court

Manager: Sharon Mewis
Owner: Thurlestone Court Ltd
Contact: 4 Church Road,
Dartmouth, Devon, TQ6 9HQ
✆ 01803 832672

Situated on a quiet hill with spectacular views of the surrounding countryside and estuary, Beacon Court is located on a bus route which runs to Dartmouth. As part of The Court Group, the home produces a 'group' newsletter. As part of their activities programme, Beacon Court provides weekly outings to residents at a small charge. The programme also includes handicrafts and baking sessions.

Registered places: 34
Guide weekly rate: Between £350–£500
Specialist care: Dementia, mental disorder, physical disability
Medical services: Podiatry, dentist, optician
Qualified staff: Fails standards

Home details
Location: Rural area, 0.6 miles from Dartmouth
Communal areas: 2 lounges, dining room, conservatory, garden
Accessibility: *Floors:* 4 • *Access:* Lift and stair Lift
　　　Wheelchair access: Good
Smoking: In designated area
Pets: ✓
Routines: Flexible

Room details
Single: 34
Shared: 0
En suite: Undisclosed
Facilities: TV point

Door lock: ✓
Lockable place: ✗

Services provided
Beauty services: Hairdressing
Mobile library: ✗
Religious services: ✗
Transport: ✗
Activities: *Coordinator:* ✗ • *Examples:* Arts and crafts, baking
　　　Outings: ✓
Meetings: ✓

Registered places: 104
Guide weekly rate: £278–£533
Specialist care: Nursing, day care, dementia, physical disability, respite
Medical services: Podiatry, optician, physiotherapy
Qualified staff: Exceeds standard: 59% at NVQ level 2

Home details
Location: Residential area, 2.5 miles from Plymouth
Communal areas: Lounges, dining rooms, garden
Accessibility: *Floors:* 2 • *Access:* Lift • *Wheelchair access:* Good
Smoking: In designated area
Pets: At manager's discretion
Routines: Structured

Room details
Single: 93
Shared: 8
En suite: 95
Facilities: 0

Door lock: ✓
Lockable place: ✓

Services provided
Beauty services: Hairdressing
Mobile library: ✓
Religious services: ✗
Transport: ✗
Activities: *Coordinator:* ✓ • *Examples:* Bingo, games, quizzes
    Outings: ✗
Meetings: ✗

Bedford Park Care Centre

Manager: Sally Thornton
Owner: Aermid Health Care
Contact: Pearn Road, Mannamead, Plymouth, Devon, PL3 5JF
☏ 01752 770477
@ Manager.bedfordpark@aermid.com

A purpose-built facility, Bedford Park Care Centre is arranged in three distinct units, the nursing unit, residential unit and 'Compton Gardens'. All residents have access to the landscaped gardens, which include a raised fishpond. It is a short bus ride to Plymouth city centre and the bus stop is near to the home. Currently three cats live in the home. The home has a dedicated activities coordinator who arranges activities such as bingo and quizzes.

Registered places: 24
Guide weekly rate: £293–£357
Specialist care: Day care, respite
Medical services: Podiatry
Qualified staff: Meets standard

Home details
Location: Residential area, 1.5 miles from Torquay
Communal areas: Lounge, dining room, garden
Accessibility: *Floors:* 2 • *Access:* Lift and stair lift
    Wheelchair access: Good
Smoking: ✗
Pets: ✗
Routines: Flexible

Room details
Single: 18
Shared: 2
En suite: 19
Facilities: None

Door lock: ✗
Lockable place: ✓

Services provided
Beauty services: Hairdressing
Mobile library: ✗
Religious services: ✗
Transport: ✗
Activities: *Coordinator:* ✓ • *Examples:* Bingo • *Outings:* ✗
Meetings: ✗

Beechcroft Care Home

Manager: Julia Gow-Smith
Owner: Julia and Thornton Gow-Smith
Contact: Palermo Road, Babbacombe, Torquay, Devon, TQ1 3NW
☏ 01803 327360

A Victorian building with a modern extension, Beechcroft Residential Home is located in the Babbacombe area of Torquay from a park, shops, and tourist facilities such as a model village and the Babbacombe Downs. The residents are very much involved in the day-to-day decisions that affect them and the home. The home has a dedicated activities coordinator who arranges activities such as bingo for the residents.

Beechmount Residential Home

Manager: Emma Perkins
Owner: South West Residential Homes Ltd
Contact: Rousdown Road, Chelston, Torquay, Devon, TQ2 6PB
) 01803 605607

Beechmount Residential Home is situated one and a half miles from Torbay town centre and provides views across the bay. There are plans to make the garden more safe and accessible. The home also has a lounge and a dining room for residents to socialise in. There is an activities coordinator in the home who arranges reminiscence sessions for the residents as well as bingo and crafts. There are regular residents meetings.

Registered places: 25
Guide weekly rate: £275–£360
Specialist care: Respite, dementia, physical disability
Medical services: Podiatry, dentist, optician
Qualified staff: Exceeds standard: 58% at NVQ level 2

Home details
Location: Residential area, 1.5 miles from Torbay
Communal areas: Lounge, dining room, garden
Accessibility: *Floors:* 2 • *Access:* Lift • *Wheelchair access:* Good
Smoking: In designated area
Pets: ✓
Routines: Flexible

Room details
Single: 19
Shared: 3
En suite: 22
Facilities: TV point

Door lock: ✓
Lockable place: ✗

Services provided
Beauty services: Hairdressing
Mobile library: ✗
Religious services: ✗
Transport: ✗
Activities: *Coordinator:* ✓ • *Examples:* Arts and crafts, bingo *Outings:* ✗
Meetings: ✓

Belmont Grange Residential Home

Manager: Kerry Meldon-Dempsey
Owner: Belmont Care Ltd
Contact: Belmont Grange, Belmont Road, Ilfracombe, Devon, EX34 8DR
) 01271 863816
www.belmontgrange.co.uk

Belmont Grange is located in an urban area, one mile from Ilfracombe town centre. The home has two lounges and a dining room and is currently undergoing a refurbishment programme. There are plans to construct a sensory garden. The home offers a variety of activities to residents such as arts and crafts and quizzes. There are also outings on offer to the residents and there are regular meetings held to discuss any issues the residents may have.

Registered places: 25
Guide weekly rate: £306–£372
Specialist care: Dementia, mental disorder, respite
Medical services: Podiatry, dentist, optician
Qualified staff: Meets standard

Home details
Location: Urban area, 1 mile from Ilfracombe
Communal areas: 2 lounges, dining room
Accessibility: *Floors:* 2 • *Access:* Lift • *Wheelchair access:* Good
Smoking: ✗
Pets: At manager's discretion
Routines: Flexible

Room details
Single: 21
Shared: 2
En suite: 20
Facilities: TV point, telephone point

Door lock: ✓
Lockable place: ✓

Services provided
Beauty services: Hairdressing
Mobile library: ✗
Religious services: ✓
Transport: ✗
Activities: *Coordinator:* ✓ • *Examples:* Arts and crafts, reminiscence sessions • *Outings:* ✓
Meetings: ✓

Registered places: 20
Guide weekly rate: From £325
Specialist care: Day care, physical disability
Medical services: Podiatry, optician, physiotherapy
Qualified staff: Fails standards

Home details

Location: Residential area, 0.5 miles from Brixham
Communal areas: 2 lounges, dining room, conservatory, patio and garden
Accessibility: *Floors:* 2 • *Access:* Lift • *Wheelchair access:* Good
Smoking: ✗
Pets: At manager's discretion
Routines: Flexible

Room details

Single: 14
Shared: 3
En suite: 8
Facilities: TV point, telephone point

Door lock: ✓
Lockable place: ✓

Services provided

Beauty services: Hairdressing
Mobile library: ✓
Religious services: ✗
Transport: ✗
Activities: *Coordinator:* ✓ • *Examples:* Music and movement, quizzes • *Outings:* ✓
Meetings: ✗

Belmont House

Manager: Belinda Phillips
Owner: Patrick and Belinda Phillips
Contact: 13 Greenover Road, Brixham, Devon, TQ5 9LY

🕿 01803 856420
@ patlinbelmont@100-mph.com

Situated on the side of a hill, Belmont House has a sheltered garden at the front of building where residents can enjoy the raised pond and fountain. The home is located in a residential area, approximately half a mile from Brixham. The home has two lounges for residents to socialise in and a conservatory and patio in addition to the garden. The home arranges for a mobile library to visit and the activities coordinator arranges both outings and internal activities such as quizzes.

Registered places: 64
Guide weekly rate: £550–£600
Specialist care: Nursing, dementia, mental disorder, physical disability, respite
Medical services: Podiatry, dentist, optician
Qualified staff: Fails standards

Home details

Location: Residential area, 6 miles from Plymouth
Communal areas: 3 lounges, 3 dining rooms, 2 conservatories, 3 gardens
Accessibility: *Floors:* 2 • *Access:* Lift • *Wheelchair access:* Good
Smoking: In designated area
Pets: At manager's discretion
Routines: Flexible

Room details

Single: 64
Shared: 0
En suite: 59
Facilities: TV point, telephone point

Door lock: ✗
Lockable place: ✓

Services provided

Beauty services: Hairdressing
Mobile library: ✓
Religious services: Monthly Communion service
Transport: Minibus
Activities: *Coordinator:* ✓ • *Examples:* Barbecues, summer fêtes *Outings:* ✓
Meetings: ✓

Bickleigh Down Care Centre

Manager: Suzanne Marsh
Owner: Four Seasons Healthcare Ltd
Contact: Woolwell Road, Woolwell, Plymouth, Devon, PL6 7JW

🕿 01752 695555
@ bickleigh.down@fshc.co.uk
🖰 www.fshc.co.uk

Bickleigh Down Care Centre is a purpose-built home that lies close to Dartmoor Park. With good access to local amenities, the home is close to a shopping complex that includes a general store and medical centre and is also near a bus route. Divided into three units, the home includes one 24-bedded unit dedicated to those elderly residents suffering from mental illness. There is a residents meeting every three months and the home has its own minibus for outings. There is also a monthly Communion service.

Bindon & Elmcroft Residential Homes

Manager: C Deverenne
Owner: Bindon Care Ltd
Contact: 32–42 Winslade Road, Sidmouth, Devon, EX10 9EX
☎ 01395 514500
@ info@bindoncare.com
🖱 www.bindoncare.com

Situated approximately one mile from Sidmouth town centre and seafront, Bindon and Elmcroft are two separate properties with a single registration. The two properties share the home's secure gardens. The home arranges a monthly Communion service and there is a car used for transportation. The home arranges outings and daily activities such as arts and crafts and performances by visiting entertainers.

Registered places: 46
Guide weekly rate: £380–£700
Specialist care: Day care, dementia, mental disorder, physical disability, respite
Medical services: Podiatry, optician, physiotherapy
Qualified staff: Fails standards

Home details
Location: Residential area, 1 mile from Sidmouth
Communal areas: 3 lounges, dining room, garden
Accessibility: *Floors:* 2 • *Access:* Stair Lift • *Wheelchair access:* Limited
Smoking: ✗
Pets: At manager's discretion
Routines: Flexible

Room details
Single: 42
Shared: 2
En suite: 39
Facilities: TV point, telephone point

Door lock: ✓
Lockable place: ✓

Services provided
Beauty services: Hairdressing
Mobile library: ✗
Religious services: Monthly Communion service
Transport: Car
Activities: *Coordinator:* ✓ • *Examples:* Arts and crafts, games, visiting entertainers • *Outings:* ✓
Meetings: ✓

Bishopsteignton House

Manager: Gail Brock
Owner: Coastal Care Homes Ltd
Contact: Forder Lane, Bishopsteignton, Devon, TQ14 9SE
☎ 01626 770383

Originally a Victorian building, Bishopsteignton House is situated close to the centre of the rural Bishopsteignton village. The home is set in attractive secluded gardens and is approximately two miles from the seaside town of Teignmouth. This location provides beautiful views over the Teign river and estuary. The gardens of Bishopsteignton House are easily accessible from the conservatory. The home arranges an Anglican Communion service once a month.

Registered places: 20
Guide weekly rate: £350–£585
Specialist care: Day care, respite
Medical services: Podiatry, hygienist, optician, physiotherapy
Qualified staff: Fails standard: 25% at NVQ level 2

Home details
Location: Village location, 3 miles from Bishopsteignton
Communal areas: Lounge, dining room, conservatory, garden
Accessibility: *Floors:* 2 • *Access:* Lift • *Wheelchair access:* Good
Smoking: ✗
Pets: At manager's discretion
Routines: Flexible

Room details
Single: 16
Shared: 2
En suite: 14
Facilities: TV point, telephone point

Door lock: ✗
Lockable place: ✗

Services provided
Beauty services: Hairdressing
Mobile Library: ✓
Religious services: Monthly Anglican Communion service
Transport: Minibus
Activities: *Coordinator:* ✓ • *Examples:* Bingo, quizzes, talks *Outings:* ✗
Meetings: ✗

Registered places: 33
Guide weekly rate: £580
Specialist care: Nursing, dementia, mental disorder,
    physical disability, respite
Medical services: Podiatry, optician
Qualified staff: Exceeds standard: 87% at NVQ level 2

Home details
Location: Rural area, 3 miles from Tavistock
Communal areas: 2 lounge/dining rooms, quiet lounge,
    hairdressing salon, patio and garden
Accessibility: *Floors:* 2 • *Access:* Lift • *Wheelchair access:* Good
Smoking: ✗
Pets: ✗
Routines: Structured

Room details
Single: 33
Shared: 0
En suite: 2
Facilities: TV point

Door lock: ✗
Lockable place: ✓

Services provided
Beauty services: Hairdressing, aromatherapy, manicures
Mobile library: ✓
Religious services: ✓
Transport: Shared people carrier
Activities: *Coordinator:* ✗ • *Examples:* Bingo, films, music to movement
    Outings: ✗
Meetings: ✓

Blackdown Nursing Home

Manager: Marjorie Hoyle
Owner: Blackdown Care Ltd
Contact: Mary Tavy,
Nr Tavistock, Devon, PL19 9QB
☎ 01822 810249
🖰 www.carehomesssw.co.uk

Situated in the village of Mary Tavy, approximately three miles from Tavistock, Blackdown Nursing Home prides itself on its welcoming and homely atmosphere. Set on the borders of Dartmoor National Park, the home has large grounds with a summerhouse and a patio area. A variety of activities are organised, including pantomimes parties and visiting entertainers. There is ample communal space in the home, including two lounge/dining rooms and one quiet lounge. Residents and their relatives meet together every three months at the home to discuss their wellbeing.

Registered places: 28
Guide weekly rate: £360–£400
Specialist care: Day care, dementia, mental disorder,
    physical disability, respite
Medical services: Podiatry, dentist, optician
Qualified staff: Meets standard

Home details
Location: Residential area, 0.2 miles from Holsworthy
Communal areas: 2 lounges, 2 quiet rooms, dining room,
    conservatory, patio and garden
Accessibility: *Floors:* 2 • *Access:* Lift • *Wheelchair access:* Good
Smoking: ✗
Pets: ✗
Routines: Flexible

Room details
Single: 28
Shared: 0
En suite: 27
Facilities: TV, telephone

Door lock: ✓
Lockable place: ✓

Services provided
Beauty services: Hairdressing
Mobile library: ✗
Religious services: ✓
Transport: Shared minibus
Activities: *Coordinator:* ✗ • *Examples:* Bingo, visiting entertainers
    Outings: ✓
Meetings: Undisclosed

Bodmeyrick Residential Home

Manager: Jane Smale
Owner: Andrew and Janet Orchard
Contact: North Road,
Holsworthy, Devon, EX22 6HB
☎ 01409 253970

Bodmeyrick is a detached home situated in residential area, around half a mile from the centre of Holsworthy. The home has a specially converted vehicle for taking small groups out on weekly trips, which it shares with a nearby home. Every month an entertainer visits the home. This has included a dancing dog, giant dominoes and musical recognition games. At the front of the property there is a lawned garden which provides a pleasant seating area. The home provides day care two mornings a week.

DEVON

Brandon House

Manager: Wendy Marsh
Owner: John and Wendy Marsh
Contact: 29 Douglas Avenue,
Exmouth, Devon, EX8 2HE
☎ 01395 267581
@ Brandonhouse29@aol.com

Situated within walking distance of the Exmouth and Torbay coast, Brandon House also permits views of the surrounding Devon countryside courtesy of the large sun windows in the main communal areas. Many of the rooms overlook the enclosed gardens and courtyard. Advocating a flexible routine where there are no visiting restrictions and visitors may stay for meals free of charge, the home also operates a trial period policy. As well as having a music player and video facilities, Brandon House is currently home to two dogs.

Registered places: 35
Guide weekly rate: £400–£700
Specialist care: Physical disability, respite
Medical services: Podiatry, dentist, optician, physiotherapy
Qualified staff: Exceeds standard: 82% at NVQ level 2

Home details

Location: Avenues area of Exmouth, 0.5 miles from Littleham
Communal areas: 3 lounges, dining room, patio and garden
Accessibility: *Floors:* 2 • *Access:* Lift and stair Lift
Wheelchair access: Good
Smoking: ✗
Pets: At manager's discretion
Routines: Flexible

Room details

Single: 35
Shared: 0
En suite: 35
Facilities: TV point, telephone point

Door lock: ✓
Lockable place: ✗

Services provided

Beauty services: Hairdressing, aromatherapy
Mobile library: ✗
Religious services: Fortnightly Communion service
Transport: ✗
Activities: *Coordinator:* ✓ • *Examples:* Arts and crafts, board games
Outings: ✗
Meetings: ✓

Briarcroft

Manager: Elaine Walsh
Owner: John and Elaine Walsh
Contact: Dawlish Road,
Teignmouth, Devon, TQ14 8TG
☎ 01626 774681

Located in a residential area, just over half a mile from Teignmouth, Briarcroft offers views of the sea from some rooms. There is a secure, flat garden with flowers and shrubs for residents to enjoy. Contained within the home is a separate self-contained flat for two individuals on the lower-ground floor. This includes two bedrooms, a lounge and a kitchen. There is a residents meeting once a month and the home arranges outings to the theatre.

Registered places: 20
Guide weekly rate: £363–£430
Specialist care: Dementia
Medical services: Podiatry, optician
Qualified staff: Fails standards

Home details

Location: Residential area, 0.7 miles from Teignmouth
Communal areas: Lounge, dining room, conservatory,
patio and garden
Accessibility: Floors: 2 • *Access:* Lift • *Wheelchair access:* Good
Smoking: In designated area
Pets: ✓
Routines: Structured

Room details

Single: 18
Shared: 1
En suite: 5
Facilities: TV point

Door lock: ✗
Lockable place: ✗

Services provided

Beauty services: Hairdressing
Mobile library: ✗
Religious services: ✗
Transport: ✗
Activities: *Coordinator:* ✗ • *Examples:* Musical entertainment
Outings: ✓
Meetings: ✓

Registered places: 21
Guide weekly rate: £316–£400
Specialist care: Dementia, mental disorder, physical disability, respite
Medical services: Podiatry, optician
Qualified staff: Meets standard

Home details

Location: Residential area, 0.2 miles from Paignton
Communal areas: Dining room, garden
Accessibility: *Floors:* 3 • *Access:* Lift • *Wheelchair access:* Good
Smoking: ✗
Pets: ✓
Routines: Flexible

Room details

Single: 19
Shared: 1
En suite: 20
Facilities: TV

Door lock: ✓
Lockable place: ✓

Services provided

Beauty services: Hairdressing
Mobile library: ✗
Religious services: Monthly Anglican Communion service
Transport: ✗
Activities: *Coordinator:* ✗ • *Examples:* Exercise, games, singalongs
  Outings: ✗
Meetings: ✗

Burnside Court Care Home

Manager: Emma Hume
Owner: ABC Carehomes Ltd
Contact: 104–106 Torquay Road, Paignton, Devon, TQ3 2AA
☎ 01803 551342

Burnside Lodge is a detached property situated on level ground and easily accessible to local facilities including the library, park and local shops. The home is furnished and decorated in a homely way and benefits from a passenger lift which provides residents with access to all areas of the home. There is an Anglican Communion service held once a month and the home arranges daily activities such as games and exercise sessions.

Registered places: 40
Guide weekly rate: £300–£360
Specialist care: Dementia, physical disability, respite
Medical services: Podiatry, dentist, optician, physiotherapy
Qualified staff: Undisclosed

Home details

Location: Residential area, 1.5 miles from Plymouth centre
Communal areas: 4 lounges, 3 dining rooms, activity centre, conservatory, garden
Accessibility: *Floors:* 2 • *Access:* Stair Lift • *Wheelchair access:* Limited
Smoking: In designated area
Pets: ✗
Routines: Flexible

Room details

Single: 40
Shared: 0
En suite: 32
Facilities: TV, telephone point

Door lock: ✓
Lockable place: ✓

Services provided

Beauty services: Hairdressing
Mobile library: Library facilities
Religious services: ✗
Transport: ✗
Activities: *Coordinator:* ✗ • *Examples:* Chairobics, singalongs, videos
  Outings: ✓
Meetings: ✓

Camelot House

Manager: Linda Broad
Owner: Elizabeth Whittingham
Contact: 69–73 Mannamead Road, Plymouth, Devon, PL3 4ST
☎ 01752 661093

In a prime location close to the centre of Plymouth, this Victorian villa is set in its own grounds and overlooks the Thorn Park flower garden. With a corner shop 10 minutes' walk away, there is also a church down the road and regular buses passing through. Camelot provides an activities centre that is complete with a snooker table. There is also a registered bar area in one of the lounges. Although the home does not provide nursing care, it is willing to take in some high-dependency clients.

Cann House

Manager: Chantal King
Owner: Premiere Health Ltd
Contact: Tamerton Foliot Road,
Plymouth, Devon, PL5 4LE

☎ 01752 771742
@ Cannhousepl5@btopenworld.com
🖰 www.cannhouse.co.uk

Originally built in 1863, Cann House is set in nine acres of land in the heart of Tamerton Foliot village. Features include one of Plymouth's oldest walled gardens and a Victorian greenhouse where fruit and vegetables are grown year round. Situated close to the hospital and village amenities, a regular bus service stops by the main entrance of the house. Specialising in providing care for older individuals with physical disabilities, the home also operates a trial period policy where prospective clients can stay for a time to see if the home is right for them.

Registered places: 60
Guide weekly rate: £405–£550
Specialist care: Nursing, palliative, physical disability, respite
Medical services: Podiatry, dentist, dietician, optician, speech therapy
Qualified staff: Exceeds standard: 72% at NVQ level 2

Home details
Location: Village location, 4 miles from Plymouth centre
Communal areas: 3 lounges, 2 dining rooms, chapel, garden
Accessibility: *Floors:* 2 • *Access:* Lift • *Wheelchair access:* Good
Smoking: ✗
Pets: ✗
Routines: Flexible

Room details
Single: 38
Shared: 11
En suite: 49
Facilities: TV point, telephone point

Door lock: ✓
Lockable place: ✓

Services provided
Beauty services: Hairdressing
Mobile library: ✗
Religious services: Regular chapel services and Communion service
Transport: ✗
Activities: *Coordinator:* ✓ • *Examples:* Bingo, singalongs
Outings: ✓
Meetings: ✓

Castle Grove Nursing Home

Manager: Susan Thomas
Owner: Raymon and Isabelle Kenny
Contact: Castle Street, Bampton,
Tiverton, Devon, EX16 9NS

☎ 01398 331317
@ info@castle-grove.co.uk
🖰 www.castle-grove.co.uk

A listed Georgian building set in a rural location amid four acres of gardens, Castle Grove was once the home of Sir Christopher and Lady Codrington. Castle Grove is renowned for its good cuisine: the proprietor – who oversees the menus – was a chef for many years at The Dorchester Hotel. There is a level walk to Bampton and its shops, tearooms, post office and library. Currently major building works are in progress. Six new rooms will be created, as will a new centrepiece to the house a sun lounge known as 'the Orangery'.

Registered places: 20
Guide weekly rate: £600–£900
Specialist care: Nursing
Medical services: Podiatry, dentist, optician, physiotherapy
Qualified staff: Exceeds standard: 70% at NVQ level 2

Home details
Location: Residential area, 8 miles from Tiverton
Communal areas: Lounge, dining room, garden
Accessibility: *Floors:* 2 • *Access:* Lift • *Wheelchair access:* Good
Smoking: ✗
Pets: ✓
Routines: Flexible

Room details
Single: 16
Shared: 2
En suite: 18
Facilities: TV point, telephone point

Door lock: ✗
Lockable place: ✓

Services provided
Beauty services: Hairdressing, aromatherapy, facials
Mobile library: ✗
Religious services: Fortnightly Anglican Communion service
Transport: ✗
Activities: *Coordinator:* ✓ • *Examples:* Art, exercise classes, musical entertainment • *Outings:* ✓
Meetings: ✓

Registered places: 43
Guide weekly rate: £273–£370
Specialist care: Dementia, respite
Medical services: Podiatry, dentist, optician, physiotherapy
Qualified staff: Exceeds standard: 68% at NVQ level 2

Home details
Location: Residential area, 1 mile from Plymouth centre
Communal areas: 5 lounges, 3 dining rooms, garden
Accessibility: *Floors:* 3 • *Access:* Lift and stair lift
   Wheelchair access: Good
Smoking: ✗
Pets: At manager's discretion
Routines: Flexible

Room details
Single: 39
Shared: 2
En suite: 34
Facilities: TV point, telephone point

Door lock: ✓
Lockable place: ✓

Services provided
Beauty services: Hairdressing
Mobile library: Library facilities
Religious services: Monthly nondenominational Communion service
Transport: ✗
Activities: *Coordinator:* ✓ • *Examples:* Card making, musical
   entertainment, reminiscence • *Outings:* ✓
Meetings: ✓

Charlton House

Manager: Tonya Gerry
Owner: Gill Boyes and Tonya Gerry
Contact: 55 Mannamead Road,
Plymouth, Devon, PL3 4SR
☏ 01752 661405
@ info@charltonhouse.eclipse.co.uk

Charlton House is a large Victorian house that, though adapted, retains many of its original features. Set in its own grounds away from the main road, the home's gardens contain water features and a fountain. With a bus stop opposite that can take residents into the centre of Plymouth, Charlton House is also located 200 yards from local shops. Outings are arranged weekly and often include activities such as going out for lunches. Recently introduced is a quarterly relatives coffee morning where relatives of residents living in the home can meet up to chat.

Registered places: 20
Guide weekly rate: From £363
Specialist care: Dementia, physical disability, mental disorder
Medical services: Podiatry
Qualified staff: Undisclosed

Home details
Location: Residential area, 0.5 miles from Teignmouth
Communal areas: Lounge, dining room, garden
Accessibility: *Floors:* 2 • *Access:* Lift • *Wheelchair access:* Good
Smoking: ✗
Pets: At manager's discretion
Routines: Flexible

Room details
Single: 16
Shared: 2
En suite: 14
Facilities: TV

Door lock: ✓
Lockable place: ✓

Services provided
Beauty services: Hairdressing, manicures
Mobile library: ✗
Religious services: ✗
Transport: ✗
Activities: *Coordinator:* ✓ • *Examples:* Videos, games, reading
   Outings: ✓
Meetings: ✓

Charterhouse Residential Care Home

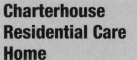

Manager: Margaret Brett
Owner: Mr and Mrs Brett
Contact: Second Drive, Dawlish Road,
Teignmouth, Devon, TQ14 8TL
☏ 01626 774481
@ margaretbrett@btinternet.com

Charterhouse Residential Care Home has been adapted from a large, detached property set in its own grounds. The home is in an elevated position and enjoys good views of the sea and the surrounding countryside. The home is located in a residential area, approximately half a mile from Teignmouth. The home has an activities coordinator and takes the residents on outings. There are also regular residents meetings.

Chatsworth House

Manager: Sally Colwill
Owner: Mr and Mrs Rhodes,
Mr and Mrs Davey
Contact: Dormy Avenue, Mannamead,
Plymouth, Devon, PL3 5BE
) 01752 660048
@ Chatsworthreshomepl3@btopenworld.com

Situated close to Thorn Park, Chatsworth House is set in an acre of landscaped gardens and only a few minutes' walk away from local amenities. The home is also serviced by buses running frequently to the city centre from near the home's main entrance. Chatsworth House is also home to a cat and other pets would be allowed at the manager's discretion. Visiting hours are flexible and relatives can stay as late as they wish.

Registered places: 26
Guide weekly rate: £339–£370
Specialist care: Dementia, emergency admissions, physical disability, respite
Medical services: Podiatry, dentist, optician, physiotherapy
Qualified staff: Exceeds standard: 65% at NVQ level 2

Home details
Location: Residential area, 1 mile from Plymouth centre
Communal areas: Lounge, dining room, garden
Accessibility: *Floors:* 3 • *Access:* Stair lift *Wheelchair access:* Good
Smoking: In designated area
Pets: At manager's discretion
Routines: Flexible

Room details
Single: 22
Shared: 2
En suite: 7
Facilities: TV point, telephone point

Door lock: ✓
Lockable place: ✓

Services provided
Beauty services: Hairdressing
Mobile library: ✓
Religious services: ✗
Transport: Car
Activities: *Coordinator:* ✗ • *Examples:* Armchair aerobics, bingo, darts • *Outings:* ✗
Meetings: ✗

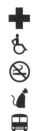

The Check House

Manager: Chaslyn Bryant
Owner: The Check House Ltd
Contact: Beer Road,
Seaton, Devon, EX12 2PR
) 01297 21858
@ checkhouse1@aol.com
⌂ www.checkhouse.co.uk

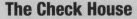

The Check House is a Grade II listed house set in raised landscaped grounds permitting views of the sea. Having recently expanded, the development of the Rossetti Wing won the home a prestigious Heathcare Design Award for the best extension to an existing home in the UK in 2005. The home has its own library facilities as well as a car and a minibus. As well as offering a flexible visiting policy, guests are also welcomed at mealtimes where they may stay free of charge for either of the two sittings offered to residents at lunch and suppertime.

Registered places: 49
Guide weekly rate: £650–£995
Specialist care: Nursing, day care, respite
Medical services: Podiatry, dentist, optician, physiotherapy
Qualified staff: Exceeds standard 70% st NVQ level 2

Home details
Location: Residential area, 0.7 miles from Seaton
Communal areas: 3 lounges, dining room, hairdressing salon, library, conservatory, garden
Accessibility: *Floors:* 3 • *Access:* Lift • *Wheelchair access:* Good
Smoking: ✗
Pets: At manager's discretion
Routines: Flexible

Room details
Single: 43
Shared: 3
En suite: 46
Facilities: TV point, telephone point

Door lock: ✓
Lockable place: ✓

Services provided
Beauty services: Hairdressing, aromatherapy, massage
Mobile library: Library facilities
Religious services: Monthly Anglican and Baptist Communion service:
Transport: Minibus and car
Activities: *Coordinator:* ✓ • *Examples:* Art, bingo, exercise *Outings:* ✓
Meetings: ✗

Registered places: 10
Guide weekly rate: £385–£407
Specialist care: Respite
Medical services: Podiatry, dentist, optician
Qualified staff: Undisclosed

Home details

Location: Residential area, 1 mile from Exmouth
Communal areas: Lounge, dining room, garden
Accessibility: *Floors:* 1 • *Wheelchair access:* Good
Smoking: ✗
Pets: At manager's discretion
Routines: Flexible

Room details

Single: 10
Shared: 0
En suite: 10
Facilities: TV, telephone

Door lock: ✗
Lockable place: ✗

Services provided

Beauty services: Hairdressing
Mobile library: ✓
Religious services: ✗
Transport: Car
Activities: *Coordinator:* ✓ • *Examples:* Bingo, games • *Outings:* ✓
Meetings: ✗

Chestnuts

Manager: Christine Nield
Owner: John and Christine Nield
Contact: 65 Salterton Road,
Exmouth, Devon, EX8 2EJ
☏ 01395 277198

A small, family-run home where the owners live on the premises, Chestnuts is situated on the main bus route into Exmouth. With gardens at the front and rear of the property, each of the home's bedrooms has doors which lead directly out to them. The home has its own transport for outings and also arranges for a mobile library to visit. The daily activities the activities coordinator arranges include bingo and games.

Registered places: 24
Guide weekly rate: £300–£385
Specialist care: Dementia, physical disability, respite
Medical services: Podiatry, optician
Qualified staff: Undisclosed

Home details

Location: Residential area, 1.5 miles from Torquay
Communal areas: Lounge, dining room, 2 conservatories, garden
Accessibility: *Floors:* 3 • *Access:* Stair lift *Wheelchair access:* Good
Smoking: In designated area
Pets: At manager's discretion
Routines: Flexible

Room details

Single: 18
Shared: 3
En suite: 19
Facilities: None

Door lock: ✓
Lockable place: ✓

Services provided

Beauty services: Hairdressing
Mobile library: ✗
Religious services: ✗
Transport: ✗
Activities: *Coordinator:* ✓ • *Examples:* Arts and crafts, one-to-one sessions *Outings:* ✗
Meetings: ✗

Choice Care Home

Manager: Lorraine Cunningham
Owner: Rosepost Healthcare Ltd
Contact: Cary Avenue, Babbacombe,
Torquay, Devon, TQ1 3QT
☏ 01803 403026

A large property set in its own grounds, Choice Care Home is located in a residential area near to local facilities, one and a half miles from Torquay. The home has its own activities coordinator who arranges group activities such as craft sessions, as well as one-to-one activities. The home allows smoking in a designated area and pets would be allowed at the manager's discretion.

Clayfield

Manager: Lynette Hollick
Owner: Lynette and Antony Hollick
Contact: 3-4 Clayfield Villas,
Victoria Road, Barnstaple,
Devon, EX32 8NP
) 01271 374066
@ clayfield@piltonia.supanet.com

Clayfield is comprised of two converted Victorian houses with an enclosed courtyard, approximately half a mile from Barnstaple. It is a family-run home that is situated close to a bus stop where there is a regular service to the centre of Barnstaple. The home produces a newsletter every month that keeps residents informed about events in the home. There is a residents meeting every quarter and the home has its own library facilities. The home also has a garden for residents to enjoy in the warmer months.

Registered places: 13
Guide weekly rate: £325–£440
Specialist care: Day care, dementia, emergency admissions, mental disorder
Medical services: Podiatry, dentist, optician, physiotherapy
Qualified staff: Exceeds standard: 75% at NVQ level 2

Home details
Location: Residential area, 0.6 miles from Barnstaple
Communal areas: Lounge, dining room, library, garden
Accessibility: *Floors:* 2 • *Access:* Lift • *Wheelchair access:* Good
Smoking: ✗
Pets: ✗
Routines: Flexible

Room details
Single: 9
Shared: 2   **Door lock:** ✓
En suite: 2   **Lockable place:** ✓
Facilities: TV, telephone point

Services provided
Beauty services: Hairdressing, aromatherapy
Mobile library: Library facilities
Religious services: Weekly Communion service
Transport: ✗
Activities: *Coordinator:* ✓ • *Examples:* Reminiscence • *Outings:* ✓
Meetings: ✓

Coombes Wood House

Manager: Louis Cook
Owner: Louis and Marjorie Cook
Contact: Coombesend Road East,
Kingsteignton, Newton Abbot,
Devon, TQ12 3DZ
) 01626 365101

Set in a rural location, approximately two and a half miles from Newton Abbot, Coombes Wood House is owned by Mr and Mrs Cook, both registered nurses. The location of the home allows attractive views of the surrounding countryside. Every year the home holds a summer fête, and throughout the year residents enjoy trips to locations such as Dartmoor, often having cream tea. The home also has two lounges and a quiet room for residents to relax in.

Registered places: 36
Guide weekly rate: £400–£450
Specialist care: Day care, dementia, mental disorder, physical disability, respite
Medical services: Podiatry, dentist
Qualified staff: Meets standard

Home details
Location: Rural area, 2.5 miles from Newton Abbot
Communal areas: 2 lounges, quiet room, 2 dining rooms, conservatory, garden
Accessibility: *Floors:* 2 • *Access:* Lift • *Wheelchair access:* Good
Smoking: ✗
Pets: ✗
Routines: Flexible

Room details
Single: 34
Shared: 1   **Door lock:** ✓
En suite: 35   **Lockable place:** ✓
Facilities: TV point

Services provided
Beauty services: Hairdressing, massage, reflexology
Mobile library: ✗
Religious services: ✗
Transport: ✗
Activities: *Coordinator:* ✓ • *Examples:* Bingo, games, musical entertainment • *Outings:* ✓
Meetings: ✗

Registered places: 30
Guide weekly rate: £287–£530
Specialist care: Undisclosed
Medical services: Podiatry, physiotherapy
Qualified staff: Meets standard

Home details

Location: Rural area, 0.2 miles from Moretonhampstead
Communal areas: Lounge, dining room, conservatory, garden
Accessibility: *Floors:* 2 • *Access:* Lift • *Wheelchair access:* Good
Smoking: ✗
Pets: ✗
Routines: Flexible

Room details

Single: 30
Shared: 0
En suite: 30
Facilities: TV

Door lock: ✓
Lockable place: ✓

Services provided

Beauty services: Hairdressing
Mobile library: ✗
Religious services: ✗
Transport: ✗
Activities: *Coordinator:* ✓ • *Examples:* Bingo, musical exercise
  Outings: ✓
Meetings: ✗

Coppelia House

Manager: Michelle Butt
Owner: Peninsula Care Homes Ltd
Contact: Court Street,
Moretonhampstead, Devon, TQ13 8LZ
) 01647 440729
@ coppelia@peninsulacarehomes.
  co.uk
🖱 www.peninsulacarehomes.com

An attractive house situated in a rural area close to Dartmoor National Park, Coppelia House is located less than half a mile from Moretonhampstead. The home's gardens have an allotment as well as an area to grow tomatoes. The home has its own activities coordinator who arranges bingo and musical exercises as well as a sherry event on a Sunday. The home also organises outings for the residents.

Registered places: 20
Guide weekly rate: £320–£350
Specialist care: Dementia, physical disability, respite
Medical services: Podiatry, optician
Qualified staff: Exceeds standard: 100% at NVQ level 2

Home details

Location: Residential area, 2.8 miles from Plymouth
Communal areas: 2 lounges, dining room, garden
Accessibility: *Floors:* 2 • *Access:* Stair lift • *Wheelchair access:* Good
Smoking: In designated area
Pets: ✗
Routines: Flexible

Room details

Single: 20
Shared: 0
En suite: 6
Facilities: TV point, telephone point

Door lock: ✓
Lockable place: ✗

Services provided

Beauty services: Hairdressing
Mobile library: ✗
Religious services: Monthly Anglican service
Transport: ✗
Activities: *Coordinator:* ✗ • *Examples:* Art, visiting entertainers
  Outings: ✓
Meetings: ✗

Copper Beeches

Manager: Susan Carthy
Owner: Steven and Tui Shirley
Contact: 90 Plymstock Road,
Plymstock, Plymouth, Devon, PL9 7PJ
) 01752 403836
@ s.carthy@21stcenturycare.co.uk
🖱 www.21stcenturycare.co.uk

Located in the ex-fishing village of Oreston, Copper Beeches is currently undergoing building works. Once this work is complete, the complete capacity of the home will be 35. One bedroom is reserved for respite use only. The home organises twice daily activities and there are plans to employ an activities coordinator in the near future. The activities programme can include performances from visiting entertainers and craft sessions. There are also outings planned for the residents.

The Corners Residential Home

Manager: Kathleen Newton
Owner: Kathleen Newton
Contact: 34 The Avenue,
Tiverton, Devon, EX16 4HW
) 01884 253682

The Corners Residential Home is set within its own landscaped gardens in a quiet residential area of Tiverton. Residents regularly participate in activities such as quizzes, skittles and bingo, and occasionally go out on trips in the car. In the home itself there is a lounge and a conservatory for residents to relax in.

Registered places: 8
Guide weekly rate: From £340
Specialist care: None
Medical services: Podiatry
Qualified staff: Undisclosed

Home details
Location: Residential area, 1 mile from Tiverton
Communal areas: Lounge, dining room, conservatory
Accessibility: *Floors:* 2 • *Access:* Stair Lift • *Wheelchair access:* Good
Smoking: ✗
Pets: ✓
Routines: Flexible

Room details
Single: 6
Shared: 1
En suite: Undisclosed
Facilities: None

Door lock: ✓
Lockable place: ✓

Services provided
Beauty services: Hairdressing
Mobile library: ✗
Religious services: ✗
Transport: ✓
Activities: *Coordinator:* ✗ • *Examples:* Bingo, skittles, quizzes
   Outings: ✓
Meetings: ✗

Cornerways

Manager: Gillian Plastow
Owner: Peninsula Care Homes Ltd
Contact: 14–16 Manor Road,
Paignton, Devon, TQ3 2HS
) 01803 551207
@ cornerways@peninsulacarehomes.co.uk
www.peninsulacarehomes.co.uk

Cornerways is located on the seafront in Paignton and was formerly a hotel.
Although the home has limited outdoor space, its proximity to the seafront means residents can enjoy walks along the front and visit Paignton's shops easily. The activities coordinator has organised a small mobile shop for the home. Outings include visiting a donkey sanctuary. The home also has three lounges for residents to relax in.

Registered places: 50
Guide weekly rate: £289–£510
Specialist care: Nursing, mental disorder, dementia, physical disability, respite
Medical services: Podiatry
Qualified staff: Meets standard

Home details
Location: Residential area, 0.7 miles from Paignton
Communal areas: 3 lounges, dining room
Accessibility: *Floors:* 3 • *Access:* Lift • *Wheelchair access:* Good
Smoking: ✗
Pets: ✓
Routines: Flexible

Room details
Single: 44
Shared: 3
En suite: 50
Facilities: TV point

Door lock: ✓
Lockable place: ✓

Services provided
Beauty services: Hairdressing
Mobile library: ✗
Religious services: ✗
Transport: ✗
Activities: *Coordinator:* ✓ • *Examples:* Barbecues, cream teas
   Outings: ✓
Meetings: ✗

Registered places: 25
Guide weekly rate: From £450
Specialist care: Day care, physical disability, respite
Medical services: Podiatry, optician, physiotherapy
Qualified staff: Exceeds standard: 70% at NVQ level 2

Home details
Location: Residential area, 0.6 miles from Tavistock
Communal areas: 3 lounges, dining room, conservatory, garden
Accessibility: *Floors:* 2 • *Access:* Stair Lift • *Wheelchair access:* Good
Smoking: In designated area
Pets: At manager's discretion
Routines: Flexible

Room details
Single: 25
Shared: 0
En suite: 11
Facilities: TV point, telephone point

Door lock: ✓
Lockable place: ✓

Services provided
Beauty services: Hairdressing
Mobile library: ✓
Religious services: Fortnightly Anglican Communion service
Transport: ✗
Activities: *Coordinator:* ✓ • *Examples:* Music and movement, bingo
Outings: ✓
Meetings: ✗

Crelake House

Manager: Patricia Hall
Owner: Crelake Care Ltd
Contact: 4 Whitchurch Road,
Tavistock, Devon, PL19 9BB
☎ 01822 616224
@ jwast@aol.com

Situated around half a mile from the town's facilities, Crelake House boasts landscaped gardens with patio areas which residents can enjoy in the warmer months. The home arranges a fortnightly Anglican Communion service for the residents and also arranges for a mobile library to visit the home. The activities coordinator at the home organises a range of activities including music and movement and bingo, as well as outings in the local area.

Registered places: 21
Guide weekly rate: £400
Specialist care: Day care, respite
Medical services: Podiatry, optician, physiotherapy
Qualified staff: Exceeds standard: 66% at NVQ level 2

Home details
Location: Residential area, 1 mile from Teignmouth
Communal areas: 2 lounges, dining room, conservatory,
    patio and garden
Accessibility: *Floors:* 2 • *Access:* Lift • *Wheelchair access:* Good
Smoking: ✗
Pets: ✓
Routines: Flexible

Room details
Single: 21
Shared: 0
En suite: 20
Facilities: TV point, telephone point

Door lock: ✓
Lockable place: ✓

Services provided
Beauty services: Hairdressing, reflexology
Mobile library: ✓
Religious services: ✗
Transport: Car
Activities: *Coordinator:* ✓ • *Examples:* Film afternoons,
    musical entertainment, quizzes • *Outings:* ✓
Meetings: ✓

Croft Lodge

Manager: Pauline Southey
Owner: Carole Fryer
Contact: 26 Haldon Avenue,
Teignmouth, Devon, TQ14 8LA
☎ 01626 775991
@ Croft.lodge@hotmail.co.uk

Situated in a quiet residential area on a bus route to Teignmouth, Croft Lodge has an accessible level garden with a number of benches and parasols. The home's manager lives on the premises. A handyman is employed by the home to respond to maintenance issues quickly. The home also employs two gardeners. There are residents meetings every three to four months to discuss any issues the residents may have. The home also has its own car for transport and offers a range of services including reflexology and tai chi.

The Croft Residential Home

Manager: Cheryl Howe
Owner: Cheryl Howe
Contact: 22 College Road,
Newton Abbot, Devon, TQ12 1EQ
) 01626 207265
@ thecroftresidentialhome@blueyonder.co.uk

With a front garden that includes an ornamental stream and pond and permits views across the valley, The Croft Residential Home also has a sloping back garden, where seasonal vegetables may be grown. Currently, the home is being extended. When this is complete all the bedrooms will have en suite facilities, there will be a passenger lift as well as the stair lift and there will be two more day rooms. The home has its own car and uses this to take residents on outings in the local area.

Registered places: 14
Guide weekly rate: £306–£400
Specialist care: Day care, dementia
Medical services: Podiatry, dentist, optician, physiotherapy
Qualified staff: Exceeds standard: 75% at NVQ level 2

Home details

Location: Residential area, 1.7 miles from Newton Abbot
Communal areas: Lounge, dining room, garden
Accessibility: *Floors:* 2 • *Access:* Stair Lift *Wheelchair access:* Good
Smoking: In designated area
Pets: At manager's discretion
Routines: Flexible

Room details

Single: 8
Shared: 3
En suite: 0
Facilities: TV point, telephone point

Door lock: ✓
Lockable place: ✓

Services provided

Beauty services: Hairdressing, aromatherapy
Mobile library: ✗
Religious services: Monthly Communion service
Transport: Car
Activities: *Coordinator:* ✓ • *Examples:* Cooking, games
Outings: ✓
Meetings: ✗

Cross Park House

Manager: Arleathea Mead
Owner: Stonehaven Healthcare Ltd
Contact: Monksbridge Road,
Brixham, Devon, TQ5 9NB
) 01803 856619
@ info@stone-haven.co.uk
⊕ www.stone-haven.co.uk

The home is on the outskirts of Brixham, on a hill facing open countryside and overlooking the town centre. It is an attractive Edwardian house with purpose-built facilities for residential care. There are two lounge areas of the home, one that has an accessible patio leading from it. A large conservatory is used as a dining room and has garden views. In the garden, sturdy furniture enables residents to sit outside in comfort and there is a fishpond. There is a monthly newsletter produced.

Registered places: 23
Guide weekly rate: £303–£390
Specialist care: Nursing, dementia, physical disability, respite
Medical services: Podiatry, dentist, optician, physiotherapy
Qualified staff: Fails standards

Home details

Location: Residential area, 0.8 miles from Brixham
Communal areas: 2 lounges, dining room/conservatory,
patio and garden
Accessibility: *Floors:* 3 • *Access:* 2 lifts • *Wheelchair access:* Good
Smoking: ✗
Pets: ✓
Routines: Flexible

Room details

Single: 23
Shared: 0
En suite: 1
Facilities: TV

Door lock: ✓
Lockable place: ✓

Services provided

Beauty services: Hairdressing
Mobile library: ✗
Religious services: ✗
Transport: ✗
Activities: *Coordinator:* ✗ • *Examples:* Arts and crafts, discussion
Outings: ✓
Meetings: ✗

Registered places: 14
Guide weekly rate: Undisclosed
Specialist care: Day care, respite
Medical services: Podiatry, optician, physiotherapy
Qualified staff: Fails standard

Home details
Location: Rural area, 1.3 miles from Totnes
Communal areas: 2 lounges, dining room, garden
Accessibility: *Floors:* 3 • *Access:* Lift • *Wheelchair access:* Good
Smoking: ✗
Pets: ✓
Routines: Flexible

Room details
Single: 13
Shared: 1
En suite: 14
Facilities: TV point, telephone point

Door lock: ✓
Lockable place: ✓

Services provided
Beauty services: Hairdressing
Mobile library: ✗
Religious services: Monthly Anglican Communion service
Transport: Minibus
Activities: *Coordinator:* ✓ • *Examples:* Exercise sessions, walks •
  Outings: ✓
Meetings: ✗

Dawn Residential Home

Manager: Gillian Barker
Owner: Kenneth and Gillian Barker
Contact: Cott Lane, Dartington,
Totnes, Devon, TQ9 6HE
) 01803 862964
@ dawnresthome@hotmail.com

Set in an acre of land with attractive views of the countryside, Dawn Residential Home is situated about 10 minutes from the village amenities. A family business, the owners of Dawn Residential Home live in the grounds and are heavily involved with the running of the home. The home has its own minibus for outings and regularly takes residents on walks in the local area. The home also arranges an Anglican Communion service once a month.

Registered places: 31
Guide weekly rate: £420
Specialist care: Dementia, mental disorder, physical disability, respite
Medical services: Podiatry, dentist, optician
Qualified staff: Undisclosed

Home details
Location: Residential area, 0.5 miles from Heavitree
Communal areas: 3 Lounges, dining room, garden
Accessibility: *Floors:* 2 • *Access:* Stair Lift *Wheelchair access:* Good
Smoking: ✗
Pets: ✓
Routines: Flexible

Room details
Single: 23
Shared: 5
En suite: 0
Facilities: TV

Door lock: ✓
Lockable place: ✗

Services provided
Beauty services: Hairdressing, manicures
Mobile library: ✗
Religious services: ✗
Transport: ✗
Activities: *Coordinator:* ✗ • *Examples:* Games, entertainment
  Outings: ✗
Meetings: Undisclosed

Dene Court

Manager: John Hall
Owner: John Hall
Contact: Butts Road, Heavitree,
Exeter, Devon, EX2 5HU
) 01392 274651

Dene Court is located in a residential area, half a mile from Heavitree and is near to local shops and public transport links. Some activities are organised, including games and outside entertainment. There are several communal areas around the home, all with ornaments and a homely feel to them. These communal areas include three lounges and a garden.

Dene House

Manager: John De'Ath
Owner: John and Madeleine De'Ath
Contact: 12 Cleveland Road,
Torquay, Devon, TQ2 5BE
) 01803 293077

Dene House is located in a residential area, just over half a mile from Torquay. The home arranges a variety of activities for residents to participate in, including exercise sessions and musical entertainment. The home also takes the residents on outings in the local area. The home has a lounge and a garden for residents to relax in, as well as a separate dining room.

Registered places: 12
Guide weekly rate: £250–£450
Specialist care: Dementia, mental disorder
Medical services: Undisclosed
Qualified staff: Undisclosed

Home details
Location: Residential area, 0.7 miles from Torquay
Communal areas: Lounge, dining room, garden
Accessibility: *Floors:* 2 • *Access:* Lift • *Wheelchair access:* Limited
Smoking: Undisclosed
Pets: Undisclosed
Routines: Undisclosed

Room details
Single: 12
Shared: 0
En suite: Undisclosed
Facilities: None

Door lock: ✕
Lockable place: ✕

Services provided
Beauty services: Hairdressing
Mobile library: ✕
Religious services: ✕
Transport: ✕
Activities: *Coordinator:* ✕ • *Examples:* Exercise sessions, musical entertainment, quizzes • *Outings:* ✓
Meetings: Undisclosed

Devonia House Nursing Home

Manager: Jean Sherriff
Owner: Anthony Bloom
Contact: Leg O'mutton Corner,
Yelverton, Devon, PL20 6DJ
) 01822 852081

Devonia House is a converted Victorian property in a rural location, just over half a mile from Yelverton. The home is also situated on the edge of Dartmoor National Park. The home has a conservatory and a garden for residents to enjoy in the warmer months and inside the home there is a lounge with a separate dining room. Some of the activities on offer include board games and reading.

Registered places: 32
Guide weekly rate: Undisclosed
Specialist care: Nursing, physical disability
Medical services: Podiatry, dentist, optician
Qualified staff: Exceeds standard: 75% at NVQ level 2

Home details
Location: Rural area, 0.7 miles from Yelverton
Communal areas: Lounge, dining room, conservatory, garden
Accessibility: *Floors:* 3 • *Access:* 2 lifts • *Wheelchair access:* Good
Smoking: ✕
Pets: ✕
Routines: Flexible

Room details
Single: 23
Shared: 4
En suite: 21
Facilities: None

Door lock: ✕
Lockable place: ✓

Services provided
Beauty services: Hairdressing
Mobile library: ✕
Religious services: ✕
Transport: ✕
Activities: *Coordinator:* ✕ • *Examples:* Board games, reading *Outings:* ✕
Meetings: ✕

Registered places: 34
Guide weekly rate: £273–£330
Specialist care: Day care, dementia, respite
Medical services: Podiatry, hygienist, optician, physiotherapy
Qualified staff: Exceeds standard: 98% at NVQ level 2

Home details
Location: Residential area, 2 miles from Plymouth
Communal areas: 2 lounges, dining room, conservatory, garden
Accessibility: *Floors:* 3 • *Access:* Stair Lift *Wheelchair access:* Limited
Smoking: ✗
Pets: At manager's discretion
Routines: Flexible

Room details
Single: 34
Shared: 0
En suite: 0
Facilities: TV point, telephone point

Door lock: ✓
Lockable place: ✓

Services provided
Beauty services: Hairdressing
Mobile library: ✓
Religious services: Monthly Communion service
Transport: ✗
Activities: *Coordinator:* ✓ • *Examples:* Armchair exercises,
    visiting entertainers • *Outings:* ✗
Meetings: ✓

Dewi Sant

Manager: Jennie Preston
Owner: Jennie Preston
Contact: 32 Eggbuckland Road,
Mannamead, Plymouth,
Devon, PL3 5HG
☎ 01752 664923

Located close to Mutley Plain shopping centre, Dewi Sant has an enclosed garden for residents to enjoy. The home's activities coordinator puts on a wide variety of activities for residents, including armchair exercises and performances from visiting entertainers. Dewi Sant has two lounges, a conservatory and dining room on the ground floor. The home also arranges a monthly Communion service and for a mobile library to visit.

Registered places: 17
Guide weekly rate: £325–£395
Specialist care: Day care, respite
Medical services: Podiatry, dentist, optician, physiotherapy
Qualified staff: Exceeds standard: 70% at NVQ level 2

Home details
Location: Residential area, 2 miles from Torquay centre
Communal areas: Lounge, conservatory, dining room/coffee lounge,
    garden
Accessibility: *Floors:* 3 • *Access:* Lift • *Wheelchair access:* Good
Smoking: In designated area
Pets: At manager's discretion
Routines: Flexible

Room details
Single: 15
Shared: 1
En suite: 16
Facilities: TV point, telephone point

Door lock: ✓
Lockable place: ✓

Services provided
Beauty services: Hairdressing
Mobile library: Library facilities
Religious services: ✗
Transport: 7-seater vehicle
Activities: *Coordinator:* ✗ • *Examples:* Armchair aerobics, bingo,
    board games • *Outings:* ✓
Meetings: ✓

Didsbury Court

Manager: Mrs Matthews
Owner: Mr and Mrs Watson
Contact: 17–19 Park Road,
St Marychurch, Torquay,
Devon, TQ1 4QR
☎ 01803 329735

Didsbury Court is a large detached Victorian house three minutes' walk from the shops and close to the medical centre as well as the natural beauty of the Downs. Decorated in a homely fashion, many of the bedrooms overlook the home's gardens which feature a summerhouse and wishing well. With a low staff turnover, the home prides itself on creating an atmosphere that 'is both friendly and informal'. With a comprehensive activities programme on offer that includes clergy visits on request, the home also provides DVD facilities and can take residents on various trips including expeditions to the nearby shopping precinct.

Doneraile

Manager: Graham Jones
Owner: Graham and Karen Jones
Contact: 24 College Road,
Newton Abbot, Devon, TQ12 1EQ
📞 01626 354540

Doneraile is situated in a quiet, residential area, which permits attractive views of the surrounding countryside. The home boasts a large terrace at the front and landscaped gardens to the rear. The home arranges for a Communion service to take place once a month and also has its own car to use as transportation for outings. The activities, which take place inside the home, include musical entertainment and singalongs. The home also arranges for residents to have access to a mobile library.

Registered places: 25
Guide weekly rate: £287–£400
Specialist care: Dementia, physical disability, respite
Medical services: Podiatry, optician
Qualified staff: Exceeds standard: 68% at NVQ level 2

Home details
Location: Residential area, 1 mile from Netwon Abbot
Communal areas: Lounge, dining room, garden
Accessibility: *Floors:* 2 • *Access:* Lift and stair Lift
  Wheelchair access: Good
Smoking: ✗
Pets: At manager's discretion
Routines: Flexible

Room details
Single: 23
Shared: 1
En suite: 13
Facilities: TV point, telephone point

Door lock: ✓
Lockable place: ✓

Services provided
Beauty services: Hairdressing
Mobile library: ✓
Religious services: Monthly Communion service
Transport: Car
Activities: *Coordinator:* ✗ • *Examples:* Musical entertainment, singalongs • *Outings:* ✓
Meetings: ✗

Donnington House

Manager: Jennifer Burrows
Owner: Stonehaven Healthcare Ltd
Contact: 47 Atlantic Way, Westward Ho,
Bideford, Devon, EX39 1JD
📞 01237 475001

Donnington House is located in a residential area, two and a half miles from Bideford. The activities are varied and are sometimes funded by residents or fundraising. These include bingo and performances by visiting entertainers. Residents or visitors are encouraged to bring pets to the home such as cats and rabbits. Once a month a trained Pets As Therapy dog is also brought in. The home has a garden with a patio area for residents to enjoy in the warmer months.

Registered places: 25
Guide weekly rate: £274–£395
Specialist care: Dementia, physical disability
Medical services: Podiatry, dentist, optician
Qualified staff: Exceeds standard: 67% at NVQ level 2

Home details
Location: Residential area, 2.5 miles from Bideford
Communal areas: 3 lounges, 2 dining rooms, patio and garden
Accessibility: *Floors:* 3 • *Access:* Stair Lift • *Wheelchair access:* Good
Smoking: ✗
Pets: ✓
Routines: Flexible

Room details
Single: 26
Shared: 5
En suite: 10
Facilities: None

Door lock: ✓
Lockable place: ✓

Services provided
Beauty services: Hairdressing
Mobile library: ✗
Religious services: ✗
Transport: ✗
Activities: *Coordinator:* ✗ • *Examples:* Arts and crafts, bingo, visiting entertainers • *Outings:* ✗
Meetings: ✗

Registered places: 19
Guide weekly rate: £300–£600
Specialist care: Day care, physical disability, respite
Medical services: Podiatry, dentist, optician
Qualified staff: Undisclosed

Home details

Location: Residential area, in Seaton
Communal areas: 2 lounges, 2 dining rooms, conservatory, garden
Accessibility: *Floors:* 2 • *Access:* Lift • *Wheelchair access:* Good
Smoking: ✗
Pets: At manager's discretion
Routines: Flexible

Room details

Single: 13
Shared: 3
En suite: 9

Door lock: ✓
Lockable place: ✓

Facilities: TV point, telephone point

Services provided

Beauty services: Hairdressing, manicures
Mobile library: Library facilities
Religious services: Fortnightly nondenominational Communion service
Transport: ✗
Activities: *Coordinator:* ✓ • *Examples:* Bingo, quizzes, singalongs
    Outings: ✓
Meetings: ✓

Dove Court

Manager: Maureen Goddard
Owner: Doveleigh Care Ltd
Contact: Seaton Down Hill,
Seaton, Devon, EX12 2JD
📞 01297 22451
@ admin@doveleighcourt.co.uk
🖱 www.doveleighcare.co.uk

Situated on the main route into Seaton and overlooking the town and the coast, Dove Court is also easily accessed by the A3052. Although situated 500 yards from shops, the home is located on a hill, which may restrict some less-mobile residents. Outings tend to run on a fortnightly basis and the home provides a list of useful addresses and telephone numbers that include the local library and taxi service. With views overlooking the coast, Dove Court also has gardens and seating areas surrounding the home and fresh fruit is readily available in the lounge.

Registered places: 49
Guide weekly rate: £326–£490
Specialist care: Nursing, physical disability, respite
Medical services: Podiatry, dentist
Qualified staff: Meets standard

Home details

Location: Residential area, 4.3 miles from Plymouth
Communal areas: 2 lounges, dining room, library facilities, garden
Accessibility: *Floors:* 2 • *Access:* Stair lift • *Wheelchair access:* Good
Smoking: In designated area
Pets: At manager's discretion
Routines: Structured

Room details

Single: 29
Shared: 5
En suite: 28

Door lock: ✓
Lockable place: ✓

Facilities: TV point, telephone point

Services provided

Beauty services: Hairdressing
Mobile library: ✗
Religious services: ✗
Transport: Minibus
Activities: *Coordinator:* ✗ • *Examples:* Musical entertainers, slide shows
    Outings: ✓
Meetings: ✗

Down House

Manager: Mr Sutherland
Owner: Mayhaven Healthcare Ltd
Contact: 277 Tavistock Road,
Derriford, Plymouth, Devon, PL6 8AA
📞 01752 789393
@ down.hs@btinternet.com
🖱 www.mayhaven.co.uk

Situated in a residential area near Plymouth City Centre, Down House is located on a bus route and a short walk from a mini market. As well as a piano in the main lounge, the home offers broadband at a reduced rate for residents. Down House offers regular outings for residents: twice weekly during summer and once weekly in winter. Currently major building works are underway at Down House. A dining room is being built and a lift will be installed to replace the stair lift. Some rooms are also being refurbished.

Dunmore Residential Care Home

Manager: Mrs Snow
Owner: Buckland Care Ltd
Contact: 30 Courtenay Road, Newton Abbot, Devon, TQ12 1HE
☎ 01626 352470
@ dunmorecare@aol.com
🖱 www.bucklandcare.co.uk

Situated in a raised position on a hill, Dunmore is in a prime position to provide panoramic views of the town and its surrounding countryside. The home has been designed accordingly with all the communal rooms offset by large windows which show well the natural beauty of Dartmoor. Although the lawn is inaccessible to most residents as it is on a slope, a patio with garden furniture provides pleasant outdoor surroundings. A comprehensive activities programme provides much enjoyment with bus outings proving particularly popular with residents.

Registered places: 28
Guide weekly rate: £400–£500
Specialist care: Day care, dementia, physical disability, respite
Medical services: Podiatry, dentist, optician
Qualified staff: Undisclosed

Home details
Location: Residential area, 1 mile from Newton Abbot
Communal areas: 2 lounges, dining room, patio and garden
Accessibility: *Floors:* 4 • *Access:* Lift • *Wheelchair access:* Good
Smoking: ✗
Pets: At manager's discretion
Routines: Structured

Room details
Single: 22
Shared: 3
En suite: 25
Facilities: TV

Door lock: ✓
Lockable place: ✗

Services provided
Beauty services: Hairdressing
Mobile library: ✓
Religious services: Monthly nondenominational church service
Transport: ✗
Activities: *Coordinator:* ✗ • *Examples:* Armchair exercises, bingo, musical entertainment • *Outings:* ✓
Meetings: ✗

Durnsford Lodge Residential Home

Manager: Carole Scott
Owner: Ernest and Iris Bertie
Contact: 90 Somerset Place, Stoke, Plymouth, Devon, PL3 4BG
☎ 01752 562872
@ care@durnsfordlodge.co.uk
🖱 www.durnsfordlodge.co.uk

Situated in a residential area, Durnsford Lodge is located a short walk from the nearest shops and around two miles from Plymouth. It is about a 10-minute drive to the coast. While some rooms overlook views of the home's garden, others look out towards Plymouth Sound and the coastline. The home has two lounges and two gardens for residents to relax in and the activities coordinator provides a varied programme for their enjoyment. This programme includes armchair exercises, reminiscence sessions and musical afternoons.

Registered places: 28
Guide weekly rate: £275–£333
Specialist care: Day care, dementia, physical disability, respite
Medical services: Podiatry, optician, physiotherapy
Qualified staff: Exceeds standard: 98% at NVQ level 2

Home details
Location: Residential area, 2 miles from Plymouth
Communal areas: 2 lounges, dining room, 2 gardens
Accessibility: *Floors:* 2 • *Access:* Lift • *Wheelchair access:* Good
Smoking: In designated area
Pets: At manager's discretion
Routines: Flexible

Room details
Single: 20
Shared: 4
En suite: 6
Facilities: TV point, telephone point

Door lock: ✓
Lockable place: ✓

Services provided
Beauty services: Hairdressing
Mobile library: ✓
Religious services: ✗
Transport: ✗
Activities: *Coordinator:* ✓ • *Examples:* Bingo, musical afternoons *Outings:* ✗
Meetings: ✗

Registered places: 27
Guide weekly rate: £400
Specialist care: Day care, dementia, respite
Medical services: Podiatry, hygienist, optician
Qualified staff: Meets standard

Home details

Location: Residential area, 1 mile from Torquay
Communal areas: 3 lounges, dining room, hairdressing salon, garden
Accessibility: *Floors:* 3 • *Access:* Stair Lift • *Wheelchair access:* Good
Smoking: ✗
Pets: At manager's discretion
Routines: Structured

Room details

Single: 23
Shared: 2
En suite: Undisclosed
Facilities: TV point, telephone point

Door lock: ✓
Lockable place: ✗

Services provided

Beauty services: Hairdressing
Mobile library: ✓
Religious services: Monthly Anglican Communion service
Transport: Minibus
Activities: *Coordinator:* ✓ • *Examples:* Quizzes, bingo, gardening
   Outings: ✓
Meetings: ✗

Eclipse Lodge

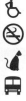

Manager: Janet Jenkins
Owner: Crocus Care Ltd
Contact: Rawlyn Road,
Torquay, Devon, TQ2 6PQ
☎ 01803 607604
@ clare@crocuscare.co.uk
🖱 www.crocuscare.co.uk

Close to the Torquay seafront, Eclipse Lodge is set in a residential location 10 minutes' walk from the train station. The home prides itself on the range of activities and outings on offer. Currently there are three activities coordinators on the staff, with two on duty each day. Residents go on a weekly outing and day trips also take place frequently. Eclipse Lodge has a locked door policy, which means that residents can't leave the site unaccompanied. The home also has its own minibus to take residents on outings.

Registered places: 16
Guide weekly rate: From £350
Specialist care: Respite
Medical services: Podiatry, dentist, optician, physiotherapy
Qualified staff: Exceeds standard: 90% at NVQ level 2

Home details

Location: Residential area, 2 miles from Plymouth centre
Communal areas: Lounge, dining room, conservatory,
   patio and garden
Accessibility: *Floors:* 2 • *Access:* Stair Lift • *Wheelchair access:* ✗
Smoking: In designated area
Pets: At manager's discretion
Routines: Flexible

Room details

Single: 14
Shared: 1
En suite: 13
Facilities: TV

Door lock: ✗
Lockable place: ✓

Services provided

Beauty services: Hairdressing
Mobile library: ✗
Religious: ✗
Transport: ✗
Activities: *Coordinator:* ✗ • *Examples:* Film shows, armchair aerobics
   Outings: ✓
Meetings: ✗

Evergreen Residential Home

Manager: Jacqueline Tope
Owner: Mr and Mrs Tope
Contact: 2–3 Brandeth Road,
Mannamead, Plymouth,
Devon, PL3 5HQ
☎ 01752 665042

A specially adapted home created from two internally combined Victorian villas, Evergreen Residential Home is a modest-size building with a homely, 'non-institutional' atmosphere. While the owners live on the premises five days a week, the home also currently has a dog. Situated five minutes' walk from local amenities such as a general store and post office, the home is well serviced by buses and residents may also enjoy the nearby parks and bowling green. Apart from the main lounge, Evergreen's conservatory offers a place to relax whatever the weather, as is fully glazed with central heating.

Falkland Lodge

Manager: Teresa Warwick
Owner: Westcarehomes Ltd
Contact: Falkland Road,
Torquay, Devon, TQ2 5JR
☎ 01803 292476

Situated close to the seafront, some of the rooms in Falkland Lodge permit views of the sea. Staff take residents on one-to-one trips to Torquay, either to the shops or to the seaside. The home also has an activities coordinator who arranges internal activities such as bingo and quizzes. There is an Anglican Communion service held every fortnight and the home has visits from a mobile library.

Registered places: 31
Guide weekly rate: £298–£386
Specialist care: Dementia, mental disorder, respite
Medical services: Podiatry, hygienist, optician, physiotherapy
Qualified staff: Meets standard

Home details
Location: Residential area, 0.5 miles from Torquay
Communal areas: Lounge, dining room, conservatory, garden
Accessibility: *Floors:* 3 • *Access:* Lift • *Wheelchair access:* Good
Smoking: In designated area
Pets: At manager's discretion
Routines: Flexible

Room details
Single: 23
Shared: 4
En suite: 19
Facilities: TV point

Door lock: ✓
Lockable place: ✓

Services provided
Beauty services: Hairdressing, aromatherapy, massage
Mobile library: ✓
Religious services: Fortnightly Anglican Communion service
Transport: ✗
Activities: *Coordinator:* ✓ • *Examples:* Bingo, quizzes, storytelling
 Outings: ✓
Meetings: ✗

Fanshawe Nursing Home

Manager: Mrs Watts
Owner: RMJJ Healthcare Ltd
Contact: 53 Hooe Road, Hooe,
Plymouth, Devon, PL9 9QS
☎ 01752 481663
@ fanshawe@talktalk.net

Fanshawe Nursing Home is a Victorian house set back from the main road and a five-minute walk from Hooe village where there are amenities such as pubs, a post office and general store. Approximately five miles from the city centre, the home is also well served by a regular bus service. Fanshawe has been modernised and refurbished to offer comfort for older individuals, often with a physical disability. Completing its homely feel, the home has a cat and budgie that live alongside the residents.

Registered places: 23
Guide weekly rate: £580
Specialist care: Nursing, physical disability, respite
Medical services: Podiatry, dentist, optician, physiotherapy
Qualified staff: Undisclosed

Home details
Location: Residential area, 5 miles from Plymouth centre
Communal areas: 3 lounges, dining room, patio and garden
Accessibility: *Floors:* 2 • *Access:* Lift • *Wheelchair access:* Good
Smoking: ✗
Pets: ✗
Routines: Flexible

Room details
Single: 11
Shared: 6
En suite: 8
Facilities: TV point

Door lock: ✗
Lockable place: ✗

Services provided
Beauty services: Hairdressing, manicures
Mobile library: ✗
Religious services: Monthly church service
Transport: ✗
Activities: *Coordinator:* ✗ • *Examples:* Cards, skittles • *Outings:* ✗
Meetings: ✗

Registered places: 11
Guide weekly rate: Undisclosed
Specialist care: Dementia, mental disorder
Medical services: Podiatry, optician, physiotherapy
Qualified staff: Fails standard

Home details

Location: Residential area, 1 mile from Ilfracombe
Communal areas: Lounge, dining room, conservatory, garden
Accessibility: *Floors:* 3 • *Access:* Stair Lift • *Wheelchair access:* Good
Smoking: ✗
Pets: At manger's discretion
Routines: Flexible

Room details

Single: 9
Shared: 2
En suite: 7
Facilities: TV point, telephone point

Door lock: ✓
Lockable place: ✓

Services provided

Beauty services: Hairdressing
Mobile library: ✓
Religious services: Monthly Communion service
Transport: ✗
Activities: *Coordinator:* ✓ • *Examples:* Bingo • *Outings:* ✓
Meetings: ✓

Fernbank House

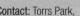

Manager: Susan Leek
Owner: Trevor and Susan Leek
Contact: Torrs Park,
Ilfracombe, Devon, EX34 8AZ
) 01271 866166

A detached Edwardian villa set in a conservation area, Fernbank House offers views over Ilfracombe's hills and the sea. The home has a garden with a pond. There is a residents meeting every quarter to discuss any issues the residents may have and the home also organises a monthly Communion service. The home has an activities coordinator who arranges outings for the residents as well as internal activities such as bingo.

Registered places: 14
Guide weekly rate: Undisclosed
Specialist care: Nursing, day care, dementia, physical disability
Medical services: Podiatry, occupational therapy, optician, physiotherapy
Qualified staff: Undisclosed

Home details

Location: Residential area, 1 mile from Newton Abbot
Communal areas: Lounge, dining room, conservatory, patio and garden
Accessibility: *Floors:* 2 • *Access:* None • *Wheelchair access:* Limited
Smoking: ✗
Pets: At manager's discretion
Routines: Flexible

Room details

Single: 7
Shared: 4
En suite: Undisclosed
Facilities: TV point

Door lock: ✗
Lockable place: ✗

Services provided

Beauty services: Hairdressing
Mobile library: ✓
Religious services: Weekly Communion service
Transport: Minibus
Activities: *Coordinator:* ✗ • *Examples:* Games, reminiscence, woodwork *Outings:* ✓
Meetings: Undisclosed

Forde Park Care Home

Manager: Barbara Underhill
Owner: The Wilson Crawford Partnership
Contact: 18 Keyberry Park,
Newton Abbot, Devon, TQ12 1BZ
) 01626 352904
@ info@fordepark.co.uk
www.fordepark.co.uk

Forde Park Care Home is an attractive Victorian building close to Forde Park is approximately one mile from Newton Abbot. The home is paired with Forde Park Nursing Home where residents can be transferred if their needs change. Activities organised at the home include gardening, basic cookery, flower arranging painting, musical activities and outings. The home also has its own minibus and arranges a weekly Communion service.

The Fourways Residential Home

Manager: Rachel White
Owner: Fourways Ltd
Contact: Glen Road,
Sidmouth, Devon, EX10 8RW
) 01395 513932
@ white615@btinternet.com

Situated 10 minutes from the beach, Fourways is located half a mile from the centre of Sidmouth. Each room has en suite bathrooms and windows from floor to ceiling. The home provides free timetabled visits to Sidmouth in a bus while an in-house shop ensures less active residents have access to confectionary, toiletries and magazines. The residents can request trip locations. Such outings have included trips to the beach and to an otter sanctuary.

Registered places: 19
Guide weekly rate: From £625
Specialist care: Day care, physical disability, respite
Medical services: Podiatry, hygienist, optician, physiotherapy
Qualified staff: Exceeds standard: 90% at NVQ level 2

Home details
Location: Residential area, 0.6 miles from Sidmouth
Communal areas: Lounge, dining room, library facilities,
2 patios and garden
Accessibility: *Floors:* 2 • *Access:* Stair lift • *Wheelchair access:* Good
Smoking: ✗
Pets: ✗
Routines: Flexible

Room details
Single: 17
Shared: 2
En suite: 19
Facilities: TV, telephone

Door lock: ✓
Lockable place: ✓

Services provided
Beauty services: Hairdressing, aromatherapy, manicures
Mobile library: ✗
Religious services: Weekly Catholic visits,
monthly Anglican Communion service
Transport: Free bus to town
Activities: *Coordinator:* ✓ • *Examples:* Quizzes, scrabble
Outings: ✓
Meetings: ✗

Frensham House

Manager: Nicholas Ross
Owner: Stonehaven Healthcare Ltd
Contact: 125 New Road,
Brixham, Devon, TQ5 8BY
) 01803 857476
@ frensham@stone-haven.co.uk
⌂ www.stone-haven.co.uk

Built on a hillside on the main road leading to Brixham town centre, Frensham House is set in its own secluded walled garden with exotic trees and flowers. It is a manageable five-minute walk to the town centre. The home produces a newsletter twice a month which includes details of activities, staff training and birthdays. The home has its own car for transport and there is an Anglican Communion service every fortnight.

Registered places: 14
Guide weekly rate: £350–£450
Specialist care: Day care, dementia, physical disability, respite
Medical services: Podiatry, hygienist, optician, physiotherapy
Qualified staff: Exceeds standard: 90% at NVQ level 2

Home details
Location: Residential area, 0.5 miles from Brixham
Communal areas: Lounge, dining room, conservatory, garden
Accessibility: *Floors:* 2 • *Access:* Stair Lift • *Wheelchair access:* Good
Smoking: In designated area
Pets: ✗
Routines: Flexible

Room details
Single: 8
Shared: 3
En suite: 0
Facilities: TV point, telephone point

Door lock: ✓
Lockable place: ✓

Services provided
Beauty services: Hairdressing
Mobile library: ✗
Religious services: Fortnightly Anglican Communion service
Transport: Car
Activities: *Coordinator:* ✓ • *Examples:* Harpist visits • *Outings:* ✗
Meetings: ✗

Registered places: 39
Guide weekly rate: £488–£520
Specialist care: Nursing, respite
Medical services: Podiatry, dentist, physiotherapy
Qualified staff: Exceeds standard: 65% at NVQ level 2

Home details

Location: Residential area, 5 miles from Plymouth
Communal areas: Lounge, dining room, patio and garden
Accessibility: *Floors:* 2 • *Access:* Lift • *Wheelchair access:* Good
Smoking: ✕
Pets: ✕
Routines: Flexible

Room details

Single: 37
Shared: 1
En suite: 38
Facilities: TV point

Door lock: ✓
Lockable place: ✓

Services provided

Beauty services: Hairdressing
Mobile library: ✓
Religious services: ✕
Transport: Minibus
Activities: *Coordinator:* ✓ • *Examples:* Arts and crafts, games, musical entertainers • *Outings:* ✓
Meetings: ✓

Freshfields Nursing Home

Manager: Hyang Teasdale
Owner: Freshfields Management Company Ltd
Contact: Agaton Road, St Budeaux, Plymouth, Devon, PL5 2EW
☏ 01752 360000
@ freshfield@talktalkbusiness.net

A purpose-built home that is managed by one of the directors of Freshfield Management Company Ltd, Freshfields Nursing Home has a large garden with a summerhouse and decking area for residents to enjoy in good weather. There is currently a rabbit living in the home. There is a residents meeting once a month to discuss any issues the residents may have. The home has its own minibus for transport and arranges outings for the residents.

Registered places: 21
Guide weekly rate: From £400
Specialist care: Day care, dementia, emergency admissions, physical disability, respite
Medical services: Podiatry, dentist, occupational therapy, optician
Qualified staff: Exceeds standard: 71% at NVQ level 2

Home details

Location: Residential area, in Brixham
Communal areas: 2 lounges, dining room, garden
Accessibility: *Floors:* 2 • *Access:* Lift • *Wheelchair access:* Good
Smoking: ✕
Pets: ✕
Routines: Flexible

Room details

Single: 19
Shared: 1
En suite: 20
Facilities: TV point, telephone point

Door lock: ✓
Lockable place: ✓

Services provided

Beauty services: Hairdressing, manicures
Mobile library: Library facilities
Religious services: ✕
Transport: ✕
Activities: *Coordinator:* ✓ • *Examples:* Bingo, one-to-one sessions *Outings:* ✓
Meetings: ✓

Furzeham Lodge

Manager: Carol Griffett
Owner: Mr and Mrs Dennis, Mr and Mrs Baker
Contact: Higher Furzeham Road, Furzeham Green, Brixham, Devon, TQ5 8BL
☏ 01803 856657
@ furzehamdask@aol.com

Situated in the fishing port town of Brixton, Furzeham Lodge is a detached building that has been designed to create a homely atmosphere. With bright, attractive gardens and outdoor seating areas, the home offers views of the surrounding Devonshire countryside and is situated on a gentle hill, 15 minutes' walk from the nearby shops and not far from the harbour. There is ample parking to the side of the home. Wine and cooked breakfasts are available.

Furzehatt Care Centre

Manager: Christine Johnson
Owner: Sanctuary Care Ltd
Contact: 59 Furzehatt Road, Plymstock, Plymouth, Devon, PL9 8QX
) 01752 484 008
@ cjohnson@sancturay-housing.co.uk
⌂ www.sanctuary-housing.co.uk

Located in a residential area, Furzehatt is a purpose-built care home with a recently installed sensory garden. Throughout the year the home organises coach trips to locations such as the nearby moors. The home produces a monthly newsletter containing details on resident and staff achievements, birthdays and upcoming activities. The home also a residents meeting once a month.

Registered places: 62
Guide weekly rate: Undisclosed
Specialist care: Nursing, dementia, physical disability
Medical services: Podiatry, dentist, occupational therapy, optician, physiotherapy
Qualified staff: Meets standard

Home details
Location: Residential area, 3.5 miles from Plymouth
Communal areas: 3 lounges, 2 dining rooms, 2 conservatories, garden
Accessibility: *Floors:* 2 • *Access:* Lift • *Wheelchair access:* Good
Smoking: In designated area
Pets: ✓
Routines: Flexible

Room details
Single: 62
Shared: 0
En suite: 59
Facilities: TV point, telephone point
Door lock: ✓
Lockable place: ✓

Services provided
Beauty services: Hairdressing
Mobile library: ✓
Religious services: Monthly Anglican Communion
Transport: ✗
Activities: *Coordinator:* ✓ • *Examples:* Bingo, carpet bowls, visiting entertainers • *Outings:* ✓
Meetings: ✓

Georgian House

Manager: Rachel Coleman
Owner: Elizabeth Feller
Contact: Park Hill Road, Torquay, Devon, TQ1 2DZ
) 01803 295196

Georgian House is a detached Grade II listed mansion, with a recently built annex. It is situated in a quiet residential area of Torquay and is within walking distance of Meadsfoot beach and Daddyhole Plain. The town centre and harbour are less than a mile away and a regular bus service stops outside the home. The home has hosted piano concerts, charity raffles, cream teas, clothes shows, shoe shows and make-up demonstrations and has provided reminiscence sessions, music therapy, handicraft and art sessions and quizzes. The home has been involved in raising money for charities.

Registered places: 40
Guide weekly rate: £485–£850
Specialist care: Dementia , mental disorder, physical disability
Medical services: Podiatry
Qualified staff: Fails standard

Home details
Location: Residential area, 0.5 miles from Torquay
Communal areas: 2 lounges, dining room, conservatory, library/computer room, chapel
Accessibility: *Floors:* 3 • *Access:* Lift • *Wheelchair access:* Good
Smoking: ✗
Pets: ✗
Routines: Flexible

Room details
Single: 40
Shared: 0
En suite: 0
Facilities: TV point
Door lock: ✓
Lockable place: ✗

Services provided
Beauty services: Hairdressing
Mobile library: ✗
Religious services: ✗
Transport: ✗
Activities: *Coordinator:* ✗ • *Examples:* Arts and crafts, reminiscence, music therapy • *Outings:* ✗
Meetings: ✓

Registered places: 30
Guide weekly rate: £380–£600
Specialist care: Day care, dementia, respite
Medical services: Podiatry, physiotherapy
Qualified staff: Fails standard

Home details

Location: Residential area, 1 mile from Honiton
Communal areas: Undisclosed
Accessibility: *Floors:* 2 • *Access:* Stair Lift • *Wheelchair access:* Good
Smoking: Undisclosed
Pets: ✗
Routines: Undisclosed

Room details

Single: 26
Shared: 2
En suite: Undisclosed
Facilities: None

Door lock: ✓
Lockable place: ✗

Services provided

Beauty services: Hairdressing
Mobile library: ✗
Religious services: ✗
Transport: Minibus
Activities: *Coordinator:* ✗ • *Examples:* Arts and crafts, games,
 musical entertainment • *Outings:* ✓
Meetings: ✓

Gittisham Hill House

Manager: Carol White
Owner: Gittisham Care Ltd
Contact: Sidmouth Road,
Honiton, Devon, EX14 3TY
☎ 01404 42083
@ gittishamcare@aol.com

Situated in 10 acres of parkland and surrounded by Gittisham offers vast opportunities for relaxation outdoors in a secure environment. A minibus makes daily trips to places of interest while a monthly newsletter details the resident and family meetings which take place twice a month, as well as the forthcoming programme of activities and events. These activities include arts and crafts sessions and musical entertainment.

Registered places: 24
Guide weekly rate: £390–£430
Specialist care: None
Medical services: Podiatry, dentist, optician
Qualified staff: Exceeds standard: 61% at NVQ level 2

Home details

Location: Residential area, 0.5 miles from Teignmouth centre
Communal areas: Lounge, dining room, conservatory, garden
Accessibility: *Floors:* 2 • *Access:* Stair Lift • *Wheelchair access:* Good
Smoking: ✗
Pets: At manager's discretion
Routines: Flexible

Room details

Single: 22
Shared: 1
En suite: 19
Facilities: TV point, telephone point

Door lock: ✓
Lockable place: ✗

Services provided

Beauty services: Hairdressing
Mobile library: ✗
Religious services: Monthly Anglican visits
Transport: 7-seater vehicle
Activities: *Coordinator:* ✗ • *Examples:* Bingo, quizzes, scrabble
 Outings: ✓
Meetings: ✗

Glendale Court

Manager: Gloria Taylor
Owner: Glenn and Gloria Taylor
Contact: Third Drive, Landscore Road,
Teignmouth, Devon, TQ14 9JT
☎ 01626 774229
@ Glendale1@btinternet.com

Glendale Court is a modern building that is situated in a quiet residential area of Teignmouth approximately half a mile from the local shops. Because of this and some public transport restrictions, the home is flexible with the use of its transport to take residents outside of the home. There is a fountain in the garden and the home is not far from Teignmouth seafront, which provides a lovely location for visitors wishing to take relatives out on trips. Although Glendale Court is not currently home to any animals, small pets are welcome.

Glenkealey Residential Home

Manager: Kristine Fitzpatrick
Owner: Kristine Fitzpatrick
Contact: Upper Hermosa Road, Teignmouth, Devon, TQ14 9JW
☎ 01626 774214

Situated on a bus route in a residential area, Glenkealy boasts views of the coast and the countryside. The home is located approximately half a mile from Teignmouth. The home arranges a residents meeting once a month and there is a religious service every week. The home has its own car and regularly takes the residents on outings. There are also internal activities organised by the activities coordinator, such as quizzes and exercise sessions.

Registered places: 14
Guide weekly rate: Undisclosed
Specialist care: Day care
Medical services: Podiatry, dentist, optician, physiotherapy
Qualified staff: Fails standard

Home details
Location: Residential area, 0.5 miles from Teignmouth
Communal areas: 2 lounges, dining room, garden
Accessibility: *Floors:* 2 • *Access:* Lift and stair Lift *Wheelchair access:* Good
Smoking: In designated area
Pets: At manager's discretion
Routines: Flexible

Room details
Single: 12
Shared: 1
En suite: 13
Facilities: TV point, telephone point

Door lock: ✓
Lockable place: ✓

Services provided
Beauty services: Hairdressing
Mobile library: ✗
Religious services: Weekly
Transport: Car
Activities: *Coordinator:* ✓ • *Examples:* Quizzes, exercises • *Outings:* ✓
Meetings: ✓

Golden Sands

Manager: Jackie Bateman
Owner: Mr and Mrs Thisby
Contact: 10 Nelson Road, Westward Ho, Bideford, Devon, EX39 1LF
☎ 01237 477730

Golden Sands is located in a residential area approximately 12 miles from Barnstaple. The home is set on the beachfront, giving it lovely views, and providing a nearby place for residents to take short walks. There is a bus route right outside the house, with routes into Barnstaple town centre. The home is pet-friendly, with Pets As Therapy visits and the owner has two labradors. Outings are organised into Barnstable or to other nearby towns. The home also arranges for Methodist and Anglican ministers to visit the home.

Registered places: 17
Guide weekly rate: From £405
Specialist care: None
Medical services: Podiatry, dentist, optician, physiotherapy
Qualified staff: Meets standard

Home details
Location: Residential area, 12 miles from Barnstaple
Communal areas: 2 lounges, dining room, conservatory, patio and garden
Accessibility: *Floors:* 2 • *Access:* Lift • *Wheelchair access:* Good
Smoking: ✗
Pets: ✓
Routines: Flexible

Room details
Single: 15
Shared: 1
En suite: 5
Facilities: TV, telephone point

Lockable place: ✓
Door lock: ✓

Services provided
Beauty services: Hairdressing, manicures
Mobile library: ✓
Religious services: Methodist and Anglican visits
Transport: ✗
Activities: *Coordinator:* ✓ • *Examples:* Reminiscence therapy, sponsored knitting, puzzles • *Outings:* ✓
Meetings: ✓

Registered places: 32
Guide weekly rate: £380–£420
Specialist care: Day care, respite
Medical services: Podiatry, dentist, optician, physiotherapy
Qualified staff: Undisclosed

Home details

Location: Residential area, in Torbay
Communal areas: 3 lounges, dining room, computer room, garden
Accessibility: *Floors:* 3 • *Access:* Lift and stair Lift
   Wheelchair access: Good
Smoking: ✗
Pets: At manager's discretion
Routines: Flexible

Room details

Single: 32
Shared: 0   Door lock: ✗
En suite: 32   Lockable place: ✓
Facilities: TV point, telephone point

Services provided

Beauty services: Hairdressing
Mobile library: Library facilities
Religious services: Monthly visits from all denominations
Transport: Car
Activities: *Coordinator:* ✗ • *Examples:* Bingo, skittles, quizzes
   Outings: ✓
Meetings: ✓

Grange-Lea Residential Home

Manager: Eleanor Morgan
Owner: Mr and Mrs Baker
Contact: 38 Preston Down Road, Preston, Paignton, Devon, TQ3 2RL
) 01803 522342
@ info@grange-lea.co.uk
🖰 www.grange-lea.co.uk

Grange-Lea is a detached property set in an elevated position on the side of a hill and overlooking Torbay. Approximately half a mile from the seafront, the home is a five-minute walk from the local shops. While some of the bedrooms have patio doors leading onto the gardens, most rooms also permit sea and bay views. There is level access into the home and Grange-Lea cares for its day care residents by providing transport to and from the home. There are garden parties in the summer and around five outings a year.

Registered places: 17
Guide weekly rate: £380–£450
Specialist care: Day care, dementia, physical disability, respite
Medical services: Podiatry, hygienist, optician, physiotherapy
Qualified staff: Exceeds standard: 60% at NVQ level 2

Home details

Location: Village location, 4.5 miles from Newton Abbot
Communal areas: Lounge, dining room, conservatory, garden
Accessibility: *Floors:* 2 • *Access:* Lift • *Wheelchair access:* Good
Smoking: In designated area
Pets: ✓
Routines: Flexible

Room details

Single: 11
Shared: 3   Door lock: ✓
En suite: 14   Lockable place: ✓
Facilities: TV point, telephone point

Services provided

Beauty services: Hairdressing
Mobile library: ✓
Religious services: Fortnightly Anglican Communion service
Transport: Car
Activities: *Coordinator:* ✓ • *Examples:* Arts and crafts,
   flower arranging, visiting entertainers • *Outings:* ✓
Meetings: ✗

The Grange Residential Hotel

Manager: Victoria Kay
Owner: Ogwell Grange Ltd
Contact: Townsend Hill, Ipplepen, Newton Abbot, Devon, TQ12 5RU
) 01803 813656
@ suttonr@btconnect.com

A Grade II listed building, the Grange Residential Hotel is well positioned a few miles from Torbay and Newton Abbot and approximately 150 yards from the town centre's shops. For less mobile residents, the home has a 'tuck shop' where individuals can purchase small items such as sweets. The home has its own car for transport and offers the residents the chance to go on outings as well as internal activities such as arts and crafts.

Greycliffe Residential Care Complex

Manager: Shirley Kirkcaldy
Owner: Alexander and Shirley Kirkcaldy
Contact: Lower Warberry Road, Wellswood, Torquay, Devon, TQ1 1QY
) 01803 292106
@ Alexander.Kirkcaldy@btinternet.com

A period property located in a quiet residential area, Greycliffe has one and a half acres of beautiful, flat, gardens. The home is situated approximately half a mile from Torquay town centre. As well as the standard accommodation, the home also has two apartments with extras including a lounge, kitchenette and bathroom. There are plans to add a conservatory to the home. The home has its own car for transport and takes the residents on regular outings in the local area.

Registered places: 25
Guide weekly rate: £400–£475
Specialist care: Dementia, respite
Medical services: Podiatry, dentist
Qualified staff: Exceeds standard: 70% at NVQ level 2

Home details
Location: Residential area, 0.5 miles from Torquay
Communal areas: Lounge, dining room, garden
Accessibility: *Floors:* 2 • *Access:* Stair lift • *Wheelchair access:* Good
Smoking: ✗
Pets: At manager's discretion
Routines: Flexible

Room details
Single: 21
Shared: 2   **Door lock:** ✓
En suite: 19   **Lockable place:** ✓
Facilities: TV point, telephone point

Services provided
Beauty services: Hairdressing
Mobile library: ✓
Religious services: Weekly service, monthly Communion service
Transport: Car
Activities: *Coordinator:* ✓ • *Examples:* Bingo, visiting entertainers
   Outings: ✓
Meetings: ✓

Halsdown Nursing Home

Manager: Amanda Allison
Owner: Ronald and Margaret Blake
Contact: 243 Exeter Road, Exmouth, Devon, EX8 3NA
) 01395 272390

Halsdown House is conveniently located for bus services, situated in a residential area just over a mile from Exmouth. The home has a conservatory and a garden for residents to relax in, as well as a lounge. The home has its own activities coordinator who arranges bingo and musical entertainment for the residents.

Registered places: 17
Guide weekly rate: £622–£697
Specialist care: Nursing
Medical services: Podiatry
Qualified staff: Fails standard

Home details
Location: Residential area, 1.3 miles from Exmouth
Communal areas: Lounge, dining room, conservatory, garden
Accessibility: *Floors:* 2 • *Access:* Lift • *Wheelchair access:* Good
Smoking: ✗
Pets: ✓
Routines: Flexible

Room details
Single: Undisclosed
Shared: Undisclosed   **Door lock:** ✗
En suite: Undisclosed   **Lockable place:** ✓
Facilities: TV

Services provided
Beauty services: Hairdressing
Mobile library: ✗
Religious services: ✗
Transport: ✗
Activities: *Coordinator:* ✓ • *Examples:* Bingo, musical entertainment
   Outings: ✗
Meetings: ✗

Registered places: 32
Guide weekly rate: £333–£368
Specialist care: Dementia
Medical services: Podiatry
Qualified staff: Exceeds standard: 90% at NVQ level 2

Home details
Location: Urban area, 1 mile from Plymouth
Communal areas: 3 lounges, 2 dining rooms, conservatory
Accessibility: *Floors:* 3 • *Access:* Lift • *Wheelchair access:* Limited
Smoking: At manager's discretion
Pets: ✗
Routines: Flexible

Room details
Single: 29
Shared: 3
En suite: Undisclosed
Facilities: TV

Door lock: ✓
Lockable place: ✗

Services provided
Beauty services: Hairdressing, aromatherapy
Mobile library: ✗
Religious services: ✗
Transport: ✗
Activities: *Coordinator:* ✗ • *Examples:* Games, quizzes, musical entertainment • *Outings:* ✗
Meetings: ✓

Hamilton House Residential Home

Manager: Elizabeth Glover
Owner: Penton Homes Ltd
Contact: 23 Houndiscombe Road, Mutley, Plymouth, Devon, PL4 6HG
☎ 01752 265691
@ lizglover@yahoo.co.uk

Hamilton House is made up of two large houses converted into one care home for 32 residents. It is within walking distance from Mutley Plain shopping centre and is one mile from Plymouth town centre. Activities are organised regularly and are adapted to be suitable for those with dementia. One-to-one activities, such as hand massage, ensure that each residents benefits from some individual time with the carers. Two lounges and the dining rooms are found on the lower ground floor. There is also a conservatory and lounge on the ground floor.

Registered places: 26
Guide weekly rate: £303–£375
Specialist care: Day care, dementia, emergency admissions, physical disability, respite
Medical services: Podiatry, hygienist, optician, physiotherapy
Qualified staff: Meets standard

Home details
Location: Residential area, 1 mile from Paignton
Communal areas: 2 lounge, dining room, gardens
Accessibility: *Floors:* 4 • *Access:* Lift and stair lift
Wheelchair access: Good
Smoking: ✗
Pets: ✓
Routines: Flexible

Room details
Single: 18
Shared: 4
En suite: 22
Facilities: TV point, telephone point

Door lock: ✗
Lockable place: ✓

Services provided
Beauty services: Hairdressing, aromatherapy, massage
Mobile library: ✓
Religious services: Monthly Communion service
Transport: Minibus
Activities: *Coordinator:* ✓ • *Examples:* Pets as Therapy, exercise *Outings:* ✓
Meetings: ✓

Harbour Rise Rest Home

Manager: Alison Hardie
Owner: Harbour Rise Ltd
Contact: 18 Roundham Road, Paignton, Devon, TQ4 6DN
☎ 01803 551834
@ enquiries@harbourrise.co.uk
🖰 www.harbourrise.co.uk

Harbour Rise Rest Home is a semi-detached building with gardens at the front and side of the home. It is located close to a post office, shop and bus stop and is about one mile from the train station and the centre of Paignton. The home has visits from a mobile library and also arranges a Communion service every month. There is a minibus which is used to take residents on outings and there is a residents meeting every three months. The home also arranges Pets As Therapy visits and exercise sessions.

Hatt House

Manager: Patricia Oaten
Owner: Michael and Patricia Oaten
Contact: 14 Park Road, St Marychurch, Torquay, Devon, TQ1 4QR
) 01803 326316
@ Hatt.house@virgin.net

A period property Hatt House is set in an acre of its own grounds, approximately two miles from Torquay. The home has a garden for residents to enjoy in the summer and there is a minibus available for transportation. There is an Anglican Communion service every month and the home arranges for a mobile library to come to the home. The home has a dedicated activities coordinator who arranges armchair aerobics and performances from visiting entertainers for the residents.

Registered places: 24
Guide weekly rate: Undisclosed
Specialist care: Dementia, mental disorder
Medical services: Podiatry, hygienist, optician, physiotherapy
Qualified staff: Meets standard

Home details
Location: Residential area, 2 miles from Torquay
Communal areas: 2 lounges, dining room, garden
Accessibility: *Floors:* 2 • *Access:* Lift • *Wheelchair access:* Good
Smoking: ✗
Pets: ✓
Routines: Flexible

Room details
Single: 17
Shared: 3
En suite: 6
Facilities: TV point, telephone point

Door lock: ✓
Lockable place: ✓

Services provided
Beauty services: Hairdressing
Mobile library: ✓
Religious services: Monthly Anglican Communion service
Transport: Minibus
Activities: *Coordinator:* ✓ • *Examples:* Armchair aerobics, quizzes, visiting entertainers • *Outings:* ✗
Meetings: ✗

Hembury Fort House

Manager: Caroline White
Owner: Agnes Taylor and Caroline White
Contact: Awliscombe, Honiton, Devon, EX14 3LD
) 01404 841334

A Georgian house set in eight acres of grounds, Hembury Fort is situated outside the village of Awliscombe. Many of the rooms in the home permit beautiful views across the Otter Valley. The home also has expansive gardens. Although not in walking distance of local facilities, the home is on a bus route and has an on-site shop which is open once or twice a week. The home's lounge is split into two distinct areas with one dedicated to quiet. Offering a comprehensive activities programme, the home will hire a minibus to take residents on outings.

Registered places: 25
Guide weekly rate: £306–£415
Specialist care: Dementia
Medical services: Podiatry, dentist, optician
Qualified staff: Fails standard

Home details
Location: Rural area, 3.5 miles from Honiton
Communal areas: Lounge, dining room, garden
Accessibility: *Floors:* 3 • *Access:* Lift • *Wheelchair access:* Good
Smoking: ✗
Pets: At manager's discretion
Routines: Flexible

Room details
Single: 25
Shared: 0
En suite: 23
Facilities: TV point, telephone point

Door lock: ✓
Lockable place: ✓

Services provided
Beauty services: Hairdressing
Mobile library: ✓
Religious services: Monthly Communion service
Transport: ✗
Activities: *Coordinator:* ✓ • *Examples:* Bingo, musical entertainment, reminiscence therapy • *Outings:* ✓
Meetings: ✓

Registered places: 17
Guide weekly rate: £385–£400
Specialist care: Nursing, dementia, mental disorder
Medical services: Podiatry, hygienist, optician, physiotherapy
Qualified staff: Meets standard

Home details

Location: Residential area, 2.2 miles from Bideford
Communal areas: 2 Lounges, dining room, patio and garden
Accessibility: *Floors:* 3 • *Access:* Stair lift • *Wheelchair access:* Good
Smoking: In designated area
Pets: ✓
Routines: Structured

Room details

Single: 16
Shared: 1
En suite: 6
Facilities: TV point, telephone point

Door lock: ✓
Lockable place: ✗

Services provided

Beauty services: Hairdressing, aromatherapy, manicures
Mobile Library: ✓
Religious services: ✓
Transport: ✗
Activities: *Coordinator:* ✗ • *Examples:* Arts and crafts,
    exercise sessions, games • *Outings:* ✓
Meetings: ✓

Herons Lea

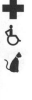

Manager: Glenys Quill
Owner: Herons Lea Residential Home Ltd
Contact: Silford Cross, Abbotsham,
Bideford, Devon, EX39 3PT
☎ 01237 476176

Situated in a rural location within three acres of grounds, Herons Lea is just over two miles from Bideford. The home has a resident cat, and would allow other pets. Visits from religious leaders can be requested. Although a small fee is charged for activities, this is mentioned in the home's Service User's Guide. These activities include performances by visiting entertainers, arts and crafts and exercise sessions.

Registered places: 25
Guide weekly rate: Undisclosed
Specialist care: Dementia, respite
Medical services: Podiatry, dentist, occupational therapy, optician
Qualified staff: Meets standard

Home details

Location: Urban area, 2 miles from Plymouth
Communal areas: 2 lounges, dining room, patio
Accessibility: *Floors:* 3 • *Access:* Lift • *Wheelchair access:* Good
Smoking: In designated area
Pets: At manager's discretion
Routines: Flexible

Room details

Single: 23
Shared: 1
En suite: Undisclosed
Facilities: TV point

Door lock: ✓
Lockable place: ✓

Services provided

Beauty services: Hairdressing
Mobile library: ✓
Religious services: ✗
Transport: ✗
Activities: *Coordinator:* ✗ • *Examples:* Bingo, exercise sessions
    Outings: ✓
Meetings: ✗

Higher Park Lodge

Manager: Deborah Norman
Owner: Higher Park Lodge Ltd
Contact: Devonport Park, Stoke,
Plymouth, Devon, PL1 4BT
☎ 01752 606066

A large building with an attached purpose-built extension, Higher Park Lodge is situated close to the village of Stoke and neighbouring Devonport Park. Although the home does not have a garden, residents may take advantage of this location. The home does have a patio area for residents to sit outside. There are also two lounges for residents to socialise in. The home arranges outings for the residents and internal activities such as bingo and exercise sessions.

Hillbrow House

Manager: **Rosemarie Heard**
Owner: Hillbrow Residential Care
Home Ltd
Contact: 1 Park Road,
Crediton, Devon, EX17 3BS
) 01363 773055
@ hillbrow@shears.eclipse.co.uk

An extended 18th-century building, Hillbrow House is situated in a residential area and boasts a sheltered garden with flowerbeds and a pond. Located on a main bus route, for independent residents with a reasonable degree of fitness, the shops are located within a mile radius. The home is less than a mile from Crediton. The home has its own car for transport and often takes the residents on outings. The activities coordinator also arranges activities in the home, for example arts and crafts and gardening.

Registered places: 24
Guide weekly rate: £400
Specialist care: Day care, respite
Medical services: Podiatry, hygienist, optician, physiotherapy
Qualified staff: Meets standard

Home details
Location: Residential area, 0.3 miles from Crediton
Communal areas: 2 lounges, dining room, conservatory, garden
Accessibility: *Floors:* 2 • *Access:* Lift • *Wheelchair access:* Good
Smoking: In designated area
Pets: ✓
Routines: Flexible

Room details
Single: 24
Shared: 0
En suite: 5
Facilities: TV point, telephone point

Door lock: ✓
Lockable place: ✓

Services provided
Beauty services: Hairdressing
Mobile library: ✓
Religious services: Monthly Anglican Communion service
Transport: Car
Activities: *Coordinator:* ✓ • *Examples:* Arts and crafts, gardening
  Outings: ✓
Meetings: ✓

Holwell Villa

Manager: Christina Burridge
Owner: Ronald and Barbara Marlow
Contact: 119 New Road,
Brixham, Devon, TQ5 8BY
) 01803 854103

Holwell Villa is a detached property situated within walking distance of Brixham town centre with its range of shops and amenities. The home has its own greenhouse which residents are allowed to use freely. There is also a patio area in the garden for residents to enjoy in summer. The home arranges bingo sessions for the residents in the lounge. There is also a separate dining room. Pets would be allowed in the home at the manager's discretion.

Registered places: 17
Guide weekly rate: Undisclosed
Specialist care: Day care, dementia, physical disability, respite
Medical services: Podiatry, optician
Qualified staff: Undisclosed

Home details
Location: Residential area, 0.5 miles from Brixham
Communal areas: Lounge, dining room, patio and garden
Accessibility: *Floors:* 3 • *Access:* Lift • *Wheelchair access:* Good
Smoking: In designated area
Pets: At manager's discretion
Routines: Flexible

Room details
Single: 11
Shared: 3
En suite: 4
Facilities: None

Door lock: ✓
Lockable place: ✓

Services provided
Beauty services: Hairdressing
Mobile library: ✗
Religious services: ✗
Transport: ✗
Activities: *Coordinator:* ✗ • *Examples:* Bingo • *Outings:* ✗
Meetings: ✗

Registered places: 24
Guide weekly rate: £392–£499
Specialist care: Day care, physical disability
Medical services: Podiatry, optician, physiotherapy
Qualified staff: Meets standard

Home details

Location: Residential area, 1 mile from Exmouth
Communal areas: 2 lounges, dining room, conservatory, garden
Accessibility: *Floors:* 3 • *Access:* Lift • *Wheelchair access:* Good
Smoking: In designated area
Pets: ✓
Routines: Flexible

Room details

Single: 18
Shared: 3
En suite: 18
Facilities: TV point, telephone point

Door lock: ✓
Lockable place: ✓

Services provided

Beauty services: Hairdressing
Mobile library: ✓
Religious services: Monthly Communion service
Transport: Car
Activities: *Coordinator:* ✗ • *Examples:* Visiting entertainers
   Outings: ✓
Meetings: ✓

The Homestead

Manager: Hazel Neville
Owner: Homestead Homes Ltd
Contact: 6 Elwyn Road,
Exmouth, Devon, EX8 2EL
☎ 01395 263778
@ call.us@homesteadhomes.co.uk

Situated in a residential area in its own well-kept gardens, The Homestead is an Edwardian property. It is a short, flat walk to the local shops and a short bus ride to Exmouth town centre, one mile away. The home has its own car for transport and often takes the residents on outings. There is Communion service once a month and there are visits from a mobile library.

Registered places: 33
Guide weekly rate: £500–£640
Specialist care: Day care, dementia, physical disability
Medical services: Podiatry, hygienist, optician, physiotherapy
Qualified staff: Exceeds standard: 80% at NVQ level 2

Home details

Location: Village location, 5 miles from Dartmouth
Communal areas: Lounge, 2 dining rooms, garden room,
   patio and garden
Accessibility: *Floors:* 3 • *Access:* Lift • *Wheelchair access:* Good
Smoking: ✗
Pets: ✗
Routines: Flexible

Room details

Single: 27
Shared: 3
En suite: 27
Facilities: TV, telephone point

Door lock: ✓
Lockable place: ✓

Services provided

Beauty services: Hairdressing
Mobile library: ✓
Religious services: Monthly Communion service
Transport: Car
Activities: *Coordinator:* ✓ • *Examples:* Exercise classes, games,
   musical entertainment • *Outings:* ✓
Meetings: ✓

Hyne Town House

Manager: Jean White
Owner: Stephen and Yvonne Mould
Contact: Strete, Dartmouth,
Devon, TQ6 0RU
☎ 01803 770011
@ info@hynetownhouse.co.uk
🖰 www.hynetownhouse.co.uk

Situated behind the Parish Church and on a bus route which runs to Kingsbridge and Dartmouth, Hyne Town House is a Georgian house with purpose-built wing. Although the home does not allow pets, it has two lovebirds that live in the home's garden room. This room is an attractive sunny space where residents may relax and enjoy the home's sea views in comfort. The home has its own car for transport and often takes the residents on outings. There is a regular residents meeting and a Communion service takes place on a monthly basis.

Innisfree Residential Home

Manager: Linda Wilbraham
Owner: Jacqueline Glenning
Contact: 15–17 Polsham Park, Paignton, Devon, TQ3 2AD
☎ 01803 552269

Innisfree Residential Home is a large property that is situated close to Paignton's local facilities as well as the beach. The home produces a newsletter which informs residents of upcoming activities. The home has an activities coordinator who arranges daily activities such as bingo as well as outings for the residents. There are regular residents meetings to allow residents to voice any issues or suggestions they may have.

Registered places: 16
Guide weekly rate: £325–£421
Specialist care: Respite
Medical services: Podiatry
Qualified staff: Exceeds standard: 80% at NVQ level 2

Home details
Location: Village location, 0.5 miles from Paignton
Communal areas: 2 lounges, dining room, conservatory, garden
Accessibility: *Floors:* 2 • *Access:* Stair lift • *Wheelchair access:* Good
Smoking: ✗
Pets: ✓
Routines: Flexible

Room details
Single: 16
Shared: 0
En suite: 16
Facilities: None

Door lock: ✓
Lockable place: ✓

Services provided
Beauty services: Hairdressing
Mobile library: ✗
Religious services: ✗
Transport: ✗
Activities: *Coordinator:* ✓ • *Examples:* Bingo • *Outings:* ✓
Meetings: ✓

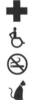

Ivydene Care Home

Manager: Janet Smith
Owner: Sanctuary Care Ltd
Contact: 21 Staniforth Drive, Ivybridge, Devon, PL21 0UJ
☎ 01752 894888
🖥 www.ivydenecarehome.co.uk

Ivydene is a purpose-built care home located approximately half a mile from Ivybridge. Seven bedrooms in the home are dedicated to NHS-funded short-term nursing care. The home publishes a monthly newsletter for group social activities. The activities coordinator puts together a varied programme which includes exercise sessions and a book club. There are three lounges in the home in addition to a garden with a patio area.

Registered places: 56
Guide weekly rate: £267–£569
Specialist care: Nursing, physical disability
Medical services: Podiatry, physiotherapy
Qualified staff: Meets standard

Home details
Location: Residential area, 0.5 miles from Ivybridge
Communal areas: 3 lounges, dining room, patio and garden
Accessibility: *Floors:* 2 • *Access:* Lift • *Wheelchair access:* Good
Smoking: ✗
Pets: At manager's discretion
Routines: Flexible

Room details
Single: 55
Shared: 1
En suite: 56
Facilities: None

Door lock: ✓
Lockable place: ✓

Services provided
Beauty services: Hairdressing
Mobile library: ✗
Religious services: ✗
Transport: ✗
Activities: *Coordinator:* ✓ • *Examples:* Bingo, book club, exercise *Outings:* ✗
Meetings: ✓

Registered places: 28
Guide weekly rate: £294–£345
Specialist care: Respite
Medical services: Podiatry, physiotherapy
Qualified staff: Undisclosed

Home details

Location: Residential area, 1 mile from Torquay
Communal areas: Lounge, dining room, conservatory
Accessibility: *Floors:* 2 • *Access:* Lift and stair lift
    Wheelchair access: Good
Smoking: ✗
Pets: ✗
Routines: Flexible

Room details

Single: 28
Shared: 0
En suite: 14
Facilities: TV point

Door lock: ✓
Lockable place: ✓

Services provided

Beauty services: Hairdressing
Mobile library: ✗
Religious services: ✗
Transport: ✗
Activities: *Coordinator:* ✓ • *Examples:* Bingo • *Outings:* ✗
Meetings: ✗

Jubilee House

Manager: Eileen Pope
Owner: ADL plc
Contact: Bronshill Road,
Torquay, Devon, TQ1 3HA
☎ 01803 311002
@ jubileemanager@adlcare.com

Jubilee House is a detached property surrounded by mature trees. The home is located in a residential area, approximately one mile from Torquay. There are a variety of communal areas, including a large conservatory, as well as a garden. A programme of activities is also available which includes bingo.

Registered places: 28
Guide weekly rate: £280–£400
Specialist care: Day care, respite
Medical services: Podiatry, dentist, optician, physiotherapy
Qualified staff: Exceeds standard: 80% at NVQ level 2

Home details

Location: Residential area, in Kingsbridge
Communal areas: 2 lounges, dining area, patio and garden
Accessibility: *Floors:* 2 • *Access:* Stair lift • *Wheelchair access:* Good
Smoking: In designated area
Pets: At manager's discretion
Routines: Flexible

Room details

Single: 22
Shared: 3
En suite: 4
Facilities: TV point, telephone point

Door lock: ✓
Lockable place: ✓

Services provided

Beauty services: Hairdressing
Mobile library: ✓
Religious services: Monthly nondenominational Communion service
Transport: Minibus
Activities: *Coordinator:* ✓ • *Examples:* Bingo, card making
    Outings: ✓
Meetings: ✓

Kahala Court

Manager: Sheena Ford
Owner: The Court Group
Contact: Embankment Road,
Kingsbridge, Devon, TQ7 1JN
☎ 01548 852520
@ info@thecourtgroup.co.uk
🖰 www.thecourtgroup.co.uk

A detached house set in the heart of the port town of Kingsbridge, Kahala Court is well placed to overlook the estuary. With local amenities such as shops and a library less than 10 minutes' walk away, residents who would not struggle with the home's steep drive can also enjoy leisurely walks down by the river. Residents benefit from a three monthly auditing of activities made available, while monthly outings on the home's minibus ensure that residents do not lose touch with the wider community.

Kent Farm

Manager: Pauleen Maitrise
Owner: Pauleen Maitrise
Contact: Mill Street, Uffculme,
Cullompton, Devon, EX15 3AR
☎ 01884 840144

Close to the main village square, Kent Farm enjoys a close relationship with the local community. The building is an attractive converted dairy farm with a partially enclosed courtyard. Kent Farm is situated in a village, near a river and five miles from Cullompton. Residents go on a number of outings, including trips to nearby Cullompton. The home has its own minibus to take residents on outings. There is a residents meeting once a month and there is also an Anglican Communion service once a month.

Registered places: 15
Guide weekly rate: £280–£410
Specialist care: Day care, physical disability
Medical services: Podiatry, dentist, optician
Qualified staff: Exceeds standard: 65% at NVQ level 2

Home details

Location: Village location, 5 miles from Cullompton
Communal areas: Lounge, dining room, garden
Accessibility: *Floors:* 2 • *Access:* Lift • *Wheelchair access:* Good
Smoking: ✗
Pets: At manager's discretion
Routines: Flexible

Room details

Single: 15
Shared: 0
En suite: 10
Facilities: TV point, telephone point

Door lock: ✓
Lockable place: ✓

Services provided

Beauty services: Hairdressing
Mobile library: ✗
Religious services: Monthly Anglican Communion service
Transport: Minibus
Activities: *Coordinator:* ✓ • *Examples:* Arts and crafts, musical entertainment, quizzes • *Outings:* ✓
Meetings: ✓

Kenwith Castle Retirement Residence

Manager: Rae Vanstone
Owner: Two Rivers Investments Ltd
Contact: Abbotsham, Bideford,
Devon, EX39 5BE
☎ 01237 470060
@ kenwithcastle@aol.com

Occupying an ancient historic site that is said to have been the scene of a victorious battle against the Vikings, Kenwith Castle is a renovated 18th-century building. Set in the heart of Devon's countryside and permitting beautiful views, Kenwith is set in spectacular grounds which include attractions such as putting greens, water gardens and a six-acre trout lake. Situated a few miles from Bideford town centre, there is a bus stop at the front of the house. There are kitchen facilities provided where residents and relatives can prepare snacks, with assistance if needed.

Registered places: 59
Guide weekly rate: £500–£620
Specialist care: Nursing
Medical services: Podiatry, dentist, optician
Qualified staff: Undisclosed

Home details

Location: Rural area, 2.5 miles from Bideford
Communal areas: 5 lounges, dining room, bar, kitchenette, patio and garden
Accessibility: *Floors:* 2 • *Access:* Lift • *Wheelchair access:* Good
Smoking: In designated area
Pets: At manager's discretion
Routines: Flexible

Room details

Single: 47
Shared: 6
En suite: 53
Facilities: TV, telephone

Door lock: ✓
Lockable place: ✓

Services provided

Beauty services: Hairdressing
Mobile library: ✓
Religious services: Monthly Anglican service
Transport: ✗
Activities: *Coordinator:* ✓ • *Examples:* Craft classes, piano recitals *Outings:* ✓
Meetings: ✗

Registered places: 34
Guide weekly rate: £380–£640
Specialist care: Nursing, emergency admissions, physical disability
Medical services: Podiatry, dentist, optician, physiotherapy
Qualified staff: Undisclosed

Home details
Location: Rural location, 2 miles from Ivybridge
Communal areas: 2 lounges, dining room, conservatory, garden
Accessibility: *Floors:* 3 • *Access:* Lift • *Wheelchair access:* Good
Smoking: ✗
Pets: ✗
Routines: Flexible

Room details
Single: 24
Shared: 5
En suite: 23
Facilities: TV, telephone point

Door lock: ✓
Lockable place: ✗

Services provided
Beauty services: Hairdressing
Mobile library: ✓
Religious services: Monthly Anglican Communion service
Transport: ✗
Activities: *Coordinator:* ✓ • *Examples:* Films visiting entertainers
  Outings: ✓
Meetings: ✗

Kings Acre

Manager: Georgina Linnell
Owner: Michael Leaves
Contact: Ermington, Nr Ivybridge, Devon, PL21 0LQ
☎ 01548 830076
@ kingsace@tesco.net

A former coaching inn, Kings Acre is a property set in its own grounds that now caters primarily to those elderly individuals with a physical disability. Although lacking in extensive local amenities there is a small corner shop close by. Home to a budgie and tropical fish, Kings Acre allows pets to visit and offers a flexible visiting policy with one lounge dedicated to quiet. With beautiful views over the garden and surrounding countryside, Kings Acre's conservatory is also a pleasant place in which to pass the time. As well as a weekly newsletter, twice-yearly questionnaires allow residents and relatives to comment on the care.

Registered places: 34
Guide weekly rate: From £500
Specialist care: Nursing, physical disability, respite
Medical services: Podiatry, dentist
Qualified staff: Exceeds standard: 70% at NVQ level 2

Home details
Location: Residential area, 2 miles from Plymouth centre
Communal areas: 2 lounges, dining room, library, patio and garden
Accessibility: *Floors:* 3 • *Access:* Lift • *Wheelchair access:* Good
Smoking: In designated area
Pets: ✗
Routines: Flexible

Room details
Single: 34
Shared: 0
En suite: 4
Facilities: TV point, telephone

Door lock: ✓
Lockable place: ✓

Services provided
Beauty services: Hairdressing, beautician
Mobile library: ✓
Religious services: Monthly Anglican Communion
Transport: ✗
Activities: *Coordinator:* ✗ • *Examples:* Bingo, music and movement,
  visiting singers • *Outings:* ✗
Meetings: ✓

The Kings House

Manager: Mrs Smyth
Owner: KingsCare Ltd
Contact: Paradise Road, Stoke, Plymouth, Devon, PL1 5QL
☎ 01752 607060

A purpose-built home, The Kings House is located on a bus route that passes Plymouth train station on its way into the city centre. The home is situated in a residential area, two miles from Plymouth town centre. The home arranges an Anglican Communion service once a month and every six months there is a residents meeting. There is a range of activities on offer which include music and movement and performances by visiting singers.

Lakeview Residential Home

Manager: Vacant
Owner: South West Residential Homes Ltd
Contact: 4 South Road, Newton Abbot, Devon, TQ12 1HL
☎ 01626 354181

Lakeview Residential Home consists of a main building and two smaller buildings located in the grounds. The home overlooks Decoy Lake and there are pleasant views from the garden. The home has a lounge and a dining room in the main building and there are daily activities on offer such as knitting and jigsaws. There are regular residents meetings held in the home and there are also outings on offer.

Registered places: 29
Guide weekly rate: £350–£450
Specialist care: Dementia, learning disability, physically disabled, respite
Medical services: Podiatry, dentist, optician
Qualified staff: Meets standard

Home details
Location: Residential area, 1 mile from Newton Abbot
Communal areas: Lounge, dining room, garden
Accessibility: *Floors: 2* • *Access: Lift* • *Wheelchair access:* Good
Smoking: ✗
Pets: ✗
Routines: Flexible

Room details
Single: 23
Shared: 3
En suite: 17
Facilities: TV, telephone

Door lock: ✗
Lockable place: ✓

Services provided
Beauty services: Hairdressing
Mobile library: Library facilities
Religious services: ✓
Transport: ✗
Activities: *Coordinator:* ✗ • *Examples:* Jigsaw, knitting • *Outings:* ✓
Meetings: ✓

Lambspark Residential Home

Manager: Tracey Wraighte
Owner: Richard and Tracey Wraighte
Contact: 38 Merafield Road, Plympton, Plymouth, Devon, PL7 1TL
☎ 01752 330470
@ lambspark@supanet.com

Situated in a residential area, Lambspark Residential Home is less than five minutes' walk from amenities including shops and pubs. The home is located only half a mile from Plympton. The home has a spacious garden with a pond as well as a conservatory. The home has its own transport for outings and also arranges for a mobile library to come to the home. The activities programme includes quizzes and performances from visiting entertainers.

Registered places: 33
Guide weekly rate: Undisclosed
Specialist care: Dementia, mental disorder, physical disability
Medical services: Podiatry, optician, physiotherapy
Qualified staff: Meets standard

Home details
Location: Residential area, 0.5 miles from Plympton
Communal areas: Lounge, dining room, conservatory, garden
Accessibility: *Floors: 3* • *Access:* Lift • *Wheelchair access:* Good
Smoking: In designated area
Pets: At manager's discretion
Routines: Flexible

Room details
Single: 29
Shared: 2
En suite: 31
Facilities: TV point, telephone point

Door lock: ✓
Lockable place: ✓

Services provided
Beauty services: Hairdressing
Mobile library: ✓
Religious services: ✗
Transport: 7-seater vehicle
Activities: *Coordinator:* ✗ • *Examples:* Bingo, quizzes, visiting entertainers • *Outings:* ✓
Meetings: ✗

Registered places: 14
Guide weekly rate: £287–£396
Specialist care: Respite
Medical services: Podiatry, optician, physiotherapy
Qualified staff: Exceeds standard: 70% at NVQ level 2

Home details
Location: Residential area, 0.5 miles from Teignmouth
Communal areas: Lounge, dining room, conservatory, garden
Accessibility: *Floors:* 2 • *Access:* Stair Lift • *Wheelchair access:* Good
Smoking: ✗
Pets: At manager's discretion
Routines: Flexible

Room details
Single: 14
Shared: 0
En suite: 14
Door lock: ✓
Lockable place: ✓
Facilities: TV point, telephone point

Services provided
Beauty services: Hairdressing
Mobile library: ✗
Religious services: Anglican Communion service every 3 weeks
Transport: Cars
Activities: *Coordinator:* ✗ • *Examples:* Musical entertainment, reminiscence, scrabble • *Outings:* ✓
Meetings: ✗

Landscore House

Manager: Penelope Webb
Owner: Nicholas and Penelope Webb
Contact: 3 Landscore Road, Teignmouth, Devon, TQ14 9JU
☎ 01626 770340

Situated on a hill with some good views of the town, Landscore House is a small, family-run care home where the owners live on site. The home has recently undergone major refurbishments to improve the quality of service offered. The home is located close to a library. The home has its own transportation and often takes the residents out for one-to-one trips. There is also an Anglican Communion service every three weeks.

Registered places: 22
Guide weekly rate: £325–£530
Specialist care: Nursing, day care, emergency admissions, physical disability, respite
Medical services: Podiatry, dentist, optician
Qualified staff: Undisclosed

Home details
Location: Village location, 5 miles from Plymouth
Communal areas: Lounge, dining room, conservatory, garden
Accessibility: *Floors:* 2 • *Access:* Lift and stair lift
    Wheelchair access: Good
Smoking: ✗
Pets: ✗
Routines: Flexible

Room details
Single: 16
Shared: 3
En suite: 3
Door lock: ✓
Lockable place: ✓
Facilities: TV point, telephone point

Services provided
Beauty services: Hairdressing, manicures
Mobile library: Library facilities
Religious services: Monthly Anglican Communion service
Transport: ✗
Activities: *Coordinator:* ✗ • *Examples:* Exercise, musical entertainment
    Outings: ✓
Meetings: ✗

The Lawns

Manager: Vacant
Owner: Wells House Ltd
Contact: Brixton, Plymouth, Devon, PL8 2AX
☎ 01752 880465

A detached country house set in its own grounds on the main Kingsbridge road, The Lawns is also within the South Hams area of Devon, known for its outstanding natural beauty. With a village shop five minutes' walk away, there is also a bus stop a nearby offering regular services towards Plymouth and Kingsbridge. The Lawns offers at least two outings a year in conjunction with its sister home, The Manor. Although the home does not allow pets to stay, it is home to a resident cat and pets are welcome to visit.

Le Chalet

Manager: Mr and Mrs Maxwell
Owner: Mr and Mrs Maxwell
Contact: Bickington Road,
Barnstaple, Devon, EX31 2DB
📞 01271 342083
@ legos@lechalet.freeserve.co.uk

Situated on the outskirts of Barnstaple, Le Chalet is an attractive house situated on one floor a few minutes' walk away from a post office, pub and shop. The home is also only a few minutes' walk from a bus stop and benefits from having a Pelican crossing directly outside. A small, family-run home with an atmosphere that is said to be friendly and informal, Le Chalet has been established for over 40 years and the managers live on site. In the absence of regular outings, individual activities within the home are well supported.

Registered places: 11
Guide weekly rate: £320–£363
Specialist care: Dementia, respite
Medical services: Podiatry, dentist, optician
Qualified staff: Undisclosed

Home details
Location: Residential area, 1 mile from Barnstaple centre
Communal areas: 2 lounges, dining room, garden
Accessibility: *Floors:* 1 • *Wheelchair access:* Good
Smoking: ✗
Pets: ✗
Routines: Flexible

Room details
Single: 11
Shared: 0
En suite: 0
Facilities: TV point, telephone point

Door lock: ✓
Lockable place: ✓

Services provided
Beauty services: Hairdressing
Mobile library: ✓
Religious services: Monthly Anglican Communion service
Transport: ✗
Activities: *Coordinator:* ✗ • *Examples:* Carpet bowls, games, quizzes
  Outings: ✗
Meetings: ✗

Leaze Court

Manager: Lorraine Langford
Owner: Sally Brazier and Steven Dyke
Contact: Hillside, South Brent,
Devon, TQ10 9AY
📞 01364 73267
@ info@thecourtgroup.co.uk
🖥 www.thecourtgroup.co.uk

Leaze Court is a modestly sized care home set in its own landscaped grounds in South Brent village. The home is currently undergoing a refurbishment programme. After this is finished, the home will be registered for 30 places and all rooms will have en suite facilities. A sun lounge is being built and a lift installed so that the home will have good wheelchair access throughout. The home has its own minibus and arranges an Anglican Communion service once a month.

Registered places: 21
Guide weekly rate: £350–£420
Specialist care: Dementia, physical disability, respite
Medical services: Podiatry, optician, physiotherapy
Qualified staff: Fails standard

Home details
Location: Rural area, 0.7 miles from South Brent
Communal areas: 2 lounges, dining room, garden
Accessibility: *Floors:* 2 • *Access:* Stair lift •
  Wheelchair access: Limited
Smoking: ✗
Pets: At manager's discretion
Routines: Flexible

Room details
Single: 15
Shared: 3
En suite: Undisclosed
Facilities: TV point, telephone point

Door lock: ✓
Lockable place: ✗

Services provided
Beauty services: Hairdressing
Mobile library: ✗
Religious services: Monthly Anglican Communion service
Transport: Minibus
Activities: *Coordinator:* ✗ • *Examples:* Arts and crafts,
  film afternoons, games • *Outings:* ✓
Meetings: ✓

Registered places: 25
Guide weekly rate: Undisclosed
Specialist care: Dementia, physical disability
Medical services: Podiatry, optician
Qualified staff: Exceeds standard: 75% at NVQ level 2

Home details

Location: Residential area, 1 mile from Newton Abbott
Communal areas: 2 lounges, dining room, conservatory, garden
Accessibility: *Floors:* 2 • *Access:* Stair lift • *Wheelchair access:* Good
Smoking: In designated area
Pets: At manager's discretion
Routines: Flexible

Room details

Single: 25
Shared: 0
En suite: 24
Facilities: TV

Door lock: ✓
Lockable place: ✓

Services provided

Beauty services: Hairdressing
Mobile library: ✓
Religious services: ✗
Transport: Car
Activities: *Coordinator:* ✓ • *Examples:* One-to-one sessions,
    visiting entertainers • *Outings:* ✓
Meetings: ✗

The Lindons

Manager: Theresa Pepperell
Owner: Newcare Ltd
Contact: 120 Ashburton Road,
Newton Abbot, Devon, TQ12 1RJ
) 01626 368070

Situated close to a bus stop for easy access to and from the home, The Lindons is located in a residential area, one mile from Newton Abbot. Currently home to two cats, other pets would be allowed at the manager's discretion. The home's gardens boast a pond and a greenhouse. There is also a conservatory for residents to enjoy. The home has an activities coordinator who arranges performances by visiting entertainers as well as one-to-one sessions. The home has its own car and takes the residents on outings in the local area.

Registered places: 35
Guide weekly rate: Undisclosed
Specialist care: Day care, dementia, mental disorder,
    physical disability, respite
Medical services: Podiatry, dentist, optician, physiotherapy
Qualified staff: Meets standard

Home details

Location: Residential area, 1 mile from Paignton
Communal areas: 3 lounges, dining room, conservatory,
    patio and garden
Accessibility: *Floors:* 2 • *Access:* Lift and stair lift
    Wheelchair access: Good
Smoking: ✓
Pets: ✗
Routines: Undisclosed

Room details

Single: 25
Shared: 5
En suite: Undisclosed
Facilities: TV, telephone

Door lock: ✗
Lockable place: ✗

Services provided

Beauty services: Hairdressing, manicures
Mobile library: ✓
Religious services: ✓
Transport: ✓
Activities: *Coordinator:* ✓ • *Examples:* Bingo • *Outings:* ✓
Meetings: Undisclosed

Little Oldway

Manager: Vacant
Owner: Barry and Jacqueline Privett
Contact: Oldway Road,
Paignton, Devon, TQ3 2TD
) 01803 527156

Little Oldway is a large, listed building adjacent to the stately home Oldway Mansion and its grounds. The home is surrounded by a large, level, attractive garden. The home provides accommodation for 35 residents and there is ample space in the home. A larger lounge is used for activities, while a smaller lounge and conservatory provide pleasant quiet spaces. There is also a dining room. The home is one mile from the centre of Paignton. The home has its own activities coordinator and arranges outings for the residents.

The Lodge Residential Care Home

Manager: Vacant
Owner: Glen and Sally Child
Contact: 12 Longlands,
Dawlish, Devon, EX7 9NF
) 01626 866724

A large detached property set in an elevated position above Dawlish, The Lodge permits views of the surrounding countryside and sea. With large double glazed windows, residents may sit in the conservatory and enjoy the views whatever the weather. There is also a piano. Close to local amenities, more active residents may enjoy the short walk up to the seafront and the range of shops in the town centre.

Registered places: 11
Guide weekly rate: Undisclosed
Specialist care: Day care, respite
Medical services: Podiatry, dentist, optician
Qualified staff: Undisclosed

Home details
Location: Residential area, 0.4 miles from Dawlish
Communal areas: Lounge, dining room, library, conservatory, garden
Accessibility: *Floors:* 2 • *Access:* Stair lift • *Wheelchair access:* Good
Smoking: ✗
Pets: ✗
Routines: Flexible

Room details
Single: 7
Shared: 2
En suite: 9
Facilities: TV point, telephone point

Door lock: ✓
Lockable place: ✓

Services provided
Beauty services: Hairdressing
Mobile library: Library facilities
Religious services: ✗
Transport: ✗
Activities: *Coordinator:* ✗ • *Examples:* Accompanied walks, bingo
Outings: ✓
Meetings: ✗

Lorna House

Manager: Linda Vans-Colina
Owner: Crocus Care Ltd
Contact: Devons Road,
Torquay, Devon, TQ1 3PR
) 01803 329908
@ clare@crocuscare.co.uk

Lorna House is located in a village one and a half miles from Torquay town centre. With a comprehensive activities programme which includes monthly visits from a harpist, relatives are also kept informed of events in the home with a newsletter which is produced twice a month. The home has a shop and a gazebo is erected in the garden on warm days.

Registered places: 24
Guide weekly rate: £320–£350
Specialist care: Day care, dementia, physical disability
Medical services: Podiatry
Qualified staff: Fails standard

Home details
Location: Village location, 1.4 miles from Torquay
Communal areas: Lounge, dining room, conservatory, garden
Accessibility: *Floors:* 2 • *Access:* Stair lift
Wheelchair access: Limited
Smoking: ✗
Pets: ✗
Routines: Flexible

Room details
Single: 20
Shared: 2
En suite: 11
Facilities: None

Door lock: ✓
Lockable place: ✓

Services provided
Beauty services: Hairdressing
Mobile library: ✗
Religious services: ✗
Transport: ✗
Activities: *Coordinator:* ✗ • *Examples:* Arts and crafts, discussions,
exercise sessions • *Outings:* ✓
Meetings: ✗

Registered places: 25
Guide weekly rate: From £475
Specialist care: Day care, physical disability, respite
Medical services: Podiatry, dentist, optician
Qualified staff: Exceeds standard: 78% at NVQ level 2

Home details

Location: Village location, 2.5 miles from Exmouth
Communal areas: 2 lounges, dining room, conservatory, garden
Accessibility: *Floors:* 2 • *Access:* Lift • *Wheelchair access:* Good
Smoking: ✗
Pets: At manager's discretion
Routines: Flexible

Room details

Single: 19
Shared: 3
En suite: 22
Facilities: TV point, telephone point

Door lock: ✓
Lockable place: ✗

Services provided

Beauty services: Hairdressing
Mobile library: ✓
Religious services: Monthly Communion service
Transport: Car
Activities: *Coordinator:* ✗ • *Examples:* Films, quizzes • *Outings:* ✓
Meetings: ✗

Lympstone House

Manager: Elizabeth and Leonard Sylvester
Owner: Elizabeth and Leonard Sylvester
Contact: Strawberry Hill, Lympstone, Exmouth, Devon, EX8 5JZ
☎ 01395 270004
@ lympstonehouse@hotmail.com

A detached period property with two purpose-built wings, Lympstone House is set in large gardens with tropical mature palm trees and a fruit orchard. There are also various courtyards. The home is 15 minutes' walk from the nearest shop. Although the home does not offer nursing, five of the staff are qualified nurses. Pets are allowed at the manager's discretion and the home has chickens and dogs.

Registered places: 14
Guide weekly rate: £400
Specialist care: Physical disability
Medical services: Podiatry, dentist, optician
Qualified staff: Exceeds standard: 75% at NVQ level 2

Home details

Location: Residential area, 0.5 miles from Okehampton
Communal areas: Lounge, dining room
Accessibility: *Floors:* 2 • *Access:* Lift • *Wheelchair access:* Good
Smoking: ✗
Pets: ✓
Routines: Flexible

Room details

Single: 8
Shared: 3
En suite: Undisclosed
Facilities: None

Door lock: ✓
Lockable place: ✓

Services provided

Beauty services: Hairdressing
Mobile library: ✗
Religious services: ✗
Transport: Minibus
Activities: *Coordinator:* ✗ • *Examples:* Exercise, games
    Outings: ✓
Meetings: ✓

Lyndridge

Manager: Carol Barkwell
Owner: Lyndridge Community Care Services
Contact: Ranelagh Road, Okehampton, Devon, EX20 1JG
☎ 01837 54782

Lyndridge is located in a residential area, half a mile from Okehampton. The standard of equipment to assist immobile residents is good. The home offers a variety of activities for residents with weekly outings in the minibus owned by the home, musical entertainment and exercise events. There is a residents meeting once a month.

Maddalane

Manager: Sheila Vosper
Owner: Michael Charles and
Sheila Vosper
Contact: 158 Victoria Road, St Budeaux,
Plymouth, Devon, PL5 1QY
☏ 01752 360253

Located in a residential area, Maddalane is close to local amenities, including shops and a park. The home has a bird and a dog and there are fish living in the garden pond. Although there is a stair lift to assist less mobile residents, there are three steps that need to be ascended in order to reach the first floor. The home has its own car for transport and takes residents on regular outings. There is a residents meeting every six weeks.

Registered places: 8
Guide weekly rate: £320–£360
Specialist care: Day care
Medical services: Podiatry, hygienist, optician, physiotherapy
Qualified staff: Undisclosed

Home details
Location: Residential area, 5 miles from Plymouth
Communal areas: Lounge, dining room, conservatory, garden
Accessibility: *Floors:* 2 • *Access:* Stair lift • *Wheelchair access:* Limited
Smoking: In designated area
Pets: At manager's discretion
Routines: Flexible

Room details
Single: 5
Shared: 2
En suite: 0
Facilities: TV point, telephone point

Door lock: ✓
Lockable place: ✓

Services provided
Beauty services: Hairdressing
Mobile library: ✗
Religious services: ✗
Transport: Car
Activities: *Coordinator:* ✗ • *Examples:* Bingo, crosswords, poetry readings • *Outings:* ✓
Meetings: ✓

Malden House

Manager: Julie Hawkins
Owner: Josephine Pope
Contact: 69 Sidford Road, Sidmouth,
Devon, EX10 9LR
☏ 01395 512264
@ malden@talktalkbusiness.net
🖰 www.home.clara.net/malden

Malden House is situated approximately two miles from Sidmouth seafront in its own grounds. The garden at the home contains a greenhouse and for the last two years has won prizes for 'Sidmouth in Bloom'. The home arranges an Anglican Communion service once a month and residents have access to the home's own library facilities. There is also a conservatory and a garden for residents to relax in.

Registered places: 19
Guide weekly rate: £485–£675
Specialist care: Respite
Medical services: Podiatry
Qualified staff: Meets standard

Home details
Location: Residential area, 2 miles from Sidmouth
Communal areas: 2 lounges, dining room, library, conservatory, garden
Accessibility: *Floors:* 2 • *Access:* Lift • *Wheelchair access:* Good
Smoking: In designated area
Pets: At manager's discretion
Routines: Flexible

Room details
Single: 19
Shared: 0
En suite: 18
Facilities: TV point, telephone point

Door lock: ✓
Lockable place: ✓

Services provided
Beauty services: Hairdressing
Mobile library: Library facilities
Religious services: Monthly Anglican Communion service
Transport: ✗
Activities: *Coordinator:* ✓ • *Examples:* Armchair exercises, scrabble
Outings: ✗
Meetings: ✗

Registered places: 25
Guide weekly rate: £294–£950
Specialist care: Day care, physical disability, respite
Medical services: Podiatry, dentist, optician, physiotherapy
Qualified staff: Meets standard

Home details

Location: Village location, 5 miles from Exeter
Communal areas: 2 lounges, dining room, garden
Accessibility: *Floors:* 2 • *Access:* Stair lift • *Wheelchair access:* Good
Smoking: In designated area
Pets: At manager's discretion
Routines: Flexible

Room details

Single: 25
Shared: 0
En suite: 7
Facilities: None

Door lock: ✓
Lockable place: ✓

Services provided

Beauty services: Hairdressing, manicures, massage
Mobile library: ✗
Religious services: ✗
Transport: ✗
Activities: *Coordinator:* ✓ • *Examples:* Arts and crafts, discussions, musical entertainment • *Outings:* ✓
Meetings: ✓

The Manor

Manager: Heather Whitehead
Owner: The Manor Exmins
Contact: Main Road, Exminster, Exeter, Devon, EX6 8AP
☎ 01392 824063
@ enquiries@themanorexminster.co.uk

A Georgian-style home with an attractive front that includes a fountain and benches, The Manor overlooks fields and had attractive views out to the estuary. The Mamor is set in half an acre of land, in the village of Exminster, five miles from Exeter. With outings taking place twice weekly, the home also has a comprehensive in-house activities programme. This programme includes crafts and musical entertainment.

Registered places: 18
Guide weekly rate: From £360
Specialist care: Day, respite
Medical services: Podiatry, dentist, optician
Qualified staff: Exceeds standard: 100% at NVQ level 2

Home details

Location: Residential area, 0.6 miles from Paignton
Communal areas: 2 lounges, dining room, patio and garden
Accessibility: *Floors:* 2 • *Access:* Stair lift • *Wheelchair access:* Limited
Smoking: In designated area
Pets: At manager's discretion
Routines: Flexible

Room details

Single: 17
Shared: 1
En suite: 18
Facilities: TV, telephone point

Door lock: ✓
Lockable place: ✓

Services provided

Beauty services: Hairdressing, aromatherapy, manicures
Mobile library: ✗
Religious services: Monthly Anglican service
Transport: Minibus
Activities: *Coordinator:* ✓ • *Examples:* Arts and crafts, cooking, music
Outings: ✓
Meetings: ✓

Manor Cottage Hotel

Manager: Hazel Weaver
Owner: Kenneth Peek
Contact: 1–3 Manor Crescent, Preston, Paignton, Devon, TQ3 2TN
☎ 01803 55036

Manor Cottage is situated in a residential area, just over half a mile from Paignton town centre. With a comprehensive activities programme that includes visits from Pets As Therapy, an activities coordinator organises daily activities and outings in the home's minibus. Though there is a stair lift to assist individuals on the upper floor, residents must still be able to manage a few steps. There is a residents meeting every six weeks to discuss any issues the residents may have.

The Manor

Manager: Jean Jones
Owner: Wells House Ltd
Contact: Fore Street, Yealmpton,
Nr Plymouth, Devon, PL8 2JN
☎ 01752 880510

An attractive 18th-century listed building, The Manor is located in the quiet village of Yealmpton five minutes' walk from the shops and a few minutes from a bus stop where services run to Plymouth and Kingsbridge. The home is located seven miles from the centre of Plymouth. With a conservatory that is often used as a quiet room, more active residents may enjoy the few outings the home runs each year in conjunction with the Manor's sister home, The Lawns. Although wheelchair access is generally good in the home, resident's using the second floor must be able to walk.

Registered places: 22
Guide weekly rate: £325–£530
Specialist care: Nursing, day care, dementia, emergency admissions, physical disability, respite
Medical services: Podiatry, dentist, optician
Qualified staff: Meets standard

Home details
Location: Village location, 7 miles from Plymouth
Communal areas: Lounge, dining room, conservatory, patio and garden
Accessibility: *Floors:* 3 • *Access:* Lift and stair lift *Wheelchair access:* Good
Smoking: ✗
Pets: At manager's discretion
Routines: Flexible

Room details
Single: 16
Shared: 3
En suite: 5
Facilities: TV point, telephone point

Door lock: ✓
Lockable place: ✓

Services provided
Beauty services: Hairdressing, manicures, facials
Mobile library: ✓
Religious services: Twice-weekly Anglican Communion service
Transport: ✗
Activities: *Coordinator:* ✗ • *Examples:* Exercise, music slide shows *Outings:* ✓
Meetings: ✗

The Manor House

Manager: Kathryn Daw
Owner: Welling Ltd
Contact: 135 Looseleigh Lane, Derriford, Plymouth, Devon, PL6 5JE
☎ 01752 778280

As its name suggests, The Manor House is a detached older property set in its own grounds, a quarter of a mile from the nearest bus stop. The home is located in a rural area, four miles from Plymouth. The home has a comprehensive activities programme that includes three or four outings a year. There are also internal activities such as quizzes and reminiscence sessions. There is a residents meeting every two months and a mobile library comes to the home on a regular basis.

Registered places: 30
Guide weekly rate: £350–£400
Specialist care: Respite
Medical services: Podiatry, dentist, optician
Qualified staff: Exceeds standard: 70% at NVQ level 2

Home details
Location: Rural area, 4 miles from Plymouth
Communal areas: 2 lounges, dining room, garden
Accessibility: *Floors:* 2 • *Access:* Lift • *Wheelchair access:* Good
Smoking: In designated area
Pets: At manager's discretion
Routines: Flexible

Room details
Single: 28
Shared: 1
En suite: 17
Facilities: TV point, telephone point

Door lock: ✓
Lockable place: ✓

Services provided
Beauty services: Hairdressing, aromatherapy, massage
Mobile library: ✓
Religious services: ✗
Transport: ✗
Activities: *Coordinator:* ✓ • *Examples:* Games, quizzes, reminiscence • *Outings:* ✓
Meetings: ✓

Registered places: 15
Guide weekly rate: £380–£400
Specialist care: Physical disability, respite
Medical services: Podiatry, dentist, optician
Qualified staff: Exceeds standard: 62% at NVQ level 2

Home details

Location: Residential area, 0.2 miles from Seaton
Communal areas: 2 lounges, dining room, conservatory, garden
Accessibility: *Floors:* 2 • *Access:* Stair lift • *Wheelchair access:* Limited
Smoking: ✗
Pets: ✓
Routines: Flexible

Room details

Single: 15
Shared: 0
En suite: 9
Facilities: TV point, telephone point

Door lock: ✓
Lockable place: ✓

Services provided

Beauty services: Hairdressing
Mobile library: ✓
Religious services: Monthly Communion service
Transport: Car
Activities: *Coordinator:* ✗ • *Examples:* Arts and crafts, musical entertainment • *Outings:* ✓
Meetings: ✗

The Manor House

Manager: Seldon Curry
Owner: Seldon and Susan Curry
Contact: Fore Street, Seaton, Devon, EX12 2AD
☎ 01297 22433
@ hutchc@strngarm.demon.co.uk
🖱 www.manor-house.freeuk.com

A converted Grade II listed building, The Manor House is located near the centre of Seaton, less than five minutes' walk from the shops and the seafront. The owners live on site and oversee the running of the home. The Manor House is pet-friendly and is currently home to a dog and a cat. The home has its own car for transport and takes the residents on regular outings.

Registered places: 23
Guide weekly rate: From £450
Specialist care: Day care, respite
Medical services: Podiatry, dentist, optician, physiotherapy
Qualified staff: Exceeds standard: 63% at NVQ level 2

Home details

Location: Residential area, 0.5 miles from Exmouth
Communal areas: Lounge, dining room, conservatory, patio and garden
Accessibility: *Floors:* 2 • *Access:* Lift and stair lift
Wheelchair access: Good
Smoking: ✗
Pets: Undisclosed
Routines: Flexible

Room details

Single: Undisclosed
Shared: Undisclosed
En suite: 23
Facilities: TV point, telephone point

Door lock: ✗
Lockable place: ✓

Services provided

Beauty services: Hairdressing
Mobile library: ✗
Religious services: Monthly Communion service
Transport: ✗
Activities: *Coordinator:* ✗ • *Examples:* Exercise, fashion shows, games
Outings: ✓
Meetings: ✓

Manor Lodge

Manager: Eileen O'Neill
Owner: Manor Lodge Ltd
Contact: 8 Portland Avenue, Exmouth, Devon, EX8 2BS
☎ 01395 266691
@ mail@manorlodgedevon.co.uk
🖱 www.manorlodgedevon.co.uk

A detached house in a quiet residential area known locally as the 'Avenues', Manor Lodge is an adapted Edwardian property that is situated in half an acre of land approximately half a mile from Exmouth town centre. Many of the rooms have pleasant sea views or patio doors onto the south facing garden. Facilities are available for residents to make their own drinks and snacks while a monthly newsletter also includes activities that have been arranged. The residents have a gardening club and part of the garden is dedicated as a 'garden of remembrance' to friends and loved ones.

Mardon House

Manager: Brenda Forte
Owner: Angelo Forte
Contact: 10 Higher Brimley,
Teignmouth, Devon, TQ14 8JS
☏ 01626 772911
@ basforte@aol.com

Mardon House is located in a residential street around half a mile from Teignmouth town centre. There is a sun terrace and level garden to the rear of the home, both accessed via some steps. An activities organiser visits the home once a week to provide in-house games and stimulation for residents. Events organised in the home include quizzes, a clothes show, singalongs and external entertainment.

Registered places: 15
Guide weekly rate: £281–£372
Specialist care: Respite
Medical services: Podiatry, physiotherapy
Qualified staff: Meets standard

Home details
Location: Residential area, 0.2 miles from Teignmouth
Communal areas: Patio and garden
Accessibility: *Floors:* Undisclosed • *Access:* Undisclosed
    Wheelchair access: Limited
Smoking: ✗
Pets: ✓
Routines: Flexible

Room details
Single: 13
Shared: 2
En suite: 5
Facilities: TV point

Door lock: ✓
Lockable place: ✓

Services provided
Beauty services: Hairdressing
Mobile library: ✗
Religious services: ✗
Transport: ✗
Activities: *Coordinator:* ✓ • *Examples:* Clothes show, singalongs
    Outings: ✓
Meetings: ✗

Mayfield Hall

Manager: Elaine Sampson
Owner: Amethyst Care Ltd
Contact: 22 Bitton Park Road,
Teignmouth, Devon, TQ14 9BX
☏ 01626 772796
@ mayfieldcare@btconnect.com

Located just off a main road in Teignmouth, Mayfield Hall enjoys a good location a few hundred yards from the town's local facilities and the station. Some of the bedrooms enjoy views of the Teign Estuary. The home has a garden with a patio area for residents to enjoy in the summer and there is a range of activities on offer, including flower arranging and musical entertainment.

Registered places: 20
Guide weekly rate: £315–£415
Specialist care: Dementia, respite
Medical services: Podiatry, optician, physiotherapy
Qualified staff: Fails standards

Home details
Location: Residential area, 0.3 miles from Teignmouth
Communal areas: Lounge, dining room, patio and garden
Accessibility: *Floors:* 2 • *Access:* Lift • *Wheelchair access:* Good
Smoking: ✗
Pets: At manager's discretion
Routines: Flexible

Room details
Single: 18
Shared: 1
En suite: 18
Facilities: TV point, telephone point

Door lock: ✗
Lockable place: ✓

Services provided
Beauty services: Hairdressing
Mobile library: ✗
Religious services: ✗
Transport: ✗
Activities: *Coordinator:* ✗ • *Examples:* Flower arranging, games,
    musical entertainment • *Outings:* ✗
Meetings: ✗

Registered places: 40
Guide weekly rate: £650
Specialist care: Nursing, physical disability
Medical services: Podiatry, dentist, optician, physiotherapy
Qualified staff: Undisclosed

Home details
Location: Residential area, 7 miles from Plymouth
Communal areas: 2 lounges, dining room, conservatory, garden
Accessibility: *Floors:* 3 • *Access:* Lift • *Wheelchair access:* Good
Smoking: ✗
Pets: ✗
Routines: Flexible

Room details
Single: 40
Shared: 0
En suite: 30
Facilities: TV point, telephone point

Door lock: ✗
Lockable place: ✗

Services provided
Beauty services: Hairdressing
Mobile library: ✗
Religious services: ✓
Transport: ✗
Activities: *Coordinator:* ✓ • *Examples:* Armchair exercises, bingo,
   musical entertainment • *Outings:* ✓
Meetings: ✓

Merafield View Nursing Home

Manager: Sally Philipson
Owner: Stagecare Ltd
Contact: Underlane, Plympton,
Plymouth, Devon, PL7 1ZB
) 01752 348070
@ merafield@bmlhealthcare.co.uk
🖱 www.merafieldview-nh.co.uk

A purpose-built home, Merafield View is located near local shops and facilities, seven miles from Plymouth. The home has two lounges, a dining room and a garden with a conservatory. There is a communal lockable place available for valuables. The home has its own activities coordinator and the home tries to arrange outings every six weeks. Daily activities include bingo and visiting entertainers and the residents are taken on outings to the local garden centre. Pets are allowed to visit. Smoking is not permitted inside. There are residents meetings every quarter.

Registered places: 24
Guide weekly rate: £333–£380
Specialist care: Dementia, physical disability
Medical services: Podiatry, optician
Qualified staff: Exceeds standard: 80% at NVQ level 2

Home details
Location: Residential area, 1 mile from Plympton
Communal areas: 2 lounges, dining room, conservatory, garden
Accessibility: *Floors:* 3 • *Access:* Lift • *Wheelchair access:* Good
Smoking: In designated area
Pets: ✗
Routines: Flexible

Room details
Single: 24
Shared: 0
En suite: 24
Facilities: TV, telephone

Door lock: ✓
Lockable place: ✓

Services provided
Beauty services: Hairdressing, aromatherapy
Mobile library: Library facilities
Religious services: ✓
Transport: ✗
Activities: *Coordinator:* ✓ • *Examples:* Games, music, quizzes
   Outings: ✓
Meetings: ✓

Michaelstowe Residential Home

Manager: Maria Golden
Owner: South West Residential
Homes Ltd
Contact: 211 Ridgeway, Plympton,
Plymouth, Devon, PL7 2HP
) 01752 339096
@ Maria.michaelstowe@
   southwestcarehome.co.uk

Located on a main road in a residential area, Michaelstowe resides close to The Ridgeway Shopping Centre. There is a bus service to the local shops. The home has an activities coordinator who arranges musical entertainment and quizzes as well as one-to-one sessions. There are also outings to the local moors, for cream teas and for fish and chips. There is a hairdressing service once a week and aromatherapy once a month. There are books in the home which are changed regularly and religious services once a month. Pets are allowed to visit.

Moors Park House

Manager: Nicole Haywood-Lloyd
Owner: Moors Park Ltd
Contact: Moors Park, Bishopsteignton, Teignmouth, Devon, TQ14 9RH
☎ 01626 775465
@ nhl@moorspark.co.uk

Set in its own grounds with views across the estuary, Moors Park is a detached property that has been run as a care home for more than two decades. With a comprehensive activities programme, the home produces a monthly newsletter detailing the activities on offer for residents. Home to three cats and a dog, there are currently plans to add a further 10 rooms to the home and to extend both the lounge and dining room.

Registered places: 37
Guide weekly rate: £372–£470
Specialist care: Day care, dementia, mental disorder, physical disability, respite
Medical services: Podiatry, hygienist, optician, physiotherapy
Qualified staff: Meets standard

Home details
Location: Village location, 2.5 miles from Teignmouth
Communal areas: 2 lounges, dining room, conservatory, garden
Accessibility: *Floors:* 2 • *Access:* Lift • *Wheelchair access:* Good
Smoking: In designated area
Pets: ✓
Routines: Flexible

Room details
Single: 33
Shared: 2
En suite: 33
Facilities: TV point, telephone point

Door lock: ✓
Lockable place: ✓

Services provided
Beauty services: Hairdressing, aromatherapy
Mobile library: ✓
Religious services: Monthly Anglican Communion service
Transport: Car
Activities: *Coordinator:* ✓ • *Examples:* Animal lectures, dances, music afternoons • *Outings:* ✗
Meetings: ✗

Mount Olivet Nursing Home

Manager: Alison Homer
Owner: Grayareas Ltd
Contact: 2 Great Headland Road, Preston, Paignton, Devon, TQ3 2DY
☎ 01803 522148
@ mountolivet@grayareas.co.uk
🖰 www.mountolivet.co.uk

Situated in the Preston area of Paignton with panoramic views of Torbay, Mount Olivet is an Edwardian mansion that is five minutes from Preston's shops and 10 minutes from the seafront. The home produces a quarterly newsletter and regularly takes in student nurses from the University of Plymouth as part of their work experience. The home promotes social interaction amongst residents and for those to whom this does not come naturally and who do not receive regular visitors, a professional 'tea-time visitor' is arranged.

Registered places: 30
Guide weekly rate: £385–£550
Specialist care: Nursing, emergency admissions, palliative, physical disability, respite
Medical services: Podiatry, dentist, optician, occupational therapy
Qualified staff: Undisclosed

Home details
Location: Residential area, in Torbay
Communal areas: Lounge/dining room, library, garden
Accessibility: *Floors:* 3 • *Access:* Lift • *Wheelchair access:* Good
Smoking: ✗
Pets: ✗
Routines: Flexible

Room details
Single: 20
Shared: 5
En suite: 12
Facilities: TV, telephone point

Door lock: ✗
Lockable place: ✗

Services provided
Beauty services: Hairdressing, aromatherapy
Mobile library: Library facilities
Religious services: ✗
Transport: ✗
Activities: *Coordinator:* ✓ • *Examples:* Arts and crafts, reminiscence *Outings:* ✓
Meetings: ✓

Registered places: 14
Guide weekly rate: £400
Specialist care: Day care, dementia, mental disorder, physical disability
Medical services: Podiatry, hygienist, optician, physiotherapy
Qualified staff: Exceeds standard: 80% at NVQ level 2

Home details

Location: Residential area, 1 mile from Newton Abbot
Communal areas: Lounge, dining room, garden
Accessibility: *Floors:* 3 • *Access:* Stair lift • *Wheelchair access:* Good
Smoking: ✗
Pets: ✓
Routines: Structured

Room details

Single: 10
Shared: 2   Door lock: ✓
En suite: 4   Lockable place: ✓
Facilities: TV point, telephone point

Services provided

Beauty services: Hairdressing, aromatherapy, massage
Mobile library: ✗
Religious services: Monthly Communion service
Transport: ✗
Activities: *Coordinator:* ✗ • *Examples:* Arts and crafts,
   music and movement, reminiscence • *Outings:* ✓
Meetings: ✗

Mount Pleasant

Manager: Alan Peters
Owner: Alan and Frances Peters
Contact: 26 Mount Pleasant Road,
Newton Abbot, Devon, TQ12 1AS
☎ 01626 353351

A semi-detached property located in a residential area of Newton Abbot, Mount Pleasant sits in an elevated position on the top of a hill. Permitting spectacular views of the surrounding countryside the home also has a flat, secure garden which residents can enjoy. The home arranges a monthly Communion service and there is a varied activities programme on offer, including music and movement and reminiscence sessions.

Registered places: 60
Guide weekly rate: From £454–£1,000
Specialist care: Nursing, day care, emergency admissions,
   physical disability, respite
Medical services: Podiatry, dentist, optician
Qualified staff: Undisclosed

Home details

Location: Residential area, 1.5 miles from Torquay
Communal areas: 2 lounges, dining room, activities room,
   bar, garden
Accessibility: *Floors:* 2 • *Access:* Lift • *Wheelchair access:* Good
Smoking: In designated area
Pets: At manager's discretion
Routines: Flexible

Room details

Single: 60
Shared: 0   Door lock: ✗
En suite: 60   Lockable place: ✓
Facilities: TV, telephone point

Services provided

Beauty services: Hairdressing, manicures, massage
Mobile library: ✓
Religious services: Monthly Anglican church service
Transport: Minibus
Activities: *Coordinator:* ✓ • *Examples:* Arts and crafts, garden club,
   musical entertainment • *Outings:* ✓
Meetings: ✓

Mount Tryon

Manager: Carol Robins
Owner: Barchester Healthcare Ltd
Contact: Higher Warberry Road,
Toquay, Devon, TQ1 1RR
☎ 01803 292 077
@ Mounttryon@barchester.net
🖱 www.barchester.com

Situated on a hill in a quiet residential area of Torquay named 'The Warberries', Mount Tryon is a Hospitality Assured purpose-built home half a mile from the nearest bus stop and not ideally located for local amenities. The home holds weekly Friday meetings for residents to discuss matters within the home. Set in landscaped gardens, the home permits good views over Torquay and its bay – something that is drawn upon by the positioning of the lounge on the first floor, which has its own balcony.

Netherhayes Residential Home

Manager: Shirley Fitter
Owner: Adelaide Lodge Care Home LLP
Contact: Fore Street, Seaton, Devon, EX12 2LE
) 01297 21646
⌐ www.adelaidelodge.co.uk

With an interesting history that has seen the home converted from a doctor's surgery to a hotel, Netherhayes is situated 10 minutes' walk from the seafront. The home is also positioned on the main shopping street in Seaton and sits alongside a wide array of local amenities including shops, a post office and the town hall. With views of the surrounding countryside, the home takes advantage of this and encourages those with a horticultural interest to use the home's gardens. Netherhayes also holds a yearly garden party in conjunction with Age Concern.

Registered places: 28
Guide weekly rate: £450–£500
Specialist care: Dementia, day care, physical disability, respite
Medical services: Podiatry, dentist, optician
Qualified staff: Undisclosed

Home details
Location: Residential area, in Seaton
Communal areas: 2 lounges, 2 dining rooms, garden
Accessibility: *Floors:* 3 • *Access:* Stair lift • *Wheelchair access:* Limited
Smoking: In designated area
Pets: At manager's discretion
Routines: Flexible

Room details
Single: 26
Shared: 1
En suite: 16
Facilities: TV point, telephone point

Door lock: ✗
Lockable place: ✗

Services provided
Beauty services: Hairdressing
Mobile library: ✗
Religious services: Monthly Communion service
Transport: ✗
Activities: *Coordinator:* ✓ • *Examples:* Arts and crafts, exercise *Outings:* ✓
Meetings: ✓

Norfolk Villa

Manager: Robert Teasdale
Owner: Robert Teasdale
Contact: 45 Alma Road, Pennycomequick, Plymouth, Devon, PL3 4HE
) 01752 661979

Norfolk Villa is a large detached building that is over 150 years old. It is located in the Pennycomequick area of Plymouth. Local amenities and a bus route are within walking distance from the home. There are two dining areas in the home – one found in the old part of the home, the other making up part of the lounge. The home also has garden which the residents can enjoy in the summer months.

Registered places: 19
Guide weekly rate: £273–£320
Specialist care: Respite
Medical services: Podiatry, dentist,
Qualified staff: Exceeds standard: 75% at NVQ level 2

Home details
Location: Urban area, 1.2 miles from Plymouth
Communal areas: Lounge, 2 dining rooms, gardens
Accessibility: *Floors:* 2 • *Access:* Lift • *Wheelchair access:* Limited
Smoking: ✗
Pets: At manager's discretion
Routines: Flexible

Room details
Single: 19
Shared: 0
En suite: 11
Facilities: None

Door lock: ✓
Lockable place: ✗

Services provided
Beauty services: Hairdressing
Mobile library: ✗
Religious services: ✗
Transport: ✗
Activities: *Coordinator:* ✗ • *Examples:* Newspapers • *Outings:* ✓
Meetings: ✗

Registered places: 18
Guide weekly rate: £425–£525
Specialist care: Respite
Medical services: Podiatry, dentist, optician
Qualified staff: Exceeds standard: 100% at NVQ level 2

Home details
Location: Residential area, 1 mile from Dartmouth
Communal areas: Lounge, garden, dining room
Accessibility: *Floors:* 3 • *Access:* Lift and stair lift
  Wheelchair access: Good
Smoking: ✗
Pets: ✓
Routines: Flexible

Room details
Single: 18
Shared: 0
En suite: 14
Facilities: TV

Door lock: ✓
Lockable place: ✓

Services provided
Beauty services: Hairdressing
Mobile library: ✗
Religious services: ✗
Transport: ✗
Activities: *Coordinator:* ✗ • *Examples:* Relaxation therapy, reminiscence
  Outings: ✓
Meetings: ✗

Northernhay

Manager: Jane Garland
Owner: Jane Garland
Contact: Townstal, Pathfields,
Dartmouth, Devon, TQ6 9HL
☏ 01803 833964

Northernhay is a converted and extended house, set in a quiet residential area, just over a mile from the town of Dartmouth. Residents here enjoy a peaceful, pleasant yet varied life, with strong family and local community links. Various activities are made available on a regular basis, including relaxation therapy and reminiscence sessions.

Registered places: 16
Guide weekly rate: £320–£426
Specialist care: Dementia, respite
Medical services: Podiatry
Qualified staff: Fails standard: 25% at NVQ level 2

Home details
Location: Residential area, 0.4 miles from Paignton
Communal areas: 3 lounges, dining room, conservatory, garden
Accessibility: *Floors:* 3 • *Access:* Stair lift • *Wheelchair access:* Limited
Smoking: ✗
Pets: ✓
Routines: Flexible

Room details
Single: 14
Shared: 2
En suite: 16
Facilities: None

Door lock: ✓
Lockable place: ✓

Services provided
Beauty services: Hairdressing, manicures
Mobile library: ✗
Religious services: ✗
Transport: ✗
Activities: *Coordinator:* ✗ • *Examples:* Bingo, quizzes • *Outings:* ✗
Meetings: ✗

Oakhurst

Manager: Sara Watson
Owner: Saffron Care Ltd
Contact: 4 Courtland Road,
Paignton, Devon, TQ3 2AB
☏ 01803 524414

Oakhurst is a large detached property close to shops, a library and a park. Details of forthcoming social events are displayed in the hallway. The home gives residents a pleasant environment to live in and the three lounges allow residents to socialise and relax. There is also a garden with a conservatory. All bedrooms have en suite facilities.

Ogwell Grange Residential Care Home

Manager: Sylvia Kay
Owner: Ogwell Grange Ltd
Contact: Rectory Road, East Ogwell, Newton Abbot, Devon, TQ12 6AH
) 01626 354576
@ emailsuttonr@btconnect.com

A 19th-century Grade II listed building, Ogwell Grange is a former rectory. In a prime location 10 minutes' walk from Ogwell village where there is a church, shop and pub, the home also permits views and looks out towards the Dartmoor National Park and countryside. Set in two and a half acres of landscaped gardens, the home offers a peaceful refuge to residents whilst maintaining excellent transport links. With a regular bus service stopping by the main entrance to the home, residents are also serviced by the home's vehicle which is used on the home's monthly outings.

Registered places: 20
Guide weekly rate: Undisclosed
Specialist care: Dementia, day care, respite
Medical services: Podiatry, dentist, optician, physiotherapy
Qualified staff: Undisclosed

Home details
Location: Village location, 2 miles from Newton Abbot
Communal areas: Lounge, dining room, garden
Accessibility: *Floors:* 3 • *Access:* Lift and stair lift
    Wheelchair access: Good
Smoking: In designated area
Pets: At manager's discretion
Routines: Flexible

Room details
Single: 14
Shared: 3
En suite: 17
Facilities: TV point, telephone point

Door lock: ✓
Lockable place: ✓

Services provided
Beauty services: Hairdressing
Mobile library: ✗
Religious services: Fortnightly Christian service
Transport: Car
Activities: *Coordinator:* ✗ • *Examples:* Arts and crafts, exercise, *Outings:* ✓
Meetings: ✓

The Old Vicarage

Manager: Susan Tisdall
Owner: Michael and Patricia Parkin
Contact: Ropers Lane, Otterton, Budleigh Salterton, Devon, EX9 7JF
) 01395 568208

A converted period property of Georgian origins, The Old Vicarage permits attractive views of the surrounding countryside and is situated close to village amenities, including a church, village hall and post office. The home is located three miles from Budleigh Salterton. The home has a landscaped garden with wheelchair access. The home produces a monthly newsletter which includes news and dates for the diary. The home has its own library facilities as well as two lounges for residents to relax in.

Registered places: 26
Guide weekly rate: £650–£769
Specialist care: Physical disability, respite
Medical services: Podiatry
Qualified staff: Fails standard

Home details
Location: Village location, 3 miles from Budleigh Salterton
Communal areas: 2 lounges, 2 dining rooms, library, garden
Accessibility: *Floors:* 2 • *Access:* Lift • *Wheelchair access:* Good
Smoking: ✗
Pets: At manager's discretion
Routines: Flexible

Room details
Single: 26
Shared: 0
En suite: 26
Facilities: TV point, telephone point

Door lock: ✓
Lockable place: ✓

Services provided
Beauty services: Hairdressing
Mobile library: Library facilities
Religious services: Monthly Communion service
Transport: Car
Activities: *Coordinator:* ✗ • *Examples:* Action sport sessions *Outings:* ✓
Meetings: ✓

Registered places: 31
Guide weekly rate: £400–£700
Specialist care: Day care, mental disorder
Medical services: Podiatry, dentist, optician, physiotherapy
Qualified staff: Fails standard

Home details

Location: Residential area, 1 mile from Paignton
Communal areas: Lounge, dining room
Accessibility: *Floors:* 2 • *Access:* Lift • *Wheelchair access:* Limited
Smoking: ✓
Pets: ✗
Routines: Flexible

Room details

Single: 28
Shared: 3
En suite: Undisclosed
Facilities: None

Door lock: ✓
Lockable place: ✓

Services provided

Beauty services: Hairdressing, relaxation therapy
Mobile library: ✗
Religious services: ✗
Transport: Minibus
Activities: *Coordinator:* ✗ • *Examples:* Music, painting, summer fête
   Outings: ✓
Meetings: ✗

Oldway Heights

Manager: Barry Privett
Owner: Barry and Jacqueline Privett
Contact: 40 Headland Park Road,
Paignton, Devon, TQ3 2EL
☎ 01803 527088

Situated in Paignton close to local facilities Oldway Heights is approximately one mile from the town centre. The home predominantly cares for young adults with physical disabilities or mental disorders. Although the home makes use of a lift, four bedrooms are accessed by stairs and therefore available only to those mobile residents. The home has its own minibus and often takes the residents on outings in the local area.

Registered places: 36
Guide weekly rate: £460–£595
Specialist care: Nursing, dementia, learning disability,
   mental disorder, physical disability
Medical services: Podiatry, dentist, optician, physiotherapy,
   speech therapy
Qualified staff: Meets standard

Home details

Location: Residential area, 0.3 miles from Dawlish
Communal areas: Lounge, dining room
Accessibility: *Floors:* 3 • *Access:* Lift • *Wheelchair access:* Good
Smoking: Undisclosed
Pets: Undisclosed
Routines: Flexible

Room details

Single: 36
Shared: 0
En suite: 1
Facilities: None

Door lock: ✗
Lockable place: ✗

Services provided

Beauty services: Hairdressing
Mobile library: ✗
Religious services: ✗
Transport: ✗
Activities: *Coordinator:* ✓ • *Examples:* Bingo, exercise classes, films
   Outings: ✓
Meetings: Undisclosed

Palm Court Nursing Home

Manager: Nigel Morris
Owner: Lorraine and Graham Greenaway
Contact: 7 Marine Parade,
Dawlish, Devon, EX7 9DJ
☎ 01626 866142
@ palm.court@btinternet.com

Just 100 yards from the town's train station and park, Palm Court Nursing Home is a purpose-built property located on the seafront. There is a large dining room on the ground floor, and a lounge which permits sea views. An activities coordinator works three days a week and organises a variety of activities. The home also celebrates special occasions, such as residents' birthdays.

Park House, Little Knowle

Manager: Mabel Perry
Owner: Mabel Perry and Suzanne Pilkington
Contact: 11 Park Lane, Little Knowle, Budleigh Salterton, Devon, EX9 6QT
☎ 01395 443303
@ Perry_pilkingtonparkhouse@hotmail.com

Situated in garden grounds approximately half a mile from the town centre, Park House is located in two acres of its own land. The home has two lounges for residents to socialise in, as well as a garden. The home arranges for a mobile library to come to the home and there is a Communion service once a month. The home also arranges performances from visiting entertainers.

Registered places: 27
Guide weekly rate: £475
Specialist care: Dementia, mental disorder, physical disability, respite
Medical services: Podiatry, optician, physiotherapy
Qualified staff: Fails standard

Home details
Location: Residential area, 0.5 miles from Budleigh Salterton
Communal areas: 2 lounges, dining room, garden
Accessibility: *Floors:* 2 • *Access:* Stair lift • *Wheelchair access:* Good
Smoking: ✗
Pets: At manager's discretion
Routines: Flexible

Room details
Single: 21
Shared: 3
En suite: 24
Facilities: TV point, telephone point

Door lock: ✓
Lockable place: ✓

Services provided
Beauty services: Hairdressing
Mobile library: ✓
Religious services: Monthly Communion service
Transport: ✗
Activities: *Coordinator:* ✗ • *Examples:* Visiting entertainers
Outings: ✗
Meetings: ✗

Park View

Manager: Shirley Darling
Owner: Andrew, Geoffrey and Maria Crowe
Contact: Furze Hill Road, Ilfracombe, Devon, EX34 8HZ
☎ 01271 865657

Situated in a residential area next to Bicclescombe Park, Park View stays true to its name providing direct access to the park. Although wheelchair access is limited around the home, work is currently underway to make the whole home wheelchair friendly. The home has its own car and minibus for transportation and arranges for a mobile library to visit the home. There is also a Communion service once a month.

Registered places: 22
Guide weekly rate: £274–£383
Specialist care: Dementia, respite
Medical services: Podiatry, optician
Qualified staff: Exceeds standard: 100% at NVQ level 2

Home details
Location: Residential area, 1.2 miles from Ilfracombe
Communal areas: Lounge, dining room, conservatory, garden
Accessibility: *Floors:* 2 • *Access:* Stair lift • *Wheelchair access:* Limited
Smoking: In designated area
Pets: At manager's discretion
Routines: Flexible

Room details
Single: 22
Shared: 0
En suite: 22
Facilities: TV point, telephone point

Door lock: ✓
Lockable place: ✓

Services provided
Beauty services: Hairdressing
Mobile library: ✓
Religious services: Monthly Communion service
Transport: Minibus and car
Activities: *Coordinator:* ✗ • *Examples:* Games • *Outings:* ✗
Meetings: ✗

Registered places: 20
Guide weekly rate: £286–£390
Specialist care: Dementia, respite
Medical services: Podiatry, dentist, optician
Qualified staff: Meets standard

Home details

Location: Residential area, 1.7 miles from Plymouth
Communal areas: 2 lounges, 2 dining rooms, conservatory, patio
Accessibility: *Floors:* 2 • *Access:* Stair lift • *Wheelchair access:* Good
Smoking: ✗
Pets: ✓
Routines: Flexible

Room details

Single: 20
Shared: 0
En suite: 1
Facilities: TV, telephone

Door lock: ✓
Lockable place: ✓

Services provided

Beauty services: Hairdressing
Mobile library: ✓
Religious services: ✓
Transport: ✗
Activities: *Coordinator:* ✗ • *Examples:* Armchair aerobics, musical entertainment • *Outings:* ✗
Meetings: ✓

Park View Residential Home

Manager: Vacant
Owner: Ashley Residential Care Ltd
Contact: 70–72 Peverell Park Road, Peverell, Plymouth, Devon PL3 4NB
☏ 01752 669541

Park View Residential Care Home is located in a residential area of Plymouth, just under two miles from the city centre. The home has ample communal space with two lounges, two dining rooms, a conservatory and a patio area. The home arranges a weekly activities programme, which includes armchair aerobics and musical entertainment. There are also regular residents meetings held.

Registered places: 52
Guide weekly rate: £363–£810
Specialist care: Dementia, mental disorder, respite
Medical services: Podiatry
Qualified staff: Exceeds standard: 75% at NVQ level 2

Home details

Location: Residential area, 1.7 miles from Exeter
Communal areas: Lounge, dining room, garden
Accessibility: *Floors:* 2 • *Access:* Lift • *Wheelchair access:* Good
Smoking: ✗
Pets: ✓
Routines: Flexible

Room details

Single: 51
Shared: 1
En suite: Undisclosed
Facilities: TV point

Door lock: ✓
Lockable place: ✓

Services provided

Beauty services: Hairdressing, aromatherapy
Mobile library: ✗
Religious services: ✗
Transport: ✗
Activities: *Coordinator:* ✓ • *Examples:* Flower arranging *Outings:* ✓
Meetings: ✓

Parkland House

Manager: John Bayliss
Owner: Peninsula Care Homes Ltd
Contact: Barley Lane, Exeter, Devon, EX4 1TA
☏ 01392 251144

Parkland House is a detached, period house that has been adapted and extended. There is a separate unit, the Coach House, for those who are more independent. The home is situated near local shops and a bus route to the city centre. Opinions can be voiced at the monthly residents meetings are used to improve the service given to the residents. Strong links are maintained with peoples' families, friends and the community.

DEVON

Parkwood House

Manager: Kate Wells-McCullock
Owner: Southern Healthcare Ltd
Contact: 72–74 Exmouth Road,
Stoke, Plymouth, Devon, PL1 4QJ
☎ 01752 560000
@ admin.parkwood@
southernhealthcare.co.uk
🖰 www.southernhealthcare.co.uk

Parkwood House is located in a residential area of Stoke, approximately two miles from Plymouth town centre. The home has two activities coordinators who devise a varied activities programme for the residents. The residents enjoy a flexible daily routine and have a lounge, a dining room and a garden as communal areas. Pets are allowed in the home and smoking is permitted in a designated area. The home offers its residents a religious service and also organises a hairdressing service.

Registered places: 48
Guide weekly rate: £350–£700
Specialist care: Nursing, dementia, physical disability
Medical services: Podiatry, dentist, occupational therapy, physiotherapy
Qualified staff: Undisclosed

Home details
Location: Residential area, 2 miles from Plymouth
Communal areas: Lounge, dining room, garden
Accessibility: *Floors:* 4 • *Access:* Lift • *Wheelchair access:* Good
Smoking: In designated area
Pets: ✓
Routine: Flexible

Room details
Single: 26
Shared: 10
En suite: 10
Facilities: TV point, telephone point

Door lock: ✓
Lockable place: ✓

Services provided
Beauty services: Hairdressing
Mobile library: ✗
Religious services: ✓
Transport: ✗
Activities: *Coordinators:* ✓ • *Examples:* Bingo • *Outings:* ✗
Meetings: ✓

Pendennis Residential Home

Manager: Hilda Teale
Owner: Pendennis Ltd
Contact: 64 Dartmouth Road,
Paignton, Devon, TQ4 5AW
☎ 01803 551351
@ pendennis64@fsmail.net

A modern, attractive property set in landscaped gardens, Pendennis Residential Home is situated five minutes' walk from shops and close to the seafront. Those with an interest in gardening may enjoy pursuing their hobby with the home's raised flowerbeds and summerhouse. Pendennis also has an antiques lady who comes in once a week. With ramped access leading to the entrance, a large part of the home has also been purpose built for those residents who are not very mobile. As the manager lives on site, she is also frequently on call should she be needed.

Registered places: 22
Guide weekly rate: £291–£450
Specialist care: Dementia, day care, physical disability, respite
Medical services: Podiatry, dentist, optician
Qualified staff: Exceeds standard: 95% at NVQ level 2

Home details
Location: Residential area, 0.6 miles from Paignton
Communal areas: 2 lounges, dining room, library facilities, conservatory, garden
Accessibility: *Floors:* 3 • *Access:* Lift and stair lift *Wheelchair access:* Good
Smoking: ✗
Pets: At manager's discretion
Meetings: ✓

Room details
Single: 22
Shared: 0
En suite: 20
Facilities: TV point, telephone point

Door lock: ✓
Lockable place: ✓

Services provided
Beauty services: Hairdressing
Mobile library: Library facilities
Religious services: Monthly nondenominational Communion service
Transport: ✗
Activities: *Coordinator:* ✗ • *Examples:* Bingo, exercise *Outings:* ✗
Routines: Flexible

Registered places: 22
Guide weekly rate: Undisclosed
Specialist care: Dementia, physical disability
Medical services: Podiatry, dentist, optician
Qualified staff: Meets standard

Home details
Location: Village location, 1.6 miles from Newton Abbot
Communal areas: Lounge, dining room, garden
Accessibility: *Floors:* 2 • *Access:* Lift • *Wheelchair access:* Good
Smoking: ✗
Pets: At manager's discretion
Routines: Flexible

Room details
Single: 20
Shared: 1
En suite: 19
Facilities: TV point, telephone point

Door lock: ✓
Lockable place: ✓

Services provided
Beauty services: Hairdressing
Mobile library: Library facilities
Religious services: Monthly Communion service
Transport: ✗
Activities: *Coordinator:* ✗ • *Examples:* Arts and crafts, bingo
  Outings: ✗
Meetings: ✓

Penns Mount Residential Care Home

Manager: Elizabeth Aldridge
Owner: Penns Mount Ltd
Contact: 10 Vicarage Hill, Kingsteignton, Devon, TQ12 3BA
☎ 01626 360274
@ elizabethaldridge@btinternet.com

A picturesque Edwardian house situated on a hill and overlooking the Devonshire countryside, Penns Mount is easily accessible and 15 minutes' walk from the local shops, with a bus stop at the bottom of the drive. Although seldom offering outings for residents who prefer to stay indoors, Penn's Mount has a good array of leisure activities that include a visiting seasonal clothes shop and in-house shop selling toiletries and sweets. Penns Mount publishes a monthly newsletter which informs residents of the range of activities on offer that month.

Registered places: 25
Guide weekly rate: £297–£450
Specialist care: Dementia, learning disability, mental disorder, respite
Medical services: Podiatry, optician
Qualified staff: Fails standard

Home details
Location: Residential area, 1.2 miles from Exeter
Communal areas: 2 lounges, dining room, garden
Accessibility: *Floors:* 3 • *Access:* Lift • *Wheelchair access:* Good
Smoking: ✗
Pets: ✓
Routines: Flexible

Room details
Single: 21
Shared: 2
En suite: 15
Facilities: None

Door lock: ✓
Lockable place: ✓

Services provided
Beauty services: Hairdressing
Mobile library: ✗
Religious services: Monthly Communion service
Transport: ✗
Activities: *Coordinator:* ✗ • *Examples:* Exercise, visiting entertainers
  Outings: ✗
Meetings: ✗

Pennsylvania House

Manager: Henry Morgan
Owner: Henry Morgan
Contact: 7–9 Powderham Crescent, Exeter, Devon, EX4 6DA
☎ 01392 256346
@ henry-morgan@tiscali.co.uk

Situated in a residential area of Exeter, Pennsylvania House has just been granted planning permission for an extension at the rear of the building which will include extending the garden, 12 extra beds, a larger kitchen and a conservatory. The home organises a monthly Communion service and daily activities which includes gentle exercise and performances from visiting entertainers.

Penose Residential Home

Manager: Joyce Reed
Owner: Joyce Reed
Contact: 1–2 Tothill Avenue, St Judes, Plymouth, Devon, PL4 8PH
✆ 01752 663191
@ penvoseresident@btconnect.com

Originally comprised of two houses that have now been merged into one, Penvose Residential Home is located in an elevated position in a residential area opposite a large park. An animal-friendly home, Penvose currently has a cat, two budgies and a cockatiel. The manager and owner lives next door to the home and residents often spend time in her garden, which has a fishpond. There is a yearly carol service at the home and an Anglican Communion service once a month.

Registered places: 15
Guide weekly rate: £275–£333
Specialist care: Dementia, respite
Medical services: Podiatry
Qualified staff: Fails standard

Home details
Location: Residential area, 1.2 miles from Plymouth
Communal areas: 2 lounges, dining room, garden
Accessibility: *Floors:* 2 • *Access:* Stair lift • *Wheelchair access:* None
Smoking: In designated area
Pets: ✓
Routines: Flexible

Room details
Single: 13
Shared: 2　　　　　　　**Door lock:** ✓
En suite: 1　　　　　**Lockable place:** ✗
Facilities: TV point, telephone point

Services provided
Beauty services: Hairdressing
Mobile library: ✓
Religious services: Monthly Anglican Communion service
Transport: Car
Activities: *Coordinator:* ✗ • *Examples:* Armchair exercises, quizzes, visiting entertainers • *Outings:* ✗
Meetings: ✓

Pinewood Lodge

Manager: Tracey Sings
Owner: Margaret Rose Care Ltd
Contact: Didworthy, South Brent, Devon, TQ10 9EF
✆ 01364 72420

Set in five and a half acres of ground, Pinewood Lodge Nursing Home is set in a very rural area in Dartmoor Natural Park. Residents share the home's gardens with deer, squirrels and birds. It is around one and a half miles to the nearest shops and two and a half miles from South Brent. The home has its own car for transportation and arranges activities for the residents such as movement to music. The home also arranges for a mobile library to come to the home.

Registered places: 22
Guide weekly rate: Undisclosed
Specialist care: Nursing, day care, dementia, physical disability, respite
Medical services: Podiatry, optician, physiotherapy
Qualified staff: Fails standard

Home details
Location: Rural area, 2.5 miles from South Brent
Communal areas: Lounge, garden
Accessibility: *Floors:* 2 • *Access:* Lift • *Wheelchair access:* Good
Smoking: ✗
Pets: At manager's discretion
Routines: Flexible

Room details
Single: 18
Shared: 2　　　　　　　**Door lock:** ✓
En suite: 7　　　　　**Lockable place:** ✓
Facilities: TV point, telephone point

Services provided
Beauty services: Hairdressing, aromatherapy, massage
Mobile library: ✓
Religious services: ✗
Transport: Car
Activities: *Coordinator:* ✗ • *Examples:* Movement to music *Outings:* ✗
Meetings: ✗

Registered places: 17
Guide weekly rate: £370–£435
Specialist care: Physical disability
Medical services: Podiatry, dentist, hygienist, optician
Qualified staff: Exceeds standard: 90% at NVQ level 2

Home details

Location: Residential area, 0.6 miles from Paignton
Communal areas: 2 lounges, dining room, garden
Accessibility: *Floors:* 2 • *Access:* Lift • *Wheelchair access:* Good
Smoking: In designated area
Pets: ✓
Routines: Structured

Room details

Single: 13
Shared: 2
En suite: 15
Facilities: TV point, telephone point

Door lock: ✓
Lockable place: ✓

Services provided

Beauty services: Hairdressing
Mobile Library: ✓
Religious services: Monthly Anglican Communion service
Transport: ✗
Activities: *Coordinator:* ✓ • *Examples:* Exercise, quizzes, reminiscence • *Outings:* ✓
Meetings: ✗

Pippins

Manager: Sarah Dorling
Owner: Celia Griffiths
Contact: Mead Lane, Preston, Paignton, Devon, TQ3 2AT
☎ 01803 525757

Set in a residential area close to a park and the seafront, Pippins is a short, easy walk from the amenities of Paignton, around half a mile away. The house has a well-equipped and level garden that includes a fountain, fishpond, fruit trees and a flowerbed. There is an Anglican Communion service once a month and a mobile library comes to the home on a regular basis.

Registered places: 40
Guide weekly rate: Undisclosed
Specialist care: Day care, dementia, mental disorder, physical disability, respite
Medical services: Podiatry, optician, physiotherapy
Qualified staff: Meets standard

Home details

Location: Rural area, 6 miles from Newton Abbot
Communal areas: 2 lounges, 2 dining rooms, sensory room, garden
Accessibility: *Floors:* 2 • *Access:* Lift • *Wheelchair access:* Good
Smoking: ✗
Pets: ✓
Routines: Flexible

Room details

Single: 34
Shared: 3
En suite: 37
Facilities: TV point, telephone point

Door lock: ✓
Lockable place: ✓

Services provided

Beauty services: Hairdressing
Mobile library: ✓
Religious services: Monthly nondenominational service
Transport: Minibus
Activities: *Coordinator:* ✓ • *Examples:* Arts and crafts, games, musical entertainment • *Outings:* ✓
Meetings: ✓

Prestbury Court Residential Home

Manager: Rosalyn Nolan
Owner: Avens Care Homes Ltd
Contact: Brimley Lane, Bovey Tracey, Newton Abbot, Devon, TQ13 9JS
☎ 01626 833246
@ avenscare@aol.com
🖱 www.avenscarehomes.co.uk

Prestbury Court Residential Home is located inside a national park about two miles from Newton Abbot town centre. There is a post office one mile away. Three members of staff live on the premises in a separate property close to the home. There is a residents meeting once a month as well as a nondenominational religious service. The home has its own minibus for transport and takes the residents on regular outings.

Primley Court

Manager: Monica Gumus
Owner: Optima Care Partnership
Contact: 13 Primley Park, Paignton, Devon, TQ3 3JP
☎ 01803 555988

A modern building set in an elevated position above the coastal town of Paignton, Primley Court is close to its sister home Primley View and both are 500 yards away from the town centre where there are plenty of shops and amenities. Primley Court offers a comprehensive activities programme for those who wish to stay indoors. The home itself is simply decorated and spacious with some of the rooms overlooking sea views. A relatives group meets every six weeks.

Registered places: 51
Guide weekly rate: £625
Specialist care: Nursing, day care, dementia, mental disorder, physical disability, respite
Medical services: Podiatry, dentist, optician
Qualified staff: Meets standard

Home details
Location: Residential area, 0.8 miles from Paignton
Communal areas: 5 lounges, dining room, hairdressing salon, library, garden room, garden
Accessibility: *Floors:* 4 • *Access:* Lift • *Wheelchair access:* Good
Smoking: ✗
Pets: ✗
Routines: Flexible

Room details
Single: 43
Shared: 4
En suite: 32
Facilities: TV point

Door lock: ✓
Lockable place: ✓

Services provided
Beauty services: Hairdressing, aromatherapy
Mobile library: Library facilities
Religious services: Monthly Baptist and Methodist visits, weekly Catholic Communion service
Transport: ✗
Activities: *Coordinator:* ✓ • *Examples:* Arts and crafts, music and movement, quizzes • *Outings:* ✓
Meetings: ✓

Primley View Nursing Home

Manager: Susan Wiltshire
Owner: Optima Care Partnership
Contact: 25 Primley Park, Paignton, Devon, TQ3 3JS
☎ 01803 559229

Set in an elevated position overlooking the seaside town of Paignton, Primley View Nursing Home is a large home that offers panoramic views of the surrounding Torbay area. Situated half a mile from the town centre and close to its sister home, Primley Court, there are also bus stops nearby for those wishing to travel further afield. Comfortable and homely, Primley View has large windows which make rooms feel spacious and bright. Many of the bedrooms permit sea views and there is also the option to sit in the lounge.

Registered places: 30
Guide weekly rate: £500–£550
Specialist care: Nursing, physical disability, respite
Medical services: Podiatry, dentist, optician
Qualified staff: Meets standard

Home details
Location: Residential area, 0.5 miles from Paignton
Communal areas: 3 lounges, dining room, library, garden
Accessibility: *Floors:* 2 • *Access:* Lift • *Wheelchair access:* Good
Smoking: In designated area
Pets: At manager's discretion
Routines: Flexible

Room details
Single: 26
Shared: 2
En suite: 7
Facilities: TV point

Door lock: ✓
Lockable place: ✓

Services provided
Beauty services: Hairdressing
Mobile library: Library facilities
Religious services: ✗
Transport: ✗
Activities: *Coordinator:* ✓ • *Examples:* Arts and crafts, musical entertainment, one-to-one sessions • *Outings:* ✓
Meetings: ✗

Registered places: 38
Guide weekly rate: £350–£450
Specialist care: Day care, dementia, physical disability, respite
Medical services: Podiatry, dentist, optician, physiotherapy
Qualified staff: Exceeds standard: 85% at NVQ level 2

Home details

Location: Residential area, 1 mile from Totnes
Communal areas: 3 lounges, 2 dining rooms, conservatory, garden
Accessibility: *Floors:* 3 • *Access:* Lift • *Wheelchair access:* Good
Smoking: ✗
Pets: At manager's discretion
Routines: Flexible

Room details

Single: 36
Shared: 1
En suite: 37

Door lock: ✓
Lockable place: ✓

Facilities: TV point, telephone point

Services provided

Beauty services: Hairdressing
Mobile library: ✗
Religious services: Monthly Methodist Communion service,
   monthly Anglican Communion service
Transport: Minibus
Activities: *Coordinator:* ✗ • *Examples:* Arts and crafts, singing
   Outings: ✓
Meetings: ✓

Puddavine Court

Manager: Valerie Austin
Owner: The Court Group
Contact: Ashburton Road, Dartington, Totnes, Devon, TQ9 6EU
) 01803 866366
@ info@thecourtgroup.co.uk
🖰 www.thecourtgroup.co.uk

Situated on a site that is fabled to have once given shelter to Oliver Crowell, Puddavine Court is a grand Victorian Manor house set in two acres of attractively landscaped grounds on the outskirts of Totnes. With attractive views of the surrounding Devonshire countryside, Puddavine Court also boasts its own Italian Gardens with paving and luscious flowerbeds. Approximately 20 minutes' walk from the shops, there is also a bus stop just outside the home that may take the active resident into Totnes. Puddavine Court also provides its residents with weekly outings at a small charge.

Registered places: 30
Guide weekly rate: £370–£460
Specialist care: Dementia, mental disorder, physical disability, respite
Medical services: Podiatry, optician
Qualified staff: Meets standard

Home details

Location: Residential area, 0.2 miles from Kingsbridge
Communal areas: Lounge, dining room, garden
Accessibility: *Floors:* 3 • *Access:* Lift and stair lift
   Wheelchair access: Good
Smoking: In designated area
Pets: ✓
Routines: Structured

Room details

Single: 30
Shared: 0
En suite: 30

Door lock: ✓
Lockable place: ✓

Facilities: TV point, telephone point

Services provided

Beauty services: Hairdressing
Mobile library: ✗
Religious services: Monthly Anglican Communion service
Transport: ✗
Activities: *Coordinator:* ✗ • *Examples:* One-to-one sessions
   Outings: ✓
Meetings: ✓

Quay Court Care Centre

Manager: Susan Shute
Owner: Quay Court Care Centre Ltd
Contact: Squares Quay, Kingsbridge, Devon, TQ7 1HN
) 01548 852540

A modern building that is situated adjacent to the quay in Kingsbridge, the Quay Court Centre lies close to local facilities which include a post office and library. There is a residents meeting every three months and a monthly Anglican Communion service. The home arranges group activities for the residents such as reminiscence sessions, as well as one-to-one sessions.

Quintaville

Manager: John Murphy
Owner: L Murphy & Co Ltd
Contact: 1 Quinta Road,
Torquay, Devon, TQ1 3RJ
☎ 01803 328289

Quintaville provides a comfortable environment for the residents and has three lounges for the residents to socialise in. The home is located in an urban area, one and a half miles from Torquay. Several residents recommend the quality of the meals provided and confirmed that a varied choice was always available.

Registered places: 25
Guide weekly rate: £313–£367
Specialist care: Dementia, learning disability, mental disorder, physical disability, respite
Medical services: Podiatry, physiotherapy
Qualified staff: Meets standard

Home details
Location: Urban area, 1.5 miles from Torquay
Communal areas: 3 lounges, dining room, hairdressing salon, garden
Accessibility: *Floors:* 3 • *Access:* Lift • *Wheelchair access:* Good
Smoking: ✗
Pets: ✓
Routines: Flexible

Room details
Single: 25
Shared: 0
En suite: 0
Facilities: TV, telephone point

Door lock: ✓
Lockable place: ✓

Services provided
Beauty services: Hairdressing
Mobile library: ✗
Religious services: ✗
Transport: ✗
Activities: *Coordinator:* ✓ • *Examples:* Entertainment • *Outings:* ✗
Meetings: ✗

Radway Lodge

Manager: Karen Hellier
Owner: The Radway Partnership
Contact: Vicarage Road,
Sidmouth, Devon, EX10 8TS
☎ 01395 514015

Located in a central position in Sidmouth, Radway Lodge is a listed building which is located close to local shops, cinema and the seafront. There are two large lounges, a dining room, a large garden and a patio. The home has a flexible daily routine with breakfast served to residents in their room and lunch and supper at set times. The home has an activities coordinator who arranges activities such as visiting musical entertainment and some outings to the seafront.

Registered places: 15
Guide weekly rate: From £500
Specialist care: Nursing, day care, respite
Medical services: None
Qualified staff: Exceeds standard: 70% at NVQ level 2

Home details
Location: Residential area, 0.7 miles from Sidmouth
Communal areas: 2 lounges, dining room, patio and garden
Accessibility: *Floors:* 3 • *Access:* 2 stair lifts
Wheelchair access: Good
Smoking: In designated area
Pets: ✓
Routines: Flexible

Room details
Single: 15
Shared: 0
En suite: 0
Facilities: TV, telephone point

Door lock: ✓
Lockable place: ✓

Services provided
Beauty services: Hairdressing, manicures
Mobile library: ✓
Religious services: ✗
Transport: ✗
Activities: *Coordinator:* ✓ • *Examples:* Bingo, games, musical entertainment • *Outings:* ✓
Meetings: ✗

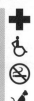

Registered places: 42
Guide weekly rate: From £300
Specialist care: Nursing, dementia, mental disorder,
    physical disability, respite
Medical services: Podiatry, optician, physiotherapy
Qualified staff: Fails standard

Home details

Location: Rural area, 1.5 miles from Buckfastleigh
Communal areas: Lounge, dining room, garden
Accessibility: *Floors:* 3 • *Access:* Lifts • *Wheelchair access:* Good
Smoking: ✗
Pets: At manager's discretion
Routines: Flexible

Room details

Single: 26
Shared: 8
En suite: Undisclosed
Facilities: TV point, telephone point

Door lock: ✓
Lockable place: ✓

Services provided

Beauty services: Hairdressing, beautician
Mobile library: ✗
Religious services: Monthly Anglican Communion service
Transport: ✗
Activities: *Coordinator:* ✗ • *Examples:* Games, exercise, singing
    Outings: ✗
Meetings: ✗

Redmount Nursing Home

Manager: Patricia K✗wling
Owner: Your Health Ltd
Contact: 21 Old Totnes Road,
Buckfastleigh, Devon, TQ11 0BY
☎ 01364 642403
@ redmount@btinternet.com
🖥 www.yourhealth.ltd.uk

Redmount Nursing Home is located on the edge of Dartmoor National Park, one and a half miles from Buckfastleigh, with a bus stop a short distance from the home. Currently the garden is being landscaped, with decking and lights being added. The home arranges for an Anglican Communion service to take place once a month in addition to daily activities such as games and gentle exercise.

Registered places: 20
Guide weekly rate: £385–£460
Specialist care: Respite
Medical services: Podiatry, dentist, optician
Qualified staff: Meet standard

Home details

Location: Residential area, 3.8 miles from Plymouth
Communal areas: Lounge, dining room, garden
Accessibility: *Floors:* 3 • *Access:* Stair lift • *Wheelchair access:* None
Smoking: ✗
Pets: ✗
Routines: Flexible

Room details

Single: 18
Shared: 1
En suite: 9
Facilities: TV, telephone

Door lock: ✓
Lockable place: ✓

Services provided

Beauty services: Hairdressing, beauty therapy
Mobile library: ✓
Religious services: ✗
Transport: 7-seater vehicle
Activities: *Coordinator:* ✗ • *Examples:* Bingo, games, exercise
    Outings: ✓
Meetings: ✓

The Retreat

Manager: Paul Constantine
Owner: Sunshine Care Ltd
Contact: Belle Vue Road, Hooe,
Plymouth, Devon, PL9 9NR
☎ 01752 402566
@ enquiries@retreatcare.co.uk
🖥 www.retreatcare.co.uk

Situated on a quiet country road in its own grounds, The Retreat is located approximately one mile from the town's shops. Residents are often taken out in the home's seven-seater vehicle. The Retreat is also on a bus route. With airy bedrooms that have big windows which allow the sun to pour in, the home also has attractive gardens with pond, greenhouse and features such as box hedging surrounding rosebeds. There is a residents meeting every six months and a mobile library comes to the home regularly.

Ridge House

Manager: Deborah Bradford
Owner: Ridge House Residential Home Ltd
Contact: Church Street, Morchard Bishop, Crediton, Devon, EX17 6PJ
☏ 01363 877335
@ ridgehouse@fsmail.net

Ridge House is located in the heart of Morchard Bishop village nine miles from the town of Crediton. The home has large gardens and has south-facing views over Dartmoor from most of the rooms and from the dining room and conservatory. The home arranges activities such as games, bingo and visiting entertainers and also organises outings which meet the individual residents needs and wishes, for example to the pub or the local garden centre.

Registered places: 15
Guide weekly rate: £400–£500
Specialist care: Day care, respite.
Medical services: Podiatry, dentist, optician, physiotherapy
Qualified staff: Exceeds standard: 70% at NVQ level 2

Home details
Location: Rural area, 9 miles from Crediton
Communal areas: Lounge, dining room, conservatory, garden
Accessibility: *Floors:* 2 • *Access:* Stair lift • *Wheelchair access:* Good
Smoking: ✗
Pets: At manager's discretion
Routines: Flexible

Room details
Single: 15
Shared: 0
En suite: 7
Facilities: TV point
Door lock: ✓
Lockable place: ✓

Services provided
Beauty services: Hairdressing, aromatherapy, manicures
Mobile library: ✓
Religious services: ✓
Transport: ✗
Activities: *Coordinator:* ✗ • *Examples:* Arts and crafts, games, visiting entertainers • *Outings:* ✓
Meetings: ✗

Ridgecourt Residential Care Home

Manager: Irene Wilson-Tancock
Owner: Ogwell Grange Ltd
Contact: Bridgetown Hill, Totnes, Devon, TQ9 5BH
☏ 01803 866152
🖥 www.ogwellgrange.co.uk

A period property set in its own grounds at the top of a hill, Ridgecourt Residential Care Home overlooks the town of Bridgetown and is located one mile from Totnes. The home has its own library facilities and also arranges for a mobile library to visit. There is an Anglican Communion service held once a month and daily activities such as art and cookery demonstrations.

Registered places: 15
Guide weekly rate: £370–£460
Specialist care: None
Medical services: Podiatry, dentist, optician
Qualified staff: Fails standard

Home details
Location: Residential area, 1 mile from Totnes
Communal areas: 2 lounges, dining room, garden
Accessibility: *Floors:* 2 • *Access:* Stair lift • *Wheelchair access:* Limited
Smoking: ✗
Pets: At manager's discretion
Routines: Flexible

Room details
Single: 15
Shared: 0
En suite: 14
Facilities: TV point, telephone point
Door lock: ✗
Lockable place: ✓

Services provided
Beauty services: Hairdresser, aromatherapy
Mobile Library: ✓
Religious services: Monthly Anglican Communion service
Transport: ✗
Activities: *Coordinator:* ✗ • *Examples:* Cookery, music • *Outings:* ✗
Meetings: ✗

Registered places: 24
Guide weekly rate: £350–£500
Specialist care: Emergency admissions, respite
Medical services: Podiatry, dentist, optician
Qualified staff: Meets standard

Home details

Location: Residential area, 0.5 miles from Dawlish
Communal areas: 2 lounges, dining room, garden
Accessibility: *Floors:* 3 • *Access:* Lift and stair lift •
Wheelchair access: Good
Smoking: ✗
Pets: At manager's discretion
Routines: Flexible

Room details

Single: 17
Shared: 2
En suite: 17
Facilities: TV point

Door lock: ✓
Lockable place: ✓

Services provided

Beauty services: Hairdressing
Mobile library: ✓
Religious services: Monthly Methodist service
Transport: ✗
Activities: *Coordinator:* ✗ • *Examples:* Arts and crafts,
visiting entertainers • *Outings:* ✓
Meetings: ✗

The Rise Care Home

Manager: Tracey Phillips
Owner: Michael and Julia Raven
Contact: Luscombe Hill,
Dawlish, Devon, EX7 0QL
☎ 01626 863245
@ therisecare@hotmail.co.uk
🖥 www.therisecarehome.co.uk

A Georgian country house set in nine acres of land and surrounded by countryside, The Rise Care Home was rebuilt in Victorian times before being converted in the 1950s' and retains many of its original features The Rise is an attractive prospect for residents who enjoy being outdoors as it has ample gardens that include a flower garden and ornamental pond area. Subject to risk assessment, residents are also welcome to access kitchen facilities where they can make themselves a small snack between meals.

Registered places: 20
Guide weekly rate: £285–£376
Specialist care: Day care, dementia, physical disability, respite
Medical services: Podiatry, dentist, optician, physiotherapy
Qualified staff: Meets standard

Home details

Location: Rural area, 6 miles from Newton Abbot
Communal areas: Lounge/dining room, patio
Accessibility: *Floors:* 2 • *Access:* Stair lift • *Wheelchair access:* Good
Smoking: In designated area
Pets: ✓
Routines: Flexible

Room details

Single: 16
Shared: 4
En suite: Undisclosed
Facilities: TV, telephone

Door lock: ✓
Lockable place: ✓

Services provided

Beauty services: Hairdressing, manicures
Mobile library: Library facilities
Religious services: ✓
Transport: ✓
Activities: *Coordinator:* ✓ • *Examples:* Games, knitting club,
visiting *Outings:* ✗
Meetings: ✗

Rosemount Residential Care Home

Manager: Rosemarie Noon
Owner: Mariarod Care Homes UK Ltd
Contact: 48 Old Exeter Street, Chudleigh,
Newton Abbot, Devon, TQ13 0JX
☎ 01626 853416
@ mariarod@btconnect.com

Set within a heritage area, Rosemount is a 400-year-old building that resides 100 yards from local facilities in the town of Chudleigh. The home has its own activities coordinator who organises activities such as musical entertainment and games as well as a knitting club. The home has a lounge, a dining room and although there is no garden there is a courtyard area. The home has its own transport and its own library facilities.

Roseville

Manager: Dianne Bradley
Owner: Underhill Care Ltd
Contact: Marine Gardens, Preston, Paignton, Devon, TQ3 2NT
) 01278 741279
@ dibradley@fsmail.net

Situated in a residential area close to the seafront, Roseville is close to local amenities and less than one mile from Paignton. The home has an enclosed garden which residents can enjoy in good weather. The home arranges a Communion service every two weeks and the residents benefit from the home's own library facilities.

Registered places: 22
Guide weekly rate: £350–£385
Specialist care: Dementia, physical disability, respite
Medical services: Podiatry, hygienist, optician, physiotherapy
Qualified staff: Exceeds standard: 90% at NVQ level 2

Home details
Location: Residential area, 0.8 miles from Paignton
Communal areas: Lounge, dining room, library facilities, conservatory, garden
Accessibility: *Floors:* 2 • *Access:* Lift • *Wheelchair access:* Limited
Smoking: In designated area
Pets: At manager's discretion
Routines: Structured

Room details
Single: 22
Shared: 0
En suite: 22
Facilities: TV point, telephone point

Door lock: ✓
Lockable place: ✓

Services provided
Beauty services: Hairdressing
Mobile library: Library facilities
Religious services: Fortnightly Communion service
Transport: Car
Activities: *Coordinator:* ✓ • *Examples:* Exercise, music, quizzes
   Outings: ✗
Meetings: ✓

Roundham Court

Manager: Denise Ellis
Owner: The Court Group
Contact: 22 Cliff Road, Paignton, Devon, TQ4 6DG
) 01803 528024

Roundham Court is a Victorian house set in ample grounds and overlooking Torbay and its harbour, five minutes' walk from a local shop. With spacious rooms, large windows and a carved oak galleried staircase, the home is well maintained. The gardens surround the home and provide ample space in which residents can relax outdoors while a maintenance man ensures all minor repairs to the building are done quickly. As well as a recently installed mobile shop, residents may benefit from the frequent outings on offer to them which are provided at a small charge.

Registered places: 35
Guide weekly rate: £325–£550
Specialist care: Day care, respite
Medical services: Podiatry, dentist, optician
Qualified staff: Undisclosed

Home details
Location: Residential area, 1 mile from Paignton centre
Communal areas: 2 lounges, dining room, garden
Accessibility: *Floors:* 2 • *Access:* Lift • *Wheelchair access:* Good
Smoking: In designated area
Pets: At manager's discretion
Routines: Flexible

Room details
Single: 33
Shared: 1
En suite: 31
Facilities: TV point, telephone point

Door lock: ✓
Lockable place: ✓

Services provided
Beauty services: Hairdressing
Mobile library: ✗
Religious services: Monthly Communion service
Transport: Minibus
Activities: *Coordinator:* ✗ • *Examples:* Bingo, visiting organist
   Outings: ✓
Meetings: ✓

Registered places: 12
Guide weekly rate: £315–£380
Specialist care: Day care, dementia, respite
Medical services: Podiatry, hygienist, optician
Qualified staff: Fails standard

Home details
Location: Residential area, 1 mile from Brixham
Communal areas: Lounge, dining room, patio and garden
Accessibility: *Floors:* 2 • *Access:* Stair lift • *Wheelchair access:* Good
Smoking: ✗
Pets: ✗
Routines: Structured

Room details
Single: 10
Shared: 1
En suite: 2
Facilities: TV

Door lock: ✗
Lockable place: ✗

Services provided
Beauty services: Hairdressing
Mobile library: ✗
Religious services: Monthly service
Transport: Car
Activities: *Coordinator:* ✓ • *Examples:* Exercise, musical entertainment
     Outings: ✓
Meetings: ✗

Rydan Lodge

Manager: Lily McCarthy
Owner: Lily and Malcolm McCarthy
Contact: 3 Nelson Road,
Brixham, Devon, TQ5 8BH
) 01803 858590
@ rydancare@tiscali.co.uk
⌨ www.torbayresidentialhomes.com/
     Rydanlodge

Situated in the fishing town of Brixham, Rydan Lodge is located in a residential area, one mile from the town centre. The home offers views of the Brixham breakwater and the surrounding coastline from some of the rooms. The home has a garden with a patio area. A religious service is held on a monthly basis and the home has its own car to use as transportation for outings. There are also daily activities in the home which include exercise sessions and musical entertainment.

Registered places: 23
Guide weekly rate: £227–£363
Specialist care: Dementia, learning disability, mental disorder
Medical services: Podiatry, optician, physiotherapy
Qualified staff: Meets standard

Home details
Location: Residential area, 0.6 miles from Bideford
Communal areas: 3 lounges, dining room, garden
Accessibility: *Floors:* 3 • *Access:* Stair lift • *Wheelchair
     access:* Good
Smoking: In designated area
Pets: ✓
Routines: Flexible

Room details
Single: 17
Shared: 2
En suite: 10
Facilities: TV point, telephone point

Door lock: ✓
Lockable place: ✓

Services provided
Beauty services: Hairdressing
Mobile library: ✓
Religious services: Weekly service, monthly Communion service
Transport: ✗
Activities: *Coordinator:* ✗ • *Examples:* Bingo, exercise sessions,
     memories afternoon • *Outings:* ✓
Meetings: ✓

Sandhurst

Manager: Kim Cox
Owner: Klaus-Jurgen and Victoria Kothe
Contact: 49–51 Abbotsham Road,
Bideford, Devon, EX39 3AQ
) 01237 477195
@ Sandhurst49@btinternet.com

Made up of two adjoining Victorian houses, Sandhurst is located on the outskirts of Bideford. The home has one flat on its second floor, comprised of a bedroom, en suite and lounge. The garden is currently being redeveloped. The garden will be levelled for wheelchair access, and raised flowerbeds will be put in. The home arranges a variety of activities for the residents including performances by visiting entertainers and exercise session. There are also regular outings in the local area.

Seaswift House

Manager: Carole Rundle-Drew
Owner: Kathryn Jackson
Contact: Sea Hill, Seaton,
Devon, EX12 2QT
☎ 01297 24493

Overlooking a bowling green, Seaswift House is located in the centre of Seaton, a two-minute walk to the local shops and the seafront. The home has a lounge, a dining room, a conservatory and a garden with a patio area. The home has an activities coordinator who arranges activities such as bingo as well as outings to the theatre and the cinema. The home has its own transport. There is also a mobile library that visits and religious services are arranged.

Registered places: 14
Guide weekly rate: Undisclosed
Specialist care: Respite
Medical services: Podiatry, dentist, optician
Qualified staff: Undisclosed

Home details
Location: Residential area, 0.4 miles from Seaton
Communal areas: Lounge, dining room, conservatory, patio and garden
Accessibility: *Floors:* 2 • *Access:* Stair lift • *Wheelchair access:* Good
Smoking: Undisclosed
Pets: ✗
Routines: Flexible

Room details
Single: 14
Shared: 0
En suite: 10
Facilities: TV

Door lock: ✓
Lockable place: ✓

Services provided
Beauty services: Hairdressing, manicures, Reiki
Mobile library: ✓
Religious services: ✓
Transport: ✓
Activities: *Coordinator:* ✓ • *Examples:* Bingo, games • *Outings:* ✓
Meetings: Undisclosed

Seaton Lodge Residential Home

Manager: Louise Evans
Owner: Geoffrey Briddick
Contact: 7–9 Seaton Avenue, Mutley, Plymouth, Devon, PL4 6QJ
☎ 01752 667077
@ seatonlodge@hotmail.co.uk

Situated in a residential area on the edge of Mutley Plain shopping precinct, Seaton Lodge is less than a mile from the centre of Plymouth and a few hundred yards from the station. The home aims to offer a non-institutional atmosphere, the home offers fortnightly trips to the pub and local beauty spots. The home has its own car to use as transport for these outings.

Registered places: 18
Guide weekly rate: £290–£310
Specialist care: Dementia, respite
Medical services: Podiatry, dentist, optician, physiotherapy
Qualified staff: Meets standard

Home details
Location: Residential area, 1 mile from Plymouth
Communal areas: 2 lounges, dining room, patio and garden
Accessibility: *Floors:* 3 • *Access:* Lift and stair lift • *Wheelchair access:* Good
Smoking: In designated area
Pets: ✓
Routines: Flexible

Room details
Single: 18
Shared: 0
En suite: 10
Facilities: TV point, telephone point

Door lock: ✓
Lockable place: ✓

Services provided
Beauty services: Hairdressing
Mobile library: ✓
Religious services: ✗
Transport: Car
Activities: *Coordinator:* ✗ • *Examples:* Bingo, games • *Outings:* ✗
Meetings: ✗

Registered places: 52
Guide weekly rate: £450–£750
Specialist care: Nursing, physical disability, respite
Medical services: Podiatry
Qualified staff: Exceeds standard: 61% at NVQ level 2

Home details

Location: Residential area, 0.5 miles from Dawlish
Communal areas: Lounge, dining room, hairdressing salon
Accessibility: *Floors:* 3 • *Access:* Lift • *Wheelchair access:* Good
Smoking: ✗
Pets: ✓
Routines: Flexible

Room details

Single: 48
Shared: 2   Door lock: ✓
En suite: 27   Lockable place: ✓
Facilities: TV point, telephone point

Services provided

Beauty services: Hairdressing
Mobile library: ✗
Religious services: ✓
Transport: ✗
Activities: *Coordinator:* ✓ • *Examples:* Arts and crafts,
    gardening and local history group • *Outings:* ✗
Meetings: ✓

Sefton Hall

Manager: Karen Bull
Owner: Southern Healthcare Ltd
Contact: Plantation Terrace,
Dawlish, Devon, EX7 9DS
☎ 01626 863125
@ karen.bolt@southernhealthcare.co.uk
🖰 www.southernhealthcare.co.uk

Sefton Hall is located in a residential area of Dawlish and provides care for 52 residents. The home also has a communal lounge, a dining room and a hairdressing salon. Pets are allowed in the home but smoking is not permitted. The home also organises a religious service for the residents. There are regular residents meetings and the residents benefit from a flexible daily routine, with activities which include arts and crafts and a local history group.

Registered places: 29
Guide weekly rate: £620–£700
Specialist care: Nursing, respite
Medical services: Podiatry, dentist, optician
Qualified staff: Meets standard

Home details

Location: Residential area, 1 mile from Sidmouth
Communal areas: Lounge, dining room, conservatory, garden
Accessibility: *Floors:* 2 • *Access:* Lift and stair lift • *Wheelchair access:* Good
Smoking: ✗
Pets: At manager's discretion
Routines: Flexible

Room details

Single: 29
Shared: 0   Door lock: ✓
En suite: 29   Lockable place: ✓
Facilities: TV point, telephone point

Services provided

Beauty services: Hairdressing
Mobile library: ✓
Religious services: Monthly Communion
Transport: ✗
Activities: *Coordinator:* ✓ • *Examples:* Drama therapy, exercise
    Outings: ✓
Meetings: ✓

The Sidmouth Nursing Home

Manager: Julie Casely
Owner: Anchorstone Services Ltd
Contact: 106–108 Winslade Road,
Sidmouth, Devon, EX10 9EZ
☎ 01395 514172
@ ebevan2@aol.com
🖰 www.sidmouthnursinghome.co.uk

The Sidmouth Nursing Home is located in a residential area, one mile from the town of Sidmouth. The home has easy access to both the town centre and the seafront. Inside the home there is ample communal space with a lounge, a dining room and a conservatory. The home also has a garden for residents to relax in. The home employs an activities coordinator who arranges a variety of activities including individual and group sessions such as an exercise class. The home also arranges outings for the residents.

Silver Threads Care Home

Manager: Robert Flynn
Owner: Angela and Robert Flynn
Contact: 1 Lyndale Terrace, Instow, Bideford, Devon, EX39 4HS

) 01271 860329
@ carehome@silverthreads.fsnet.co.uk
🖰 www.silverthreads.fsnet.co.uk

Situated in Instow village three minutes' walk from shops and a pub, Silver Threads is a small family-run care home that is next to the Taw and Torridge estuary. While wonderful views of the seafront, more able residents are also able to benefit from the fresh sea air. A private courtyard with summerhouse is also located within the grounds and offers residents an opportunity to relax outdoors.

Registered places: 14
Guide weekly rate: £385–£400
Specialist care: Dementia, mental disorder
Medical services: Podiatry, dentist, optician
Qualified staff: Fails standard

Home details
Location: Rural area, 3 miles from Bideford
Communal areas: 2 lounges, dining room, garden
Accessibility: *Floors:* 3 • *Access:* Stair lift • *Wheelchair access:* Good
Smoking: ✗
Pets: At manager's discretion
Routines: Flexible

Room details
Single: 14
Shared: 0
En suite: 10
Facilities: TV point

Door lock: ✗
Lockable place: ✓

Services provided
Beauty services: Hairdressing, manicures
Mobile library: ✓
Religious services: Weekly Methodist visits
Transport: Cars
Activities: *Coordinator:* ✓ • *Examples:* Bingo, skittles, quizzes
    Outings: ✓
Meetings: ✗

Silverleigh Cedars

Manager: Christine Brooke
Owner: Silverleigh Ltd
Contact: Silver Street, Axminster, Devon, EX13 5AF

) 01297 32611
@ sliced@freenet.co.uk
🖰 www.silverleighcedars.co.uk

Silveleigh Cedars is a converted and extended home set in its own grounds in the centre of Axminster. In a central position a few minutes from local amenities such as shops, Silverleigh Cedars also provides extensive facilities for residents in-house. As well as a piano and laptop computers, a special resident's kitchen area is provided for those with an interest in baking and at least three outings are arranged weekly. There is also a guest bedroom where visiting relatives and friends may stay free of charge.

Registered places: 54
Guide weekly rate: From £761
Specialist care: Day care, dementia, emergency admissions, mental disorder, physical disability, respite
Medical services: Podiatry, dentist, optician, physiotherapy
Qualified staff: Exceeds standard: 73% at NVQ level 2

Home details
Location: Residential area, 0.5 miles from Axminster
Communal areas: 5 lounges, 2 dining rooms, hairdressing salon, garden
Accessibility: *Floors:* 3 • *Access:* Lift and stair Lift • *Wheelchair access:* Good
Smoking: In designated area
Pets: At manager's discretion
Routines: Flexible

Room details
Single: 44
Shared: 5
En suite: 44
Facilities: TV, telephone point

Door lock: ✓
Lockable place: ✗

Services provided
Beauty services: Hairdressing
Mobile library: ✓
Religious services: Monthly combined church service
Transport: Minibus
Activities: *Coordinator:* ✓ • *Examples:* Bingo, book hour, singalongs
    Outings: ✓
Residents or relatives meetings: ✗

Registered places: 22
Guide weekly rate: £290–£430
Specialist care: Respite
Medical services: Podiatry
Qualified staff: Fails standard

Home details
Location: Village location, 3 miles from Cullompton
Communal areas: Lounge, garden, dining room
Accessibility: *Floors:* 2 • *Access:* Stair lift • *Wheelchair access:* Limited
Smoking: ✗
Pets: ✓
Routines: Flexible

Room details
Single: 21
Shared: 1
En suite: Undisclosed
Facilities: None

Door lock: ✓
Lockable place: ✓

Services provided
Beauty services: Hairdressing
Mobile library: ✗
Religious services: ✗
Transport: ✗
Activities: *Coordinator:* ✗ • *Examples:* Arts and crafts, entertainers
   Outings: ✓
Meetings: ✓

Somerville House

Manager: Sarah Kingdon
Owner: Graysar Associates Ltd
Contact: Somerville Road, Willand, Cullompton, Devon, EX15 2PP
☏ 01884 820811

Somerville House is a detached property that has been converted for its current use. The home is situated in a village, three miles from Cullompton. There is a range of activities on offer, including performances by visiting entertainers, and suggestions made by residents are considered. Visitors are always welcome in the home. The home also arranges outings for the residents in the local area.

Registered places: 24
Guide weekly rate: £275–£427
Specialist care: Physical disability, respite
Medical services: Podiatry, optician, physiotherapy
Qualified staff: Meets standard

Home details
Location: Residential area, 1.5 miles from Newton Abbot
Communal areas: 2 lounges, dining room, conservatory, garden
Accessibility: *Floors:* 2 • *Access:* Lift • *Wheelchair access:* Good
Smoking: ✗
Pets: ✗
Routines: Flexible

Room details
Single: 20
Shared: 2
En suite: 18
Facilities: TV point, telephone point

Door lock: ✓
Lockable place: ✓

Services provided
Beauty services: Hairdressing
Mobile library: ✓
Religious services: Weekly Christian service
Transport: ✗
Activities: *Coordinator:* ✗ • *Examples:* Bingo, visiting entertainers
   Outings: ✗
Meetings: ✗

Somerforde Ltd

Manager: Susan Hill
Owner: Somerforde Ltd
Contact: 2–3 Forde Park, Newton Abbot, Devon, TQ12 1DE
☏ 01626 361786

Somerforde Ltd is set in private grounds with views overlooking Forde Park, a conservation area. The home is situated in a residential area, one and a half miles from Newton Abbot. A mobile library visits the home on a regular basis and there is a Christian service once a week. The home arranges for performances by visiting entertainers and other activities such as bingo.

South Garth

Manager: Angela Westcott
Owner: Woodland Health Care Ltd
Contact: 1 Elwyn Road, Exmouth, Devon, EX8 2EL
☎ 01395 265422

A detached house with modern extension, South Garth is situated in a suburb of Exmouth, one mile from the town centre. With sheltered gardens the residents have a relaxing place to sit outside in the summer. The home also has two lounges for residents to socialise in. The home arranges a variety of activities which include armchair exercises and singalongs.

Registered places: 25
Guide weekly rate: £300–£400
Specialist care: Physical disability
Medical services: Undisclosed
Qualified staff: Meets standard

Home details
Location: Residential area, 1 mile from Exmouth
Communal areas: 2 lounges, dining room, garden
Accessibility: *Floors:* 2 • *Access:* Lift • *Wheelchair access:* Good
Smoking: ✗
Pets: ✗
Routines: Flexible

Room details
Single: 25
Shared: 0
En suite: Undisclosed
Facilities: None

Door lock: ✗
Lockable place: ✗

Services provided
Beauty services: Hairdressing
Mobile library: ✗
Religious services: ✗
Transport: ✗
Activities: *Coordinator:* ✗ • *Examples:* Armchair exercises, bingo, singalongs • *Outings:* ✗
Meetings: Undisclosed

South Lawn

Manager: Mrs Manning
Owner: Richard and Patricia Allin
Contact: 18 Hermosa Road, Teignmouth, Devon, TQ14 9JZ
☎ 01626 774117

Situated in a residential area above Teignmouth town centre, South Lawn is close to local amenities including the train station. The home is a few hundred yards away from the Teign estuary. The home's gardens have a fishpond and there is a lounge for residents to relax indoors. There is a residents meeting once a month to allow residents to voice any issues or opinions they may have.

Registered places: 20
Guide weekly rate: £306–£410
Specialist care: Physical disability
Medical services: Podiatry, hygienist, optician, physiotherapy
Qualified staff: Exceeds standard: 72% at NVQ level 2

Home details
Location: Residential area, 0.5 miles from Teignmouth
Communal areas: Lounge, dining room, garden
Accessibility: *Floors:* 2 • *Access:* Stair lift • *Wheelchair access:* Good
Smoking: ✗
Pets: ✓
Routines: Flexible

Room details
Single: 16
Shared: 2
En suite: 15
Facilities: TV point, telephone point

Door lock: ✓
Lockable place: ✓

Services provided
Beauty services: Hairdressing
Mobile library: ✓
Religious services: Fortnightly Communion service
Transport: ✗
Activities: *Coordinator:* ✓ • *Examples:* Musical entertainment, quizzes *Outings:* ✗
Meetings: ✓

Registered places: 21
Guide weekly rate: £325–£360
Specialist care: Day care, dementia, emergency admissions, physical disability, respite
Medical services: Podiatry, dentist, optician, physiotherapy
Qualified staff: Meets standard

Home details

Location: Residential area, 1 mile from Torquay
Communal areas: Lounge, dining room, patio and garden
Accessibility: *Floors:* 2 • *Access:* Stair lift
    Wheelchair access: Good
Smoking: In designated area
Pets: ✓
Routines: Flexible

Room details

Single: 17
Shared: 2
En suite: 19
Facilities: TV

Door lock: ✓
Lockable place: ✓

Services provided

Beauty services: Hairdressing, manicures
Mobile library: ✗
Religious services: ✓
Transport: ✓
Activities: *Coordinator:* ✓ • *Examples:* Games, films, exercise
    Outings: ✓
Meetings: ✗

Southbourne Residential Care Home

Manager: Vaughan Owen
Owner: Rosepost Healthcare Ltd
Contact: Cary Avenue, Babbacombe, Torquay, Devon, TQ1 3QT
☎ 01803 323502

Within walking distance of both local amenities and the Babbacombe Downs, Southbourne Residential Care Home is set in its own grounds with well-tended lawns and views of the Downs. The home is part of a group and is situated one mile from Torquay. The home employs an occupational therapist as well as an activities Coordinator who provides a varied activities program. This includes visiting entertainers, film showing and visits from the local museum with artefacts as well as outings. The home also has its own transport.

Registered places: 25
Guide weekly rate: £395–£485
Specialist care: Physical disability
Medical services: Podiatry, dentist, optician, physiotherapy
Qualified staff: Meets standard

Home details

Location: Residential area, 1 mile from Newton Abbot
Communal areas: 2 lounges, dining room, patio and garden
Accessibility: *Floors:* 2 • *Access:* Lift • *Wheelchair access:* Good
Smoking: ✗
Pets: ✓
Routines: Flexible

Room details

Single: 19
Shared: 3
En suite: 21
Facilities: TV point, telephone point

Door lock: ✓
Lockable place: ✓

Services provided

Beauty services: Hairdressing, aromatherapy
Mobile library: ✓
Religious services: Monthly Communion service
Transport: ✗
Activities: *Coordinator:* ✓ • *Examples:* Armchair exercises, musical entertainment • *Outings:* ✓
Meetings: ✓

Southlands Residential Care Home

Manager: Carol Dyke
Owner: Mark Harris and Paul Glanville
Contact: 21 Coombeshead Road, Highweek, Newton Abbot, Devon, TQ12 1PY
☎ 01626 363510

A 19th-century building that was formally the vicarage to the village church, Southlands is a large property set back from the road and situated in extensive grounds. A short drive from the main town centre, the village shops are a few minutes' walk away and the home is on a bus route. With large landscaped gardens remaining from the home's days as a rectory, outings which take advantage of the beautiful Devonshire countryside are arranged infrequently while entertainers visit the home monthly.

Southlands Court

Manager: Jennifer Hingston
Owner: Celia and Victor Goaman
Contact: Bridgerule, Holsworthy, Devon, EX22 7EW
) 01288 381631

A converted farmhouse that backs onto farmland, Southlands Court is well suited to those who like the outdoors, permitting open views of the surrounding countryside. The home's accessible gardens boast a pond and raised flowerbeds. It is a half-mile walk to the nearest shops and five miles to the town of Holsworthy. The home arranges an Anglican Communion service once a month and the home own a minibus which is used to take the residents on outings.

Registered places: 25
Guide weekly rate: £360
Specialist care: Day care, dementia, mental disorder, respite
Medical services: Podiatry, hygienist, optician, physiotherapy
Qualified staff: Fails standard

Home details
Location: Rural area, 5 miles from Holsworthy
Communal areas: 3 lounges, dining room, garden
Accessibility: *Floors:* 2 • *Access:* Stair lift • *Wheelchair access:* Limited
Smoking: In designated area
Pets: At manger's discretion
Routines: Flexible

Room details
Single: 25
Shared: 0
En suite: 25
Facilities: TV point, telephone point

Door lock: ✗
Lockable place: ✓

Services provided
Beauty services: Hairdressing
Mobile library: ✓
Religious services: Monthly Anglican Communion service
Transport: Minibus
Activities: *Coordinator:* ✓ • *Examples:* Bingo, cookery, singalongs
  Outings: ✓
Meetings: ✓

Southview

Manager: Vacant
Owner: Ashley Residential Care Ltd
Contact: Woodside, Lipson, Plymouth, Devon, PL4 8QE
) 01752 667853
@ southview@yahoo.co.uk

Situated in a residential area a few minutes' walk from local amenities and on a bus route, Southview is also a few minutes from its sister home, Park View. Having undergone refurbishment in 2006, the home is has an attractive courtyard and decked garden. Though the home does not offer locks on the bedroom doors due to the number of residents with dementia, there are electronic locks at the main doors for security.

Registered places: 19
Guide weekly rate: £275–£390
Specialist care: Dementia
Medical services: Podiatry, dentist, optician
Qualified staff: Exceeds standard: 100% at NVQ level 2

Home details
Location: Residential area, 1.5 miles from Plymouth
Communal areas: Lounge, dining room, garden
Accessibility: *Floors:* 1 • *Wheelchair access:* Good
Smoking: ✗
Pets: At manager's discretion
Routines: Flexible

Room details
Single: 17
Shared: 1
En suite: 8
Facilities: TV, telephone point

Door lock: ✗
Lockable place: ✓

Services provided
Beauty services: Hairdressing
Mobile library: ✓
Religious services: ✗
Transport: ✗
Activities: *Coordinator:* ✗ • *Examples:* Arts and crafts, musical movement, singalongs • *Outings:* ✓
Meetings: ✓

Registered places: 25
Guide weekly rate: £400–£800
Specialist care: Dementia, mental disorder
Medical services: Podiatry
Qualified staff: Meets standard

Home details
Location: Village location, 3 miles from Tavistock
Communal areas: Lounge, lounge/dining room,
    private lounge, garden
Accessibility: *Floors:* 2 • *Access:* Stair lift • *Wheelchair access:* Good
Smoking: ×
Pets: ×
Routines: Flexible

Room details
Single: 21
Shared: 2   Door lock: ×
En suite: 25   Lockable place: ×
Facilities: None

Services provided
Beauty services: Hairdressing
Mobile library: ×
Religious services: ×
Transport: ×
Activities: *Coordinator:* × • *Examples:* Bingo, musical entertainment
    Outings: ✓
Meetings: ×

Spring House

Manager: B Luckham
Owner: B Luckham
Contact: Peter Tavy, Tavistock,
Devon, PL19 9NP
) 01822 810465
@ shresidential@aol.com

Spring House, situated in the small village of Peter Tavy, lies three miles from Tavistock. There is a large paved garden in front of the house, with seating areas and a pergola. In addition to a large, bright lounge and a lounge/dining room, there is a smaller private lounge available for residents to receive phone calls or to meet with visitors. A list of planned activities is displayed on a notice board in the home and includes musical entertainment and bingo.

Registered places: 85
Guide weekly rate: £350–£500
Specialist care: Nursing, dementia, mental disorder,
    physical disability
Medical services: Podiatry
Qualified staff: Undisclosed

Home details
Location: Residential area, 4 miles from Plymouth
Communal areas: 5 lounges, 4 dining rooms, garden
Accessibility: *Floors:* 2 • *Access:* 2 lifts • *Wheelchair access:* Good
Smoking: ×
Pets: ✓
Routines: Flexible

Room details
Single: 72
Shared: 0   Door lock: ×
En suite: 72   Lockable place: ×
Facilities: None

Services provided
Beauty services: Hairdressing
Mobile library: ×
Religious services: ×
Transport: Minibus
Activities: *Coordinator:* ✓ • *Examples:* Bingo • *Outings:* ×
Meetings: ×

Springfields Care Centre

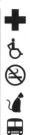

Manager: Nicola Kelly
Owner: Four Seasons Healthcare Ltd
Contact: 33 Springfield Road, Elburton,
Plymouth, Devon, PL9 8EJ
) 01752 482662
⌨ www.fshc.co.uk

Springfields Care Centre is a purpose-built home providing three units specialising in nursing care for dementia patients, general nursing care and residential care. Each unit has its own lounge and dining room areas. The home has its own minibus for transportation and an activities coordinator arranges daily activities such as bingo for the residents.

St Andrews

Manager: Angela Cunningham
Owner: Brenda and Barry Wise
Contact: 1–5 Pye Corner, Church Street, Cullompton, Devon, EX15 1JX
☎ 01884 32369

Comprised of two buildings, St Andrews is situated just off the main shopping street in Cullompton where there are shops, cafés and a health centre. The home has a garden with a patio area in addition to two lounges. The home arranges a variety of group activities such as quizzes and exercise sessions as well as one-to-one sessions. There is a residents meeting every six to eight weeks to allow residents to voice their opinions.

Registered places: 23
Guide weekly rate: £295–£400
Specialist care: Day care, dementia, mental disorder, physical disability, respite
Medical services: Podiatry, optician, physiotherapy
Qualified staff: Fails standard

Home details
Location: Residential area, 0.5 miles from Cullompton
Communal areas: 2 lounges, dining room, garden
Accessibility: *Floors:* 2 • *Access:* Lift • *Wheelchair access:* Good
Smoking: ✗
Pets: ✓
Routines: Flexible

Room details
Single: 21
Shared: 1
En suite: 15
Facilities: TV point, telephone point

Door lock: ✓
Lockable place: ✓

Services provided
Beauty services: Hairdressing
Mobile library: ✗
Religious services: Monthly Communion service
Transport: ✗
Activities: *Coordinator:* ✗ • *Examples:* Games, quizzes, exercise
　　Outings: ✓
Meetings: ✓

St Annes Residential Home

Manager: Brian Ward
Owner: Brian Ward
Contact: 4 Houndiscombe Road, Mutley, Plymouth, Devon, PL4 6HH
☎ 01752 661667
@ rod929@btinternet.com

St Annes is located an easy five to 10-minute walk from the centre of Plymouth. Residents often go on trips to nearby Peignton and Hove and the home has its own car for transport. Although there is no garden at the home, there is a secure patio area which has a canopy, making the area useable all year round. The home arranges an Anglican services to take place at the home once a month.

Registered places: 23
Guide weekly rate: £326
Specialist care: Dementia
Medical services: Podiatry, hygienist, optician, physiotherapy
Qualified staff: Meets standard

Home details
Location: Residential area, 1 mile from Plymouth
Communal areas: 2 lounges, dining room, conservatory, patio
Accessibility: *Floors:* 2 • *Access:* Stair lift • *Wheelchair access:* Good
Smoking: In designated area
Pets: ✓
Routines: Flexible

Room details
Single: 11
Shared: 6
En suite: 7
Facilities: TV point, telephone point

Door lock: ✓
Lockable place: ✓

Services provided
Beauty services: Hairdressing, manicures
Mobile library: ✓
Religious services: Monthly Anglican service
Transport: Car
Activities: *Coordinator:* ✓ • *Examples:* Bingo, chairobics
　　Outings: ✓
Meetings: ✗

Registered places: 19
Guide weekly rate: £375–£440
Specialist care: Mental disorder, physical disability
Medical services: Podiatry, dentist, optician
Qualified staff: Exceeds standard: 74% at NVQ level 2

Home details
Location: Residential area, 1 mile from Tiverton
Communal areas: 2 lounges, dining room, library, patio and garden
Accessibility: *Floors:* 2 • *Access:* None • *Wheelchair access:* Limited
Smoking: In designated area
Pets: ✗
Routines: Flexible

Room details
Single: 13
Shared: 3
En suite: 10
Facilities: TV point, telephone point

Door lock: ✓
Lockable place: ✓

Services provided
Beauty services: Hairdressing
Mobile library: Library facilities
Religious services: Monthly Catholic Communion service,
    monthly Anglican Communion service
Transport: ✗
Activities: *Coordinator:* ✗ • *Examples:* Bingo • *Outings:* ✓
Meetings: ✗

St George's Residential Care Home

Manager: Maureen Lindley
Owner: Brian and Maureen Lindley
Contact: Park Road, Tiverton, Devon, EX16 6AU
) 01884 252436
@ st.georgeshouse@virgin.net

St George's is situated in its own grounds next to Tiverton Park and five minutes' walk from Tiverton town with its range of amenities and facilities. With free parking for residents who wish to keep their own car, the home is well equipped for independent living. A paved garden at the front of the home can be used by residents with an interest in gardening while lawned gardens are at the back of the house. St George's currently has a dog and the home enjoys visits from Pets As Therapy.

Registered places: 38
Guide weekly rate: From £438
Specialist care: Nursing, physical disability, respite
Medical services: Podiatry, dentist, optician, physiotherapy
Qualified staff: Meets standard

Home details
Location: Residential area, 1.7 miles from Plymouth
Communal areas: 4 lounges, dining room, patio and garden
Accessibility: *Floors:* 2 • *Access:* Lift • *Wheelchair access:* Good
Smoking: ✗
Pets: At manager's discretion
Routines: Flexible

Room details
Single: 26
Shared: 6
En suite: 11
Facilities: TV point

Door lock: ✓
Lockable place: ✓

Services provided
Beauty services: Hairdressing
Mobile library: ✓
Religious services: ✗
Transport: Minibus
Activities: *Coordinator:* ✗ • *Examples:* Exercise, singalongs,
    visiting entertainers • *Outings:* ✓
Meetings: ✗

St James' Lodge

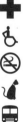

Manager: Fiona Miller
Owner: Sydney Sutherland
Contact: 74 Molesworth Road, Stoke, Plymouth, Devon, PL1 5PF
) 01752 563003
@ s.jl@btinternet.com

A large Georgian property with a level entrance, St James' Lodge is situated about 25 minutes' walk from village amenities. Well located with a bus stop just outside the home, there are services going into Plymouth city centre. The home has well-maintained gardens that include a pond and sheltered sitting area. Residents who desire to leave the home must inform the nurse in charge. While outings are not necessarily regular, bus trips are usually offered twice a week.

St Omer

Manager: Joanna Day
Owner: Ian and Joanna Day
Contact: Greenway Road, Chelston, Torquay, Devon, TQ2 6JE
) 01803 605336
@ enquiries@st-omer.org
⌐ www.st-omer.org

A detached Victorian villa situated in a quiet residential area, St Omer's location permits sea views over Torbay. The home boasts one acre of beautiful landscaped gardens, with a gazebo and specimen trees including a magnolia. Fruit and vegetables planted within the home's gardens are used for meals. There is an Anglican Communion service every two weeks in the home and a service once a month.

Registered places: 24
Guide weekly rate: £360–£400
Specialist care: Day care, dementia, physical disability, respite
Medical services: Podiatry, optician
Qualified staff: Exceeds standard: 100% at NVQ level 2

Home details
Location: Residential area, 1 mile from Torquay
Communal areas: 2 lounges, dining room, conservatory, garden
Accessibility: *Floors:* 2 • *Access:* Lift • *Wheelchair access:* Good
Smoking: ✗
Pets: ✓
Routines: Flexible

Room details
Single: 20
Shared: 4
En suite: 22
Facilities: TV point, telephone point

Door lock: ✓
Lockable place: ✓

Services provided
Beauty services: Hairdressing, manicures
Mobile library: ✓
Religious services: Fortnightly Anglican Communion service
Transport: ✗
Activities: *Coordinator:* ✓ • *Examples:* Arts and crafts, bingo, exercise
Outings: ✓
Meetings: ✓

Strand House

Manager: Mrs Pigott
Owner: Mr and Mrs Pigott
Contact: The Strand, Starcross, Exeter, Devon, EX6 8PA
) 01626 890880
@ pepigs@starcross.fsnet.co.uk

A listed building, Strand House is a small, family-run home where the owners live on the premises. Situated in the seaside town of Starcross close to its train station the home is also near the beach. Linking to the homely atmosphere, the home's dining area is in the kitchen where all residents can be accommodated at mealtimes.

Registered places: 8
Guide weekly rate: £280–£318
Specialist care: Physical disability
Medical services: Podiatry, dentist, optician
Qualified staff: Fails standard

Home details
Location: Residential area, 9 miles from Exeter
Communal areas: 2 lounges, garden
Accessibility: *Floors:* 2 • *Access:* Stair lift • *Wheelchair access:* Good
Smoking: ✗
Pets: ✗
Routines: Undisclosed

Room details
Single: 6
Shared: 1
En suite: 0
Facilities: TV point, telephone point

Door lock: ✗
Lockable place: ✗

Services provided
Beauty services: Hairdressing
Mobile library: ✓
Religious services: Monthly Anglican Communion service
Transport: ✗
Activities: *Coordinator:* ✗ • *Examples:* Games, videos
Outings: ✓
Meetings: ✗

Registered places: 20
Guide weekly rate: £306–£436
Specialist care: Day care, respite
Medical services: Podiatry, optician, physiotherapy
Qualified staff: Exceeds standard: 60% at NVQ level 2

Home details
Location: Residential area, 0.5 miles from Teignmouth
Communal areas: 2 lounges, dining room, patio and garden
Accessibility: *Floors:* 4 • *Access:* Lift • *Wheelchair access:* Good
Smoking: In designated area
Pets: ✕
Routines: Flexible

Room details
Single: 18
Shared: 1   Door lock: ✓
En suite: 19   Lockable place: ✓
Facilities: TV point, telephone point

Services provided
Beauty services: Hairdressing
Mobile library: ✓
Religious services: Monthly Anglican Communion service
Transport: ✕
Activities: *Coordinator:* ✓ • *Examples:* Chairobics, quizzes
    Outings: ✓
Meetings: ✓

Summercourt

Manager: Rebecca Coulson
Owner: Classic Care Homes Ltd
Contact: Shute Hill, Teignmouth,
Devon, TQ14 8JD
📞 01626 778580

A listed building, Summercourt is situated five minutes from the town centre, providing easy access to local amenities including a station. The home is a few hundred yards from the seafront. Summercourt is a nurse-managed home with landscaped gardens including a pond and snacks are readily available on a 24-hour basis. The home arranges an Anglican Communion service once a month.

Registered places: 14
Guide weekly rate: From £400
Specialist care: None
Medical services: Podiatry, dentist, optician, physiotherapy
Qualified staff: Meets standard

Home details
Location: Residential area, 0.5 miles from Exmouth
Communal areas: Lounge, dining room, internet café, patio
    and garden
Accessibility: *Floors:* 2 • *Access:* Stair lift • *Wheelchair access:* Good
Smoking: ✕
Pets: ✕
Routines: Flexible

Room details
Single: 14
Shared: 0   ·   Door lock: ✓
En suite: 14   Lockable place: ✓
Facilities: TV, telephone

Services provided
Beauty services: Hairdressing, aromatherapy, manicures
Mobile library: ✓
Religious services: ✓
Transport: ✓
Activities: *Coordinator:* ✓ • *Examples:* Games • *Outings:* ✓
Meetings: ✕

Summerleaze Residential Care Home

Manager: Lorraine Covell
Owner: Summerleaze Home Ltd
Contact: 79 Salterton Road, Exmouth,
Devon, EX8 2EW
📞 01395 279349
@ admin@summerleazecare.co.uk
🖱 www.summerleazecare.co.uk

Summerleaze is a small home situated half a mile from the centre of Exmouth. The home has a lounge, a dining room and a garden with a patio area. The home also has its own internet café with WIFI and broadband throughout the home. There is also a webcam for residents to keep in touch with friends and family. The home has its own activities coordinator who builds the programme around the residents' wishes. The home also has its own transport and arranges for a mobile library to visit. The home is surrounded by award winning gardens.

Sundial Lodge

Manager: Sonja Brotherton
Owner: Sundial Lodge Ltd
Contact: Park Hill Road,
Torquay, Devon, TQ1 2EA
) 01803 292889
@ Sundial.lodge@eclipse.co.uk
www.sundial-lodge.co.uk

Situated close to the seafront and 10 minutes from the town centre, Sundial Lodge is a listed Georgian building made up of self-contained apartments that include individual bathrooms and kitchens. Offering an unusual set up to maximise independence and security, residents are free to 'come and go as they please'. A three-course lunch is offered every day around midday while groceries are on offer for the remaining meals unless a resident should require meals to be prepared for them.

Registered places: 48
Guide weekly rate: From £420
Specialist care: Respite
Medical services: Podiatry, dentist, optician, physiotherapy
Qualified staff: Exceeds standard: 75% at NVQ level 2

Home details
Location: Residential area, 2 mile from Torquay
Communal areas: Lounges, dining room, patio and garden
Accessibility: *Floors:* 3 • *Access:* Lift and stair lift
Wheelchair access: Good
Smoking: ✓
Pets: Only birds allowed
Routines: Flexible

Room details
Single: 42
Shared: 3
En suite: 45
Facilities: TV, telephone

Door lock: ✓
Lockable place: ✓

Services provided
Beauty services: Hairdressing, manicures
Mobile library: ✓
Religious services: ✓
Transport: Minibus
Activities: *Coordinator:* ✓ • *Examples:* Bingo, games, quizzes, visiting entertainers • *Outings:* ✓
Meetings: ✓

Sunnymeade

Manager: Wendy Dunn
Owner: Wendy Dunn
Contact: 323 Tavistock Road, Derriford,
Plymouth, Devon, PL6 8AE
) 01752 781811

Situated in a residential area, Sunnymeade is currently in the middle of a refurbishment programme. The entire home is being upgraded, en suite facilities are being added to all the rooms and a sensory garden is being installed. The home is located close to the moors and the sea. The home has its own minibus for outings and other activities on offer include exercise sessions and performances by visiting entertainers.

Registered places: 30
Guide weekly rate: £400–£450
Specialist care: Dementia, mental disorder, physical disability, respite
Medical services: Podiatry, hygienist, optician, physiotherapy
Qualified staff: Exceeds standard: 94% at NVQ level 2

Home details
Location: Residential area, 4.5 miles from Plymouth
Communal areas: 4 lounges, 2 dining rooms, garden
Accessibility: *Floors:* 2 • *Access:* Lift • *Wheelchair access:* Good
Smoking: In designated area
Pets: ✓
Routines: Flexible

Room details
Single: 28
Shared: 1
En suite: Undisclosed
Facilities: TV point, telephone point

Door lock: ✓
Lockable place: ✓

Services provided
Beauty services: Hairdressing
Mobile library: ✓
Religious services: Monthly Communion service
Transport: Minibus
Activities: *Coordinator:* ✓ • *Examples:* Exercises, karaoke, visiting entertainers • *Outings:* ✓
Meetings: ✓

Registered places: 30
Guide weekly rate: £300–£550
Specialist care: Dementia, emergency admissions, mental disorder, physical disability, respite
Medical services: Podiatry, dentist, optician
Qualified staff: Fails standard

Home details

Location: Residential area, 0.5 miles from Seaton centre
Communal areas: 2 lounges, dining room, garden
Accessibility: *Floors:* 2 • *Access:* Stair lift • *Wheelchair access:* Good
Smoking: In designated area
Pets: ✗
Routines: Flexible

Room details

Single: 21
Shared: 3
En suite: 12
Door lock: ✓
Lockable place: ✗
Facilities: TV point, telephone point

Services provided

Beauty services: Hairdressing
Mobile library: ✗
Religious services: Monthly Anglican Communion service
Transport: Minibus
Activities: *Coordinator:* ✓ • *Examples:* Bingo, cooking, knitting
  Outings: ✓
Meetings: ✓

Swallowcliffe Retirement Hotel

Manager: Michelle Connett
Owner: Starlight Care Ltd
Contact: Old Beer Road,
Seaton, Devon, EX12 2PZ
☏ 01297 22629
@ bivianbaksh342@freeserve.co.uk

Set in a prime location overlooking beautiful coastal scenery, the Swallowcliffe Retirement Hotel began life, as its name suggests, as a hotel. Still retaining many of its original features including en suite bathrooms, it also houses one single and one double self-contained flat suited to more able individuals. Situated approximately 15 minutes' walk from the nearest shop, the home is close to Seaton's amenities which include bowling clubs and a promenade. Residents will enjoy exploring the home's gardens which have a terrace as well as flowerbeds and a variety of shrubs.

Registered places: 14
Guide weekly rate: £306–£420
Specialist care: Dementia, physical disability
Medical services: Podiatry, hygienist, optician, physiotherapy
Qualified staff: Meets standard

Home details

Location: Rural area, 3.5 miles from Okehampton
Communal areas: Lounge, dining room, conservatory, garden
Accessibility: *Floors:* 3 • *Access:* Lift • *Wheelchair access:* Good
Smoking: ✗
Pets: ✓
Routines: Flexible

Room details

Single: 10
Shared: 2
En suite: 9
Door lock: ✓
Lockable place: ✓
Facilities: TV point, telephone point

Services provided

Beauty services: Hairdressing
Mobile library: ✗
Religious services: Monthly Communion service
Transport: Car
Activities: *Coordinator:* ✓ • *Examples:* Bingo, chair aerobics
  Outings: ✗
Meetings: ✗

Tawburn House

Manager: Desmond Underwood
Owner: Desmond and Anne Underwood
Contact: Sticklepath, Okehampton,
Devon, EX20 2NL
☏ 01837 840737
⌂ www.tawburnhouse.co.uk

Situated in the centre of Sticklepath village, this Victorian property lies next to the village hall. The home is located in a rural area, three and a half miles from Okehampton. The home has been involved in an allotment project that encourages the local community to grow their own food. The home also has its own car for transport and arranges a variety of activities for residents such as bingo and chair aerobics.

DEVON

Thomas Pocklington Trust

Manager: Janis Lane
Owner: Thomas Pocklington Trust
Contact: Peirson House, Mulgrave Street, Plymouth, Devon, PL1 2RW
☎ 01752 662394

The Thomas Pocklington Trust offers care for older people with visual impairment and is situated in an urban area, just under one mile from Plymouth. The home has several lounges and dining areas as well as a garden. There are a variety of activities on offer including bingo and newspaper discussion. The home also organises outings for the residents. There are residents meetings held on a regular basis to give residents the opportunity to voice any issues they may have.

Registered places: 32
Guide weekly rate: £450
Specialist care: Dementia, respite
Medical services: Podiatry, optician
Qualified staff: Exceeds standard: 100% at NVQ level 2

Home details
Location: Urban area, 0.7 miles from Plymouth
Communal areas: Lounges, dining room, garden
Accessibility: *Floors:* 3 • *Access:* Lift • *Wheelchair access:* Good
Smoking: In designated area
Pets: ✗
Routines: Flexible

Room details
Single: 32
Shared: 0
En suite: 0
Facilities: Telephone point

Door lock: ✓
Lockable place: ✓

Services provided
Beauty services: Hairdressing
Mobile library: ✗
Religious services: ✓
Transport: ✓
Activities: *Coordinator:* ✓ • *Examples:* Bingo, newspaper discussion
　　　　　Outings: ✓
Meetings: ✓

Thornbury Villa

Manager: James Van Deijl
Owner: James and Jacqueline Van Deijl
Contact: 128 Peverell Park Road, Peverell, Plymouth, Devon, PL3 4NE
☎ 01752 262204
@ sunburyvilla@btconnect.com

Thornbury Villa is situated in a residential area, two miles from Plymouth with easy access to local shops and amenities. Visitors have said it seems like a real home, and the new conservatory is a favourite with all the residents. Thornbury Villa has a garden with a patio area in addition to the conservatory and the home arranges for a mobile library to visit. There is a varied activities programme which includes bingo and painting. There are also regular residents meetings. The home is perfect for low dependency residents, offering activities and exercise as well as independence.

Registered places: 13
Guide weekly rate: £315–£385
Specialist care: None
Medical services: Podiatry, dentist, optician, physiotherapy
Qualified staff: Exceeds standard: 90% at NVQ level 2

Home details
Location: Residential area, 2 miles from Plymouth
Communal areas: Lounge, dining room, conservatory, patio and garden
Accessibility: *Floors:* 2 • *Access:* Stair lift • *Wheelchair access:* Good
Smoking: ✗
Pets: At manager's discretion
Routines: Structured

Room details
Single: 13
Shared: 0
En suite: 13
Facilities: TV, telephone point

Door lock: ✓
Lockable place: ✓

Services provided
Beauty services: Hairdressing
Mobile library: ✓
Religious services: ✗
Transport: ✗
Activities: *Coordinator:* ✗ • *Examples:* Bingo, darts, painting
　　　　　Outings: ✗
Meetings: ✓

Registered places: 24
Guide weekly rate: Undisclosed
Specialist care: Day care, physical disability
Medical services: Podiatry
Qualified staff: Undisclosed

Home details
Location: Rural area, 6.5 miles from Newton Abbot
Communal areas: 2 lounges, dining room, 2 summerhouses,
    conservatory, garden
Accessibility: *Floors:* 2 *Access:* Lift and stair lift
    Wheelchair access: Limited
Smoking: ✗
Pets: ✓
Routines: Structured

Room details
Single: 22
Shared: 1
En suite: 21
Facilities: None

Door lock: ✓
Lockable place: ✓

Services provided
Beauty services: Hairdressing
Mobile library: ✓
Religious services: Weekly Communion service
Transport: Car
Activities: *Coordinator:* ✗ • *Examples:* Exercises, gardening, video
    afternoons • *Outings:* ✓
Meetings: ✓

Tracey House

Manager: Mrs Zakrzewski
Owner: Mr and Mrs Cooksey,
Dr and Mrs J T Zakrzewski
Contact: Haytor Road, Bovey Tracey,
Newton Abbot, Devon, TQ13 9LE
☏ 01626 833281

Set in two and half acres of attractive grounds, Tracey House is surrounded by beautiful gardens that feature fruit trees, a vegetable garden and seating areas. There are two summerhouses and a conservatory which all provide pleasant seating areas for residents in fine weather. Outings are made in cars into town, where residents can go shopping or for coffee. The home also organises internal activities such as exercise sessions and video afternoons.

Registered places: 24
Guide weekly rate: £333–£480
Specialist care: Day care, dementia, emergency admissions,
    mental disorder, respite
Medical services: Podiatry, dentist, optician
Qualified staff: Meets standard

Home details
Location: Residential area, 1.2 miles from Plymouth
Communal areas: 2 lounges, dining room, bar, library,
    conservatory, garden
Accessibility: *Floors:* 2 • *Access:* Lift • *Wheelchair access:* Good
Smoking: In designated area
Pets: At manager's discretion
Routines: Flexible

Room details
Single: 20
Shared: 2
En suite: 14
Facilities: TV point

Door lock: ✓
Lockable place: ✓

Services provided
Beauty services: Hairdressing, reflexology
Mobile library: Library facilities
Religious services: Quarterly nondenominational Communion service
Transport: Minibus
Activities: *Coordinator:* ✓ • *Examples:* Bingo, film nights, quizzes
    Outings: ✓
Meetings: ✓

Trenant House Residential Home

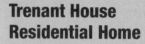

Manager: Julie Franks
Owner: Julie and Peter Franks
Contact: Queens Road, Lipson,
Plymouth, Devon, PL4 7PJ
☏ 01752 663879
@ renantpl4@btopenworld.com

A Victorian building that was originally a hotel, Trenant House is situated in its own grounds across the road from a newsagents. Just over a mile from Plymouth the city centre is easily accessed by a bus which stops just outside the home. Trenant House is a small care home which offers daily activities. The home also produces a newsletter entitled the Trenant Tribune which provides information on the activities on offer within the home. While drinks and snacks are always available, those who are capable are able to prepare their own in the bar area of the dining room.

Tudor Cottage

Manager: Christopher Love
Owner: Christopher and Norma Love
Contact: 7–8 South Street, Axminster, Devon, EX13 5AD

) 01297 33016
@ tudorcottage-carehome.co.uk

A renovated period building, Tudor Cottage is a cottage property situated in the centre of Axminster, next door to the library and a few hundred yards from the post office. With the owners living just behind the home, they are readily involved in its day-to-day running. The home has a small, enclosed garden with a fishpond. Although residents are not allowed to bring pets to the home, Tudor Cottage has its own cats and birds. The home arranges an Anglican Communion service once a month and a nondenominational service once a month.

Registered places: 19
Guide weekly rate: £485–£515
Specialist care: Day care, dementia, respite
Medical services: Podiatry, dentist, optician
Qualified staff: Fails standard

Home details
Location: Residential area, 0.3 miles from Axminster
Communal areas: 2 lounges, dining room, hairdressing salon, garden
Accessibility: *Floors:* 2 • *Access:* Stair lift • *Wheelchair access:* Good
Smoking: ✗
Pets: ✗
Routines: Flexible

Room details
Single: 15
Shared: 2
En suite: 12
Facilities: TV point, telephone point

Door lock: ✓
Lockable place: ✓

Services provided
Beauty services: Hairdressing
Mobile library: ✗
Religious services: Monthly Anglican Communion service, monthly nondenominational service
Transport: ✗
Activities: *Coordinator:* ✗ • *Examples:* Exercise, musical entertainment • *Outings:* ✓
Meetings: ✗

Tudor Court

Manager: Jean Entwistle
Owner: Royston Lock
Contact: 18–20 Midvale Road, Paignton, Devon, TQ4 5BD

) 01803 558374

Tudor Court is a large mid-terraced property that began life as two separate houses and has been renovated into a single home. The home lies close to Paignton's local amenities and the south Devon coast. Paignton town centre is only half a mile away. Residents are encouraged to treat Tudor Court as their home and many bring in their own furniture and other personal possessions. The home also arranges for musicians to come and entertain the residents and lead them in singalongs.

Registered places: 31
Guide weekly rate: £310–£400
Specialist care: Dementia, mental disorder, physical disability, respite
Medical services: None
Qualified staff: Meets standard

Home details
Location: Residential area, 0.5 miles from Paignton
Communal areas: Lounge, conservatory, patio
Accessibility: *Floors:* 4 • *Access:* Lift • *Wheelchair access:* Good
Smoking: In designated area
Pets: ✓
Routines: Flexible

Room details
Single: 27
Shared: 2
En suite: 21
Facilities: None

Door lock: ✗
Lockable place: ✗

Services provided
Beauty services: None
Mobile library: ✗
Religious services: ✗
Transport: ✗
Activities: *Coordinator:* ✗ • *Examples:* Musicians, singalongs *Outings:* ✗
Meetings: ✗

Registered places: 28
Guide weekly rate: £326
Specialist care: Dementia
Medical services: Podiatry
Qualified staff: Meets standard

Home details
Location: Residential area, 2 miles from Plymouth
Communal areas: Undisclosed
Accessibility: *Floors:* Undisclosed • *Access:* Lift
  Wheelchair access: Good
Smoking: ✗
Pets: ✗
Routines: Flexible

Room details
Single: 21
Shared: 4
En suite: Undisclosed
Facilities: None

Door lock: ✓
Lockable place: ✓

Services provided
Beauty services: Hairdressing
Mobile library: ✗
Religious services: ✗
Transport: ✗
Activities: *Coordinator:* ✗ • *Examples:* Arts and crafts, bingo,
  musical entertainment • *Outings:* ✓
Meetings: ✓

Underhill House

Manager: Linda Turner
Owner: Linda and Michael Turner
Contact: Underhill Road, Stoke,
Plymouth, Devon, PL3 4BP
☎ 01752 561638

Situated in a residential area near local facilities and close to a bus stop with routes into the city centre, Underhill House lies two miles from Plymouth. The home provides a homely environment for residents. The home arranges regular residents meetings and there are daily activities planned such as bingo and musical entertainment. The home also takes the residents on regular outings in the local area.

Registered places: 19
Guide weekly rate: £360–£400
Specialist care: Dementia, mental disorder
Medical services: Podiatry, dentist, optician
Qualified staff: Undisclosed

Home details
Location: Residential area, 1 mile from Plymouth
Communal areas: Lounge, dining room, garden
Accessibility: *Floors:* 2 • *Access:* Stair lift • *Wheelchair access:* Good
Smoking: ✗
Pets: ✗
Routines: Flexible

Room details
Single: 17
Shared: 1
En suite: 12
Facilities: TV

Door lock: ✓
Lockable place: ✓

Services provided
Beauty services: Hairdressing
Mobile library: ✗
Religious services: ✗
Transport: ✗
Activities: *Coordinator:* ✗ • *Examples:* Birthday celebrations
  Outings: ✓
Meetings: ✗

Vale Lodge Residential Home

Manager: Sheree Haswell
Owner: Sheree Haswell and Martin Atwill
Contact: 38–40 Sutherland Road,
Mutley, Plymouth, Devon, PL4 6BN
☎ 01752 220456
@ valelodgepl@btopenworld.com

Vale Lodge is within walking distance of the Mutley Plain shopping centre in Plymouth. The home is situated in a residential area, one mile from the town centre. There is a large lounge which looks out onto the back garden, a dining room on the ground floor of the home and an enclosed walled garden at the rear. The home regularly organises outings for residents, including regular trips to the sea and for afternoon tea at the local garden centre.

Valley View

Manager: Debra Sole
Owner: John and Jill Stevens
Contact: 298 Fort Austin Avenue,
Crownhill, Plymouth, Devon, PL6 5FR
) 01752 705109
@ valleyviewpl6@btopenworld.com

Named for the fantastic views it has over the surrounding countryside, Valley View is a bungalow situated in a residential area five minutes from local shops. The home is also on a bus route and only three miles from Plymouth, giving plenty of scope for the fortnightly outings the home offers. With open, sunny rooms and a lounge which overlooks the garden, residents may also enjoy the dining room with its French doors which lead out onto the terrace. The home's landscaped gardens are well maintained with level paths and a pleasant area to relax in during the summer months.

Registered places: 17
Guide weekly rate: From £350
Specialist care: Emergency admissions, respite
Medical services: Podiatry, dentist, optician, physiotherapy
Qualified staff: Meets standard

Home details
Location: Residential area, 3 miles from Plymouth
Communal areas: Lounge, dining room, library, garden
Accessibility: *Floors:* 1 • *Wheelchair access:* Good
Smoking: ✗
Pets: ✓
Routines: Flexible

Room details
Single: 17
Shared: 0
En suite: 6
Door lock: ✓
Lockable place: ✓
Facilities: TV point, telephone point

Services provided
Beauty services: Hairdressing
Mobile library: Library facilities
Religious services: ✗
Transport: ✗
Activities: *Coordinator.* ✗ • *Examples:* Bingo, keep fit • *Outings:* ✓
Meetings: ✓

Vicarage House Residential Home

Manager: Christina Czerwinsky
Owner: Dr Pepper's Care Corporation Ltd
Contact: 1 Honicknowle Lane,
Pennycross, Plymouth, Devon, PL2 3QR
) 01752 779050
@ vicaragehsepl2@btopenworld.com

Sited in a residential area, Vicarage House Residential Home is located a few hundred yards from a park and three mile from Plymouth city centre. As part of the home's extensive activities programme, a monthly newsletter is produced. The activities the home offers includes exercise sessions and musical entertainment. There are also regular outings planned. The home arranges a Communion service every six weeks and there are regular residents meetings.

Registered places: 32
Guide weekly rate: £275–£300
Specialist care: Physical disability, respite
Medical services: Podiatry, optician
Qualified staff: Fails standard

Home details
Location: Residential area, 3 miles from Plymouth
Communal areas: 2 lounges, dining room, conservatory, garden
Accessibility: *Floors:* 2 • *Access:* Lift and stair lift
Wheelchair access: Good
Smoking: In designated area
Pets: At manager's discretion
Routines: Flexible

Room details
Single: 26
Shared: 3
En suite: 0
Door lock: ✓
Lockable place: ✓
Facilities: TV point, telephone point

Services provided
Beauty services: Hairdressing
Mobile library: ✓
Religious services: Communion service every 6 weeks
Transport: ✗
Activities: *Coordinator.* ✓ • *Examples:* Bingo, keep fit, musical entertainment • *Outings:* ✓
Meetings: ✓

Registered places: 24
Guide weekly rate: £306–£445
Specialist care: Day care, dementia, mental disorder, physical disability, respite
Medical services: Podiatry, optician, physiotherapy
Qualified staff: Meets standard

Home details
Location: Residential area, 0.3 miles from Salcombe
Communal areas: 2 lounges, dining room, garden
Accessibility: *Floors:* 2 • *Access:* Lift and stair lift
Wheelchair access: Good
Smoking: ✗
Pets: At manager's discretion
Routines: Flexible

Room details
Single: 24
Shared: 0
En suite: 21
Facilities: TV point, telephone point

Door lock: ✓
Lockable place: ✓

Services provided
Beauty services: Hairdressing
Mobile library: ✓
Religious services: Monthly Anglican Communion service
Transport: Minibus
Activities: *Coordinator.* ✗ • *Examples:* Games, quizzes, visiting entertainers • *Outings:* ✓
Meetings: ✗

Wells Court
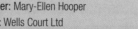

Manager: Mary-Ellen Hooper
Owner: Wells Court Ltd
Contact: Herbert Road, Salcombe, Devon, TQ8 8HD
) 01548 843484

Situated in the picturesque sailing area of Salcombe, Wells Court is very close to the Kingsbridge Estuary. The home is located in a residential area, less than half a mile from Salcombe. The home has two lounges and a garden and arranges frequent outings in the local area. There is an Anglican Communion service once a month and regular visits from a mobile library. In addition to outings the home arranges internal activities such as quizzes and performances by visiting entertainers.

Registered places: 22
Guide weekly rate: £340–£400
Specialist care: Respite
Medical services: Podiatry, dentist, optician
Qualified staff: Exceeds standard: 85% at NVQ level 2

Home details
Location: Rural area, 9 miles from Beaworthy
Communal areas: Lounge, dining room, 2 conservatories, garden
Accessibility: *Floors:* 2 • *Access:* Stair lift • *Wheelchair access:* Good
Smoking: ✗
Pets: At manager's discretion
Routines: Flexible

Room details
Single: 16
Shared: 3
En suite: 21
Facilities: TV point, telephone point

Door lock: ✓
Lockable place: ✓

Services provided
Beauty services: Hairdressing, aromatherapy
Mobile library: ✓
Religious services: Monthly Communion service
Transport: Car
Activities: *Coordinator.* ✓ • *Examples:* Painting, quizzes • *Outings:* ✓
Meetings: ✓

West Heanton

Manager: Thomas Bond
Owner: West Heanton Ltd
Contact: Buckland Filleigh, Shebbear, Beaworthy, Devon, EX21 5PJ
) 01409 281754
@ enquiries@westheanton.co.uk
www.westheanton.co.uk

An older-style property that was once an old farmhouse, West Heanton Ltd is a family-run home set in attractive grounds. The home is located in a rural area, nine miles from Beaworthy. The home has its own car for transportation and residents are taken on outings in the local area. The home also publishes a newsletter every three months and there is a residents meeting every eight weeks. The home also arranges a Communion service to take place once a month.

West View Residential Care Home

Manager: Trevor Atkinson
Owner: Peninsula Care Ltd
Contact: 72 Broad Park Road,
Bere Alston, Yelverton, Devon, PL20 7DU
☎ 01822 840674
@ west.view@tiscali.co.uk

Located in the Bere Peninsula close to Tavistock, West View Residential Care Home is situated in a village within 10 minutes' walk of local amenities and on a bus route. With attractive gardens and patio areas that include flowerpots and a greenhouse, residents may also wish to take advantage of the weekly outings on offer. A monthly newsletter gives up-to-date information on activities planned and community events. Telephone calls costing up to around £7 a month are free. The home is introducing digital TV for all televisions in resident's bedrooms. West View currently has a cat which lives on the premises.

Registered places: 28
Guide weekly rate: £380–£440
Specialist care: Day care, dementia, physical disability, sensory impairment
Medical services: Podiatry, dentist, optician
Qualified staff: Meets standard

Home details
Location: Village location, 7 miles from Tavistock
Communal areas: 3 lounges, dining room, conservatory, garden
Accessibility: *Floors:* 3 • *Access:* Stair lift • *Wheelchair access:* Good
Smoking: ✗
Pets: At manager's discretion
Routines: Flexible

Room details
Single: 24
Shared: 2
En suite: 18
Facilities: TV point, telephone point

Door lock: ✓
Lockable place: ✓

Services provided
Beauty services: Hairdressing, manicures, massage therapy
Mobile library: ✓
Religious services: Monthly Communion service, weekly fellowship service
Transport: Car
Activities: *Coordinator:* ✓ • *Examples:* Exercise, scrabble, visiting entertainers • *Outings:* ✓
Meetings: ✓

Westerlands Residential Home

Manager: Elizabeth Low
Owner: Elizabeth Low
Contact: Bellecross Road, Kingsbridge,
Devon TQ7 1NL
☎ 01548 852268

Located in a rural area, half a mile from Kingsbridge, Westerlands Residential Home offers beautiful views and quiet lounge area. There is a large garden and a swimming pool for those who enjoy outdoors. A visiting activities coordinator reads poems and shows slide shows and leads the residents in reminiscence sessions. There are also exercise sessions and games played. The home has its own seven-seater vehicle for transport and a mobile library regularly visits.

Registered places: 12
Guide weekly rate: £280–£300
Specialist care: Dementia
Medical services: Podiatry, hygienist, optician, physiotherapy
Qualified staff: Exceeds standard: 80% at NVQ level 2

Home details
Location: Rural area, 0.5 miles from Kingsbridge
Communal areas: 2 lounges, dining room, conservatory, bar, swimming pool, garden
Accessibility: *Floors:* 2 • *Access:* Stair lift *Wheelchair access:* Limited
Smoking: ✗
Pets: ✓
Routines: Flexible

Room details
Single: 10
Shared: 2
En suite: 1
Facilities: TV

Door lock: ✓
Lockable place: ✓

Services provided
Beauty services: Hairdressing
Mobile Library: ✓
Religious services: ✗
Transport: 7-seater vehicle
Activities: *Coordinator:* ✓ • *Examples:* Bingo, exercise, games *Outings:* ✓
Meetings: Undisclosed

Registered places: 37
Guide weekly rate: £360
Specialist care: Dementia, mental disorder, physical disability
Medical services: Podiatry, hygienist, optician
Qualified staff: Meets standard

Home details

Location: Residential area, 1.7 miles from Torquay
Communal areas: 2 lounges, 2 dining rooms, conservatory, library,
smoking room, garden
Accessibility: *Floors:* 3 • *Access:* Stair lift • *Wheelchair access:* Good
Smoking: In designated area
Pets: ✓
Routines: Flexible

Room details

Single: 27
Shared: 2
En suite: 19
Facilities: TV point

Door lock: ✓
Lockable place: ✓

Services provided

Beauty services: Hairdressing
Mobile library: ✓
Religious services: Monthly Communion service
Transport: People carrier
Activities: *Coordinator.* ✓ • *Examples:* Arts and crafts, visiting
entertainers • *Outings:* x
Meetings: ✓

Western Rise

Manager: Samuel Rose
Owner: John Chow
Contact: 27 Western Road, Torquay,
Devon, TQ1 4RJ
☎ 01803 312430
@ westernrise@tiscali.co.uk

Located in St Marychurch a few minutes' walk from the area's local amenities, Western Rise is also just a short bus ride from Torquay, almost two miles away. The home is located less than a mile from the coast and has its own people carrier to transport residents. The home has its own library facilities and a smoking room, as well as a conservatory and a garden. There is a residents meeting once a month and the activities coordinator leads both group and individual activities.

Registered places: 20
Guide weekly rate: Undisclosed
Specialist care: Day care, respite
Medical services: Podiatry
Qualified staff: Undisclosed

Home details

Location: Residential area, 0.5 miles from Teignmouth
Com munal areas: Lounge, conservatory, dining room,
patio and garden
Accessibility: *Floors:* 3 • *Access:* Lift • *Wheelchair access:* Good
Smoking: x
Pets: At manager's discretion
Routines: Flexible

Room details

Single: 18
Shared: 1
En suite: 19
Facilities: TV point, telephone point

Door lock: ✓
Lockable place: ✓

Services provided

Beauty services: Hairdressing
Mobile library: ✓
Religious services: Monthly Communion service
Transport: Minibus
Activities: *Coordinator.* ✓ • *Examples:* Armchair exercises, bingo,
visiting entertainers • *Outings:* ✓
Meetings: ✓

Westlands Retirement Home

Manager: Liz Feasby
Owner: Ashley and Diana Rayfield
Contact: Reed Vale, Teignmouth,
Devon, TQ14 9EH
☎ 01626 773007
🖱 www.westlandsretirementhome.co.uk

A detached house set in a quiet residential area, Westlands Retirement Home offers residents attractive views of the Devonshire countryside and Teign estuary, whilst still remaining close to local facilities. It is less than a quarter of a mile to the nearest shop, post office, chemist and bus stop, and a shopping centre and train station are a mile away. With a fish tank in the main lounge, the home's conservatory has French doors leading onto the patio where there are superb views.

The White House

Manager: Lesley Courtney
Owner: Langton Care Ltd
Contact: Woodway Road, Teignmouth, Devon, TQ14 8QB
☏ 01626 774322

Situated in a quiet, residential area of Teignmouth, The White House permits beautiful sea views and views of the town. Teignmouth town centre is one mile away and there is a regular bus service. The home arranges a monthly Communion service for the residents and there are a range of activities on offer such as armchair exercises and quizzes. The home has a garden for residents to enjoy in the summer months is addition to a lounge.

Registered places: 19
Guide weekly rate: £320–£400
Specialist care: Day care, physical disability, respite
Medical services: Podiatry, dentist, optician
Qualified staff: Meets standard

Home details
Location: Residential area, 1 mile from Teignmouth
Communal areas: Lounge, dining room, garden
Accessibility: *Floors:* 2 • *Access:* Stair lift • *Wheelchair access:* Good
Smoking: In designated area
Pets: ✗
Routines: Flexible

Room details
Single: 17
Shared: 1
En suite: 10
Facilities: TV point, telephone point

Door lock: ✓
Lockable place: ✓

Services provided
Beauty services: Hairdressing
Mobile library: ✗
Religious services: Monthly Communion service
Transport: ✗
Activities: *Coordinator:* ✗ • *Examples:* Armchair activities, quizzes
  Outings: ✗
Meetings: ✗

Windward Nursing Home

Manager: Sally Moyse
Owner: Robert Gunn
Contact: Dartmouth Road, Stoke Fleming, Dartmouth, Devon, TQ6 0QS
☏ 01803 770789
@ windwardnh@btconnect.com

Approximately two miles from the historic naval town of Dartmouth, Windward Nursing Home overlooks the countryside and the sea and is conveniently located 200 yards from local amenities including shops. Offering an unrestricted visiting policy the home also advertises that snacks and fruit are available throughout the day. Although Windward does not allow pets in the home, a neighbouring cat is a frequent visitor. There is also a piano in the home.

Registered places: 25
Guide weekly rate: £550–£650
Specialist care: Nursing, emergency admissions, physical disability, respite
Medical services: Podiatry, dentist, optician, physiotherapy
Qualified staff: Meets standard

Home details
Location: Village location, 2 miles from Dartmouth
Communal areas: 2 lounges, dining room, patio and garden
Accessibility: *Floors:* 2 • *Access:* Lift • *Wheelchair access:* Good
Smoking: ✗
Pets: ✗
Routines: Flexible

Room details
Single: 23
Shared: 1
En suite: 13
Facilities: TV point, telephone point

Door lock: ✗
Lockable place: ✓

Services provided
Beauty services: Hairdressing
Mobile library: ✓
Religious services: Monthly Anglican Communion service
Transport: Car
Activities: *Coordinator:* ✗ • *Examples:* Bingo, games • *Outings:* ✓
Meetings: ✗

Registered places: 20
Guide weekly rate: £256–£485
Specialist care: Physical disability, respite
Medical services: Podiatry, dentist, optician, physiotherapy
Qualified staff: Meets standard

Home details

Location: Village location, in South Brent
Communal areas: Lounge, dining room, garden
Accessibility: *Floors:* 2 • *Access:* Stair lift • *Wheelchair access:* Good
Smoking: ✕
Pets: ✓
Routines: Flexible

Room details

Single: 45
Shared: 0
En suite: 45
Facilities: None

Door lock: ✓
Lockable place: ✓

Services provided

Beauty services: Hairdressing, aromatherapy
Mobile library: ✕
Religious services: ✕
Transport: ✕
Activities: *Coordinator.* ✕ • *Examples*: Games, slide shows
    Outings: ✓
Meetings: ✓

Windward Retirement Home

Manager: Geraldine Swift
Owner: Thurlestone Court Ltd
Contact: Totnes Road, South Brent, Devon, TQ10 9JN
☎ 01364 72386

Windward House is a large property set in its own grounds in the village of South Brent. The accommodation is very homely and comfortable. The home has a garden for residents to enjoy in the summer as well as a lounge. The home arranges outings for the residents as well as internal activities such as games and slide shows. There are also regular residents meetings.

Registered places: 30
Guide weekly rate: £467–£575
Specialist care: Nursing, dementia, mental disorder,
    physical disability
Medical services: Podiatry, dentist, optician
Qualified staff: Exceeds standard: 80% at NVQ level 2

Home details

Location: Residential area, 1.7 miles from Torquay
Communal areas: Lounges, dining room, garden
Accessibility: *Floors:* 3 • *Access:* Lift • *Wheelchair access:* Good
Smoking: ✕
Pets: ✕
Routines: Structured

Room details

Single: 18
Shared: 6
En suite: Undisclosed
Facilities: None

Door lock: ✕
Lockable place: ✕

Services provided

Beauty services: Hairdressing, manicures
Mobile library: ✕
Religious services: ✕
Transport: ✕
Activities: *Coordinator.* ✕ • *Examples*: One-to-one sessions,
    visiting entertainers • *Outings:* ✕
Meetings: ✕

Woodland House Nursing Home

Manager: Karen Gwilliam
Owner: Woodland Healthcare Ltd
Contact: Middle Warberry Road, Torquay, Devon, TQ1 1RN
☎ 01803 296809

Situated in a residential location, approximately half an hour's walk from the facilities of Torquay, Woodland House is a nursing home that cares for people who suffer from mental health problems. The home is located approximately two miles from Torquay. The home arranges activities twice a week and offers group activities such as performances from visiting entertainers, as well as one-to-one sessions.

Woodland Park Nursing Home

Manager: Phyllis Wilton
Owner: Woodland Healthcare Ltd
Contact: Babbacombe Road, Torquay, Devon, TQ1 3SJ
) 01803 313758

An Edwardian property located 100 yards from Babbacombe Downs, Woodland Park offers its residents attractive views of the bay and its surrounding areas. It is a short, flat walk to the nearest shops and just over a mile and a half from Torquay. The home arranges group activities such as music to movement as well as one-to-one sessions. There are outings on offer to the residents in addition to the facilities of a mobile library.

Registered places: 31
Guide weekly rate: Up to £530
Specialist care: Nursing, physical disability, respite
Medical services: Podiatry, dentist, optician, physiotherapy
Qualified staff: Meets standard

Home details
Location: Residential area, 1.6 miles from Torquay
Communal areas: Lounge/dining room, conservatory, garden
Accessibility: *Floors:* 3 • *Access:* Lift • *Wheelchair access:* Good
Smoking: x
Pets: At manager's discretion
Routines: Flexible

Room details
Single: 19
Shared: 6
En suite: 8
Facilities: TV point, telephone point

Door lock: ✓
Lockable place: ✓

Services provided
Beauty services: Hairdressing, aromatherapy, massage
Mobile library: ✓
Religious services: x
Transport: x
Activities: *Coordinator:* x • *Examples:* Arts and crafts, exercise, one-to-one sessions • *Outings:* ✓
Meetings: x

The Yelverton Nursing and Residential Home

Manager: Jessica Powell
Owner: LarkCastle Ltd
Contact: 2–4 Greenbank Terrace, Yelverton, Devon, PL20 6DR
) 01822 852641
@ peter.james@
    yelverton-nursing-home.co.uk
🖰 www.yelverton-nursing-home.co.uk

A modernised Edwardian house situated on the village green. The yelverton is 10 miles from Plymouth and close to local amenities including shops, a post office and pub. Outings to Plymouth are organised regularly, visiting the sea and having fish and chips. Outdoor facilities include a paved terrace with flowerbeds for those with an interest in gardening. It is a small home, with a good staff to resident ratio that aids a friendly atmosphere. There is a TV and a piano in the lounge and an activities and exercise visitor comes to the home.

Registered places: 27
Guide weekly rate: £435–£525
Specialist care: Nursing, dementia, physical disability
Medical services: Podiatry, dentist, optician, physiotherapy
Qualified staff: Exceeds standard: 90% at NVQ level 2

Home details
Location: Village location, 10 miles from Plymouth
Communal areas: 2 lounges, dining room, patio and garden
Accessibility: *Floors:* 3 • *Access:* Lift • *Wheelchair access:* Good
Smoking: x
Pets: At manager's discretion
Routines: Flexible

Room details
Single: 25
Shared: 2
En suite: 19
Facilities: TV, telephone point

Door lock: ✓
Lockable place: ✓

Services provided
Beauty services: Hairdressing
Mobile library: ✓
Religious services: Monthly Communion service
Transport: x
Activities: *Coordinator:* x • *Examples:* Exercise, visiting entertainers *Outings:* ✓
Meetings: x

Registered places: 25
Guide weekly rate: Undisclosed
Specialist care: Day care, respite
Medical services: Podiatry, hygienist, optician, physiotherapy
Qualified staff: Exceeds standard: 100% at NVQ level 2

Home details

Location: Residential area, 2 miles from Bournemouth centre
Communal areas: 2 lounges, dining room, conservatory, garden
Accessibility:*Floors:* 2 • *Access:* Lift • *Wheelchair access:* Good
Smoking: ×
Pets: ×

Room details

Single: 17
Shared: 4
En suite: 18
Facilities: TV point, telephone point

	Door lock: ✓
	Lockable place: ✓

Services provided

Beauty services: Hairdressing
Mobile library: ✓
Religious services: Weekly Anglican Communion service
Transport: Minibus
Activities: *Coordinator:* ✓ • *Examples:* Bingo, music to movement, quizzes • *Outings:* ×
Meetings: ✓

Adamscourt Residential Care Home

Manager: Eileen Cockwell
Owner: Sheila Burden
Contact: 7 Talbot Avenue, Talbot Woods, Bournemouth, Dorset, BH3 7HP
) 01202 529855
@ burdenlodge@aol.com

Adamscourt Residential Care Home is situated in Talbot Woods close to Meyrick Park in Bournemouth. On a main route into the centre, there are good transport links for able residents. The home also has its own minibus to facilitate shopping trips. There is an activities coordinator at the home who organises weekly activities such as bingo, quizzes and occasional visiting entertainers. There is also a weekly Anglican Communion service at the home.

Registered places: 54
Guide weekly rate: £785–£940
Specialist care: Nursing
Medical services: Podiatry, dentist, optician, physiotherapy
Qualified staff: Fails standard

Home details

Location: Residential area, in Ferndown
Communal areas: 4 lounges, dining room, activity room, patio and garden
Accessibility: *Floors:* 2 • *Access:* Lift • *Wheelchair access:* Good
Smoking: ×
Pets: At manager's discretion
Routines: Flexible

Room details

Single: 54
Shared: 0
En suite: 54
Facilities: TV

	Door lock: ✓
	Lockable place: ✓

Services provided

Beauty services: Hairdressing
Mobile library: Library facilities
Religious services: ✓
Transport: Minibus
Activities: *Coordinator:* ✓ • *Examples:* Games, musical entertainment
Outings: ✓
Meetings: ×

Amberwood House

Manager: Jacqueline Roy
Owner: Colten Care Ltd
Contact: 418–424 Ringwood Road, Ferndown, Dorset, BH22 9AG
) 01202 851510
@ amberwood@coltencare.co.uk
⌂ www.coltencare.com

A new purpose-built property, Amberwood House is an attractive modern building situated near facilities which include shops, a community art centre and churches. Amberwood House is introducing the role of 'social carer', which means that residents who are unable to attend the group activities have the opportunity of one-to-one time with a member of staff. The complaints procedure assures residents that their views are significant to the home.

Avenue House

Manager: Jackie Watson
Owner: BML Healthcare
Contact: 8 Weymouth Avenue,
1 Queens Avenue, Dorchester,
Dorset, DT1 2EN
☏ 01305 265365

Allowing for easy access, Avenue House is situated on the main Dorchester to Weymouth road, a short drive from Weymouth seafront and the town centre. Although approximately 10 minutes' walk from shops and amenities this is not on the level and residents rarely walk this independently. With a lawned garden and inner courtyard, a sun terrace decorated with flower baskets and pots allows those interested in gardening to partake in their hobby.

Registered places: 33
Guide weekly rate: £420–£560
Specialist care: None
Medical services: Podiatry, dentist, optician
Qualified staff: Exceeds standard: 60% at NVQ level 2

Home details
Location: Urban area, 0.25 miles from Dorchester centre
Communal areas: 2 lounges, dining room, patio and garden
Accessibility: *Floors:* 2 • *Access:* Lift • *Wheelchair access:* Good
Smoking: ✗
Pets: At manager's discretion
Routines: Flexible

Room details
Single: 25
Shared: 4
En suite: 19
Facilities: TV point

Door lock: ✓
Lockable place: ✓

Services provided
Beauty services: Hairdressing
Mobile library: ✓
Religious services: Monthly Communion service
Transport: ✗
Activities: *Coordinator:* ✗ • *Examples:* Arts and crafts, gardening, reminiscence • *Outings:* ✗
Meetings: ✓

Avon Cliff

Manager: Tracey Thompson
Owner: Colten Care Ltd
Contact: 50–52 Christchurch Road,
Bournemouth, Dorset, BH1 3PE
☏ 01202 789998
🖱 www.coltencare.co.uk

Avon Cliff is situated in a residential area of Bournemouth, on a main road around a quarter of a mile from the seafront. The accommodation at Avon Cliff is spread over three floors, with good wheelchair access throughout. There is a main dining room on the ground floor and two smaller dining areas on the other floors. The home has safe grounds at the front and rear of the property for the enjoyment of residents. There is a director of hotel services to maintain the standards of catering.

Registered places: 52
Guide weekly rate: £722–£890
Specialist care: Respite
Medical services: Podiatry
Qualified staff: Undisclosed

Home details
Location: Residential area, 1 mile from Bournemouth centre
Communal areas: 2 lounges, dining room, 2 quiet rooms, garden
Accessibility: *Floors:* 3 • *Access:* Lift • *Wheelchair access:* Good
Smoking: ✗
Pets: ✓

Room details
Single: 48
Shared: 2
En suite: 50
Facilities: TV point
Routines: Structured

Door lock: ✓
Lockable place: ✗

Services provided
Beauty services: Hairdressing
Mobile library: ✗
Religious services: ✓
Transport: Minibus
Activities: *Coordinator:* ✓ • *Examples:* Gentle exercise, quizzes *Outings:* ✓
Meetings: ✗

Registered places: 40
Guide weekly rate: £450–£750
Specialist care: Nursing
Medical services: Podiatry, hygienist, optician
Qualified staff: Fails standard

Home details
Location: Residential area, 1 mile from Weymouth centre
Communal areas: 2 lounges, dining room, garden
Accessibility: *Floors:* 3 • *Access:* Lift • *Wheelchair access:* Good
Smoking: In designated area
Pets: ✓
Routines: Flexible

Room details
Single: 35
Shared: 5 | Door lock: ✓
En suite: 35 | Lockable place: ✓
Facilities: TV point, telephone point

Services provided
Beauty services: Hairdressing
Mobile library: ✓
Religious services: Monthly Communion service
Transport: ✗
Activities: *Coordinator.* ✓ • *Examples*: Singalongs • *Outings:* ✓
Meetings: ✗

Avon Lea
Manager: Jacqueline Whittle
Owner: Nahid Salehi
Contact: 66 Dorchester Road, Weymouth, Dorset, DT4 7JZ
☏ 01305 776094

Situated on the main road into Weymouth, Avon Lea is located on the same street as shops and within walking distance of the seafront. There are two lounges, a separate dining room and medium-sized garden for residents to enjoy. An activities coordinator organises activities such as group singalongs to encourage interaction between residents. Outings are also made into town and to the nearby seafront.

Registered places: 13
Guide weekly rate: £392–£530
Specialist care: Day care, respite
Medical services: Podiatry, dentist, occupational therapy, optician, physiotherapy
Qualified staff: Exceeds standard: 70% at NVQ level 2

Home details
Location: Rural area, 2 miles from Christchurch
Communal areas: Lounge, dining room, garden
Accessibility: *Floors:* 2 • *Access:* Lift • *Wheelchair access:* Good
Smoking: ✗
Pets: ✗
Routines: Flexible

Room details
Single: 12
Shared: 0 | Door lock: ✓
En suite: 8 | Lockable place: ✓
Facilities: TV, telephone point

Services provided
Beauty services: Hairdressing
Mobile library: ✓
Religious services: Monthly Anglican Communion service
Transport: ✗
Activities: *Coordinator.* ✓ • *Examples*: Garden parties, Nintendo wii, visiting entertainers • *Outings:* ✓
Meetings: ✗

Avon Lee Lodge
Manager: Tracy Kennedy
Owner: Leigh and Tracy Kennedy
Contact: Preston Lane, Burton, Christchurch, Dorset, BH23 7JU
☏ 01202 476736
@ enquiries@avonleelodge.co.uk
🖱 www.avonleelodge.co.uk

A converted vicarage in a quiet rural location with stunning views of local scenery, Avon Lee Lodge lies in a conservation area close to facilities which include shops, churches, clubs and post office. A bus stop is also located a short distance from the home and this provides more active residents with opportunities to travel all the way up to Christchurch and Bournemouth. As well as social events and entertainers, the activities coordinator organises for residents to play on Nintendo wii as good form of exercise. The home produces a monthly newsletter.

Batchfoot Country House

Manager: Jacqueline Johnson
Owner: M Taylor
Contact: 181 Church Street, Upwey, Weymouth, Dorset, DT3 5QE
☎ 01305 812143

Set in a listed Georgian building with its own grounds, Batchfoot Country House is situated a few hundred yards from village amenities including a teashop, craft shop, church and a wishing well. The home has received a grant to update the patio and garden area and work should be complete by spring 2008. Once this is complete residents will be able to use gardening facilities. Every bedroom has access to satellite TV.

Registered places: 16
Guide weekly rate: £353–£450
Specialist care: Respite
Medical services: Podiatry, optician
Qualified staff: Meets standard

Home details
Location: Rural area, 4 miles from Weymouth
Communal areas: 2 lounges, dining room, garden
Accessibility: *Floors:* 3 • *Access:* Stair lift
  Wheelchair access: Limited
Smoking: x
Pets: x
Routines: Flexible

Room details
Single: 16
Shared: 0
En suite: 0
Facilities: TV point, telephone point

Door lock: ✓
Lockable place: ✓

Services provided
Beauty services: Hairdressing
Mobile library: ✓
Religious services: Monthly Communion service
Transport: Car
Activities: *Coordinator.* ✓ • *Examples:* Bingo, coffee mornings, music and movement • *Outings:* x
Meetings: ✓

Birds Hill Nursing Home

Manager: Mrs Seewooruthun
Owner: Mr Seewooruthun
Contact: 25 Birds Hill Road, Poole, Dorset, BH15 2QJ
☎ 01202 671111
@ matron@birdshill.co.uk
⌂ www.birdshill.co.uk

Birds Hill Nursing Home is a family-owned home set on a hill near to Poole General Hospital. The home is set on four floors, each with a different unit. Some bedrooms and all communal lounges have views of Poole harbour. The home is located one mile from the town centre and there is a bus service. The home has its own transport and arranges one-to-one outings for the residents. The home also has two activities coordinators who arrange dancing, walks, quizzes and a gardening club.

Registered places: 72
Guide weekly rate: £625–£950
Specialist care: Nursing, day care, dementia, mental disorder, respite
Medical services: Podiatry, dentist, optician, physiotherapy
Qualified staff: Exceeds standard: 85% at NVQ Level 2

Home details
Location: Residential area, 1 mile from Poole centre
Communal areas: Lounge, dining room, conservatory, patio and garden
Accessibility: *Floors:* 4 • *Access:* Lift • *Wheelchair access:* Good
Smoking: ✓
Pets: ✓
Routines: Flexible

Room details
Single: 60
Shared: 6
En suite: 60
Facilities: TV, telephone

Door lock: ✓
Lockable place: ✓

Services provided
Beauty services: Hairdressing, manicures
Mobile library: ✓
Religious services: ✓
Transport: ✓
Activities: *Coordinator.* ✓ • *Examples:* Bingo, dancing, gardening
  Outings: ✓
Meetings: x

Registered places: 19
Guide weekly rate: £500–£650
Specialist care: None
Medical services: Podiatry, optician
Qualified staff: Fails standard

Home details

Location: Village location, 3 miles from Bridport
Communal areas: Lounge, dining room, patio and garden
Accessibility: *Floors:* 3 • *Access:* Lift • *Wheelchair access:* Good
Smoking: ×
Pets: ×
Routines: Flexible

Room details

Single: 17
Shared: 1
En suite: 16
Facilities: None

Door lock: ✓
Lockable place: ✓

Services provided

Beauty services: Hairdressing, manicures
Mobile library: ✓
Religious services: Monthly nondenominational Communion service
Transport: ×
Activities: *Coordinator.* ✓ • *Examples*: Armchair exercises, painting
   Outings: ×
Meetings: ×

Broadwindsor House

Manager: Helen Dawe
Owner: Florence Lodge Healthcare Ltd
Contact: Broadwindsor, Beaminster,
Dorset, DT8 3PX
☎ 01308 868353
@ helen.dawe@btconnect.com

Originally a rectory, House was built in the 1830s and is set in three acres of its own grounds. The house is accessed via a private driveway and is situated in the village of Broadwindsor, about three miles north of Bridport. With a piano and organ in the lounge, the home also has DVD facilities. There are plans for a heated swimming pool for the use of members.

Registered places: 30
Guide weekly rate: Undisclosed
Specialist care: Nursing, respite
Medical services: Podiatry, physiotherapy
Qualified staff: Exceeds standard: 60% at NVQ Level 2

Home details

Location: Village location, 3 miles from Lyme Regis
Communal areas: Lounge, dining room, garden
Accessibility: *Floors:* 2 • *Access:* Lift • *Wheelchair access:* Good
Smoking: ×
Pets: ×
Routines: Flexible

Room details

Single: 30
Shared: 0
En suite: 28
Facilities: TV point

Door lock: ✓
Lockable place: ✓

Services provided

Beauty services: Hairdressing
Mobile library: ×
Religious services: ×
Transport: ×
Activities: *Coordinator.* ✓ • *Examples*: Bingo • *Outings:* ✓
Meetings: ✓

Bymead House

Manager: Elizabeth Wilson
Owner: Mrs Widders
Contact: Axminster Road, Charmouth,
Bridport, Dorset, DT6 6BS
☎ 01297 560620

Bymead House is situated on the outskirts of Charmouth, approximately three miles from Lyme Regis. The home can accommodate 26 residents who need nursing care, including three NHS-funded patients. In addition four elderly people needing residential care can be accommodated. A number of the bedrooms open on to an enclosed courtyard garden.

Canford Chase

Manager: Angela Stewart
Owner: Colten Care Ltd
Contact: 40 Western Road,
Branksome Park, Poole, Dorset, BH13 6EU
☎ 01202 766182
@ canfodchase@coltencare.co.uk
🖰 www.coltencare.co.uk

Situated in a residential area of Branksome Park, Canford Chase is a large, purpose-built home. Furthermore, it is within easy reach of both Poole and Bournemouth. The reception is well furnished and the lounge has a flat wide-screen television. To add to this, the large dining room looks over the beautiful garden. Meals are available for guests at no extra charge. There is an extensive activities programme organised which includes quizzes and games and trips out in the minibus.

Registered places: 52
Guide weekly rate: Undisclosed
Specialist care: Nursing
Medical services: Podiatry, dentist, optician, physiotherapy
Qualified staff: Undisclosed

Home details
Location: Residential area, 4 miles from Poole centre
Communal areas: 3 lounges, quiet room, dining room, hairdressing salon, garden
Accessibility: *Floors:* 3 • *Access:* Lift • *Wheelchair access:* Good
Smoking: ×
Pets: At manager's discretion
Routines: Flexible

Room details
Single: 50
Shared: 1
En suite: 51
Facilities: TV point

Door lock: ×
Lockable place: ✓

Services provided
Beauty services: Hairdressing, manicures
Mobile library: ×
Religious services: Monthly Communion service
Transport: Minibus
Activities: *Coordinator:* ✓ • *Examples:* Exercises, quizzes • *Outings:* ✓
Meetings: ×

Castle Farm Residential Care Home and Farmhouse

Manager: Dawn Roessler
Owner: Castle Farm Care Ltd
Contact: Castle Farm Road,
Lytchett Matravers, Dorset, BH16 6BZ
☎ 01258 857642
@ info@castlefarmcare.co.uk
🖰 www.royalbay.co.uk

Castle Farm Residential Home and Farmhouse is a converted barn which was in agricultural use as recently as the 1980s. The home is in a rural location, on the outskirts of the village of Lytchett Matravers, six miles from Poole town centre. Set in the Dorset countryside, many residents enjoy gardening and make use of the house's greenhouse. Entertainments take place twice a week, theatre groups visit three times a year and there is a yearly fête. Rules are actively discouraged at Castle Farm. There are no set routines and residents are free to live as they please.

Registered places: 19
Guide weekly rate: £475–£550
Specialist care: Respite
Medical services: Podiatry, dentist, dietician, occupational therapy, optician, physiotherapy
Qualified staff: Exceeds standard: 90% at NVQ level 2

Home details
Location: Rural area, 6 miles from Poole
Communal areas: Lounge, dining room, conservatory, garden
Accessibility: *Floors:* • 2 *Access:* Lift • *Wheelchair access:* Good
Smoking: In designated area
Pets: ×
Routines: Flexible

Room details
Single: 15
Shared: 2
En suite: 16
Facilities: TV point, telephone point

Door lock: ✓
Lockable place: ✓

Services provided
Beauty services: Hairdressing
Mobile library: ✓
Religious services: Monthly Anglican Communion service
Transport: Minibus
Activities: *Coordinator:* ✓ • *Examples:* Drama therapy, gardening, visiting entertainers • *Outings:* ✓
Meetings: ✓

Registered places: 11
Guide weekly rate: Undisclosed
Specialist care: Respite
Medical services: Podiatry, dentist, optician
Qualified staff: Fails standard

Home details
Location: Residential area, 2 miles from Christchurch
Communal areas: Lounge, dining room, patio and garden
Accessibility: *Floors:* 2 • *Access:* Stair lift
    Wheelchair access: Limited
Smoking: ×
Pets: At manager's discretion
Routines: Flexible

Room details
Single: 8
Shared: 1   Door lock: ✓
En suite: 1   Lockable place: ✓
Facilities: TV, telephone point

Services provided
Beauty services: Hairdressing
Mobile library: ×
Religious services: ×
Transport: Car
Activities: *Coordinator:* ×• *Examples:* Walks • *Outings:* ×
Meetings: ×

Chalfont

Manager: Michael Adams and
Terence Aston
Owner: Michael Adams and
Terence Aston
Contact: 6 Southern Road, Southbourne,
Bournemouth, Dorset, BH6 3SR
☎ 01202 420957

Chalfont is situated in a quiet, residential area of Southbourne between the seafront and a shopping centre. It is a small home, which prides itself on feeling like a family home. Public transport is available within easy walking distance, with a bus stop nearby. The bus takes around 20 minutes into the centre of Bournemouth. There is a small garden at the back of the home with a patio area.

Registered places: 16
Guide weekly rate: £400–£450
Specialist care: Undisclosed
Medical services: Podiatry
Qualified staff: Exceeds standard: 100% at NVQ Level 2

Home details
Location: Rural area, 10 miles from Bournemouth centre
Communal areas: Lounge/dining room
Accessibility: *Floors:* 2 • *Access:* Lift • *Wheelchair access:* Good
Smoking: ×
Pets: ×
Routines: Flexible

Room details
Single: 12
Shared: 2   Door lock: ✓
En suite: 13   Lockable place: ×
Facilities: None

Services provided
Beauty services: Hairdressing
Mobile library: ×
Religious services: Monthly nondenominational church service
Transport: ×
Activities: *Coordinator:* × • *Examples:* Armchair exercises,
    piano concerts • *Outings:* ✓
Meetings: ×

Chaseborough House

Manager: Sally Marshall
Owner: Sally Marshall
Contact: Village Hall Lane, Wimborne,
Dorset, BH21 6SG
☎ 01202 822908

Chaseborough House is a large converted family house set in its own grounds near the village of Three Legged Cross. It is situated close to local amenities which include a pub and village hall. The owners live in the adjacent property. Residents with an interest in gardening may use the home's gardens for this purpose. The home arranges outings to nearby towns and arranges a coach to make this possible.

Chine Breeze Court

Manager: Jane Morris
Owner: Mr and Mrs Jenkins
Contact: 73 Alumhurst Road,
Westbourne, Bournemouth,
Dorset, BH4 8HP
☎ 01202 761307

Situated in a residential area of Westbourne, Chine Breeze Court is a Victorian building converted into a care home, with two floors and a lift. It is located around half a mile from shops, and less than half a mile to the seafront. There is an activities coordinator at the home who organises games, gentle exercise and visits from local entertainers, such as singers and musicians.

Registered places: 20
Guide weekly rate: £495–£650
Specialist care: Nursing, respite
Medical services: Podiatry, optician, physiotherapy
Qualified staff: Fails standard

Home details
Location: Residential area, 1.5 miles from Bournemouth centre
Communal areas: Lounge, dining room, conservatory, garden
Accessibility: *Floors:* 2 • *Access:* Lift • *Wheelchair access:* Good
Smoking: ✗
Pets: At manager's discretion
Routines: Structured

Room details
Single: 11
Shared: 4
En suite: 4
Facilities: TV point, telephone point

Door lock: ✓
Lockable place: ✓

Services provided
Beauty services: Hairdressing
Mobile library: ✓
Religious services: ✗
Transport: ✗
Activities: *Coordinator.* ✓ • *Examples*: Gentle exercise, games, visiting entertainers • *Outings:* ✗
Meetings: ✗

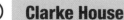

Clarke House

Manager: Wendy Erskine
Owner: Wendy Erskine
Contact: 3 Grosvenor Road,
Weymouth, Dorset, DT4 7QL
☎ 01305 773851
@ wendyerskine@wandttraining.co.uk

A period property located in a residential area, Clarke House is a small family-run Christian home. The home has daily prayer meetings, weekly services and offers Communion on request. The home is a two-minute walk from the nearest shops and a short drive from the centre of Weymouth. The home is managed by the owners, who live on the premises.

Registered places: 6
Guide weekly rate: £425–£450
Specialist care: Day care, respite
Medical services: Podiatry, hygienist, optician, physiotherapy
Qualified staff: Exceeds standard: 75% at NVQ level 2

Home details
Location: Residential area, 1 mile from Weymouth centre
Communal areas: Lounge, dining room, conservatory, garden
Accessibility: *Floors:* 2 • *Access:* None • *Wheelchair access:* Limited
Smoking: ✗
Pets: At manager's discretion
Routines: Flexible

Room details
Single: 6
Shared: 0
En suite: 6
Facilities: TV point

Door lock: ✓
Lockable place: ✓

Services provided
Beauty services: Hairdressing, aromatherapy
Mobile library: ✓
Religious services: Daily prayer meetings, weekly service
Transport: Car
Activities: *Coordinator.* ✗ • *Examples*: Exercise sessions, videos *Outings:* ✗
Meetings: ✗

Registered places: 32
Guide weekly rate: £420–£525
Specialist care: Respite
Medical services: Podiatry, dentist, optician
Qualified staff: Fails standard

Home details

Location: Residential area, 1 mile from Swanage centre
Communal areas: Lounge, dining room, garden
Accessibility: *Floors:* 3 • *Access:* Lift • *Wheelchair access:* Good
Smoking: ✓
Pets: At manager's discretion
Routines: Flexible

Room details

Single: 28
Shared: 2
En suite: 30
Facilities: None

Door lock: ✓
Lockable place: ✗

Services provided

Beauty services: Hairdressing
Mobile library: ✗
Religious services: ✗
Transport: ✗
Activities: *Coordinator.* ✓ • *Examples*: Games, exercise to music, piano afternoons • *Outings:* ✓
Meetings: ✗

Clifftop Care Home

Manager: Patricia Pride
Owner: Christine Harrison
Contact: 8 Burlington Road, Swanage, Dorset, BH19 1LS
❱ 01929 422091

A large Edwardian property set in its own grounds overlooking the sea, Clifftop Care Home is in a prime position for good views of Swanage Bay, which can be seen from the home's conservatory and gardens. There is an activities coordinator who organises outings to the seaside and in-house entertainment. Pets are allowed at the manager's discretion and the home has its own cat.

Registered places: 22
Guide weekly rate: £443–£475
Specialist care: Undisclosed
Medical services: Podiatry
Qualified staff: Meets standard

Home details

Location: Residential area, in Bridport
Communal areas: Lounge/dining room, conservatory/dining room, garden
Accessibility: *Floors:* 2 • *Access:* Stair lift
    Wheelchair access: Limited
Smoking: ✗
Pets: ✓
Routines: Flexible

Room details

Single: 22
Shared: 0
En suite: 18
Facilities: TV point

Door lock: ✓
Lockable place: ✓

Services provided

Beauty services: Hairdressing
Mobile library: ✗
Religious services: ✗
Transport: ✓
Activities: *Coordinator.* ✓ • *Examples*: Exercises, quizzes
    Outings: ✓
Meetings: ✗

Coneygar Lodge

Manager: Natily Berry
Owner: Coneygar Lodge Ltd
Contact: Coneygar Park, Bridport, Dorset, DT6 3BA
❱ 01308 427365

Coneygar Lodge is situated in a secluded area on the outskirts of Bridport, it is accessed via a private lane and is a short walk from the centre of Bridport where major bus routes and local amenities are available. Residents' accommodation is provided in four buildings grouped around a courtyard with a separate building for the laundry and kitchen. The home provides suitable transport to take small groups of residents out for afternoon tea or visits to local places of interest. The programme of events is displayed on a notice board in the Lodge.

Coniston Lodge

Manager: Katrina Bailey
Owner: Daphne Bailey
Contact: 43 Beaufort Road,
Southbourne, Bournemouth,
Dorset, BH6 5AS
) 01202 421492
@ kevin@coniston43.fsnet.co.uk

A family-run home, Coniston Lodge is sited in a residential area of Southbourne. Encouraging an independent lifestyle, bus routes are located near the home and serve both Bournemouth and Christchurch. The home also has its own car to transport residents around. A monthly Communion service is held and a mobile library also visits regularly.

Registered places: 11
Guide weekly rate: From £370
Specialist care: Respite
Medical services: Podiatry, dentist, optician, physiotherapy
Qualified staff: Meets standard

Home details
Location: Residential area, 2.5 miles from Christchurch
Communal areas: Lounge, dining room, garden
Accessibility: *Floors:* 2 • *Access:* Lift • *Wheelchair access:* Good
Smoking: ✗
Pets: At manager's discretion
Routines: Flexible

Room details
Single: 11
Shared: 0
En suite: 4
Facilities: TV point, telephone point

Door lock: ✓
Lockable place: ✓

Services provided
Beauty services: Hairdressing
Mobile library: ✓
Religious services: Monthly Communion service
Transport: Car
Activities: *Coordinator:* ✗ • *Examples:* Games, visiting entertainers
    Outings: ✗
Meetings: ✗

The Crescent

Manager: Helen Graham
Owner: Rhetor 17 Ltd
Contact: 27–29 Meyrick Park Crescent,
Bournemouth, Dorset, BH3 7AG
) 01202 553660

Located close to Meyrick Park, The Crescent overlooks the tree-lined Meyrick Park Crescent. The home is also on a bus route that runs regularly to the centre of Bournemouth. Car parking spaces are available for residents and visitors and the home has its own car to facilitate outings and shopping trips. The garden boasts a patio area with a bench and a fishpond, both easily accessible from the home. Smoking is allowed in resident's rooms.

Registered places: 40
Guide weekly rate: £450–£635
Specialist care: Nursing
Medical services: Podiatry, dentist, optician
Qualified staff: Fails standard

Home details
Location: Residential area, 1.5 miles from Bournemouth
Communal areas: Lounge, dining room, 2 conservatories, garden
Accessibility: *Floors:* 2 • *Access:* Lift • *Wheelchair access:* Good
Smoking: ✓
Pets: At manager's discretion
Routines: Flexible

Room details
Single: 26
Shared: 7
En suite: 5
Facilities: TV point

Door lock: ✓
Lockable place: ✓

Services provided
Beauty services: Hairdressing
Mobile library: ✗
Religious services: Monthly Anglican Communion service
Transport: Car
Activities: *Coordinator:* ✗ • *Examples:* Musicians, reminiscence
    Outings: ✓
Meetings: ✗

Culliford House

Manager: Suzanne Jackson
Owner: Mrs Moors
Contact: Icen Way, Dorchester, Dorset, DT1 1ET
☎ 01305 266054

Culliford House is a Victorian house within easy walking distance of all the shops and services Dorchester has to offer and staff endeavour to create a homely atmosphere for residents to enjoy. A top floor apartment is available for visitor's overnight use for individuals who have travelled far or those whose relatives are seriously ill or dying. There is a monthly Anglican Communion service and a mobile library visits the home.

Registered places: 25
Guide weekly rate: £500–£650
Specialist care: Day care, respite
Medical services: Podiatry, optician
Qualified staff: Meets standard

Home details
Location: Residential area, in Dorchester
Communal areas: Lounge, dining room, conservatory, treatment room, garden
Accessibility: *Floors:* 3 • *Access:* Lift • *Wheelchair access:* Good
Smoking: ✗
Pets: At manager's discretion
Routines: Flexible

Room details
Single: 25
Shared: 0
En suite: 25
Facilities: TV point

Door lock: ✓
Lockable place: ✓

Services provided
Beauty services: Hairdressing
Mobile library: ✓
Religious services: Monthly Anglican Communion service
Transport: ✗
Activities: *Coordinator.* ✗ • *Examples:* Musical entertainment
   Outings: ✓
Meetings: ✗

Delapre House

Manager: Judith Bell
Owner: Bell Social Work Ltd
Contact: 109 Magna Road, Bearwood, Poole, Dorset, BH11 9NE
☎ 01202 570800

Delapre House is a Christian home with regular visits from local clergy. These visits can take the form of services, Communion or one-to-one visits. On a bus route to Wimborne and Poole, the home is set back from the main road and is approximately six miles from Bournemouth town centre. There is ample communal space for this small home, including two lounges, a dining room and two conservatories.

Registered places: 10
Guide weekly rate: £550–£650
Specialist care: Nursing, day care, respite
Medical services: Podiatry, hygienist, optician, physiotherapy
Qualified staff: Exceeds standard: 75% at NVQ level 2

Home details
Location: Residential area, 6 miles from Bournemouth centre
Communal areas: 2 lounges, dining room, 2 conservatories, garden
Accessibility: *Floors:* 2 • *Access:* Lift • *Wheelchair access:* Good
Smoking: ✗
Pets: ✓
Routines: Flexible

Room details
Single: 10
Shared: 0
En suite: 10
Facilities: TV point, telephone point

Door lock: ✓
Lockable place: ✓

Services provided
Beauty services: Hairdressing
Mobile library: ✓
Religious services: Weekly Anglican service
Transport: ✗
Activities: *Coordinator.* ✗ • *Examples:* Quizzes, visiting entertainers
   Outings: ✗
Meetings: ✓

Denewood House Care Home

Manager: Caroline Bleach
Owner: Samily Care Ltd
Contact: 12–14 Denewood Road,
West Moors, Ferndown, Dorset, BH22 0LX
☏ 01202 892008

Set in a residential area of West Moors, Denewood House is situated near local shops, a pub, churches and a library. A bus stop is also situated just outside the building. Some of the bedrooms have patio doors leading out into the garden. There is no activities coordinator at the home but staff organise games for residents to participate in.

Registered places: 21
Guide weekly rate: £442–£575
Specialist care: Respite
Medical services: Podiatry, optician
Qualified staff: Fails standard: 25% at NVQ level 2

Home details
Location: Village location, 0.5 miles from West Moors centre
Communal areas: Lounge, dining room, garden
Accessibility: *Floors:* 2 • *Access:* Stair lift • *Wheelchair access:* None
Smoking: ×
Pets: At manager's discretion
Routines: Flexible

Room details
Single: 17
Shared: 2
En suite: 13
Facilities: TV

Door lock: ✓
Lockable place: ✓

Services provided
Beauty services: Hairdressing
Mobile library: ×
Religious services: ×
Transport: ×
Activities: *Coordinator.* × • *Examples*: Bingo • *Outings:* ×
Meetings: ×

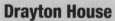

Drayton House

Manager: Andrea Quirk, Isabella Fitzgerald and Mr and Mrs Pitcher
Owner: Andrea Quirk, Isabella Fitzgerald and Mr and Mrs Pitcher
Contact: 50 West Allington, Bridport, Dorset, DT6 5BH
☏ 01308 422835

Drayton House is a small home with 19 places set near the centre of Bridport. Its size has allowed both residents and staff to build a good rapport. An activities coordinator makes sure residents are kept active and occasionally gets them to create a life scrapbook, so they can reminisce about the past.

Registered places: 19
Guide weekly rate: £417–£450
Specialist care: Respite
Medical services: Podiatry, dentist, optician
Qualified staff: Meets standard

Home details
Location: Residential area, 0.5 miles from Bridport centre
Communal areas: 2 lounges, dining room, patio and garden
Accessibility: *Floors:* 2 • *Access:* Lift • *Wheelchair access:* Good
Smoking: ×
Pets: At manager's discretion
Routines: Flexible

Room details
Single: 13
Shared: 3
En suite: 7
Facilities: None

Door lock: ✓
Lockable place: ✓

Services provided
Beauty services: Hairdressing
Mobile library: ×
Religious services: ×
Transport: ×
Activities: *Coordinator.* ✓ • *Examples*: Life scrapbooks • *Outings:* ×
Meetings: ×

Registered places: 35
Guide weekly rate: £725–£800
Specialist care: Nursing, physical disability, respite
Medical services: Podiatry, optician, physiotherapy
Qualified staff: Fails standard

Home details

Location: Residential area, 1 mile from Bournemouth centre
Communal areas: 2 lounges, dining room, garden
Accessibility: *Floors:* 3 • *Access:* Lift and stair lift
    Wheelchair access: Good
Smoking: x
Pets: At manager's discretion
Routines: Flexible

Room details

Single: 29
Shared: 1
En suite: 19
Facilities: TV point, telephone point

Door lock: x
Lockable place: ✓

Services provided

Beauty services: Hairdressing, reflexology
Mobile library: ✓
Religious services: x
Transport: x
Activities: *Coordinator.* ✓ • *Examples*: Bingo, music and movement,
    visiting entertainers • *Outings:* ✓
Meetings: x

Drumconner

Manager: Helen Colley
Owner: Drumconner Homes Ltd
Contact: 20 Poole Road, Bournemouth,
Dorset, BH4 9DR
) 01202 761420
@ info@drumconner.co.uk
⌐ www.drumconner.co.uk

Drumconner is set in a residential area approximately one mile from the centre of Bournemouth. A period property set back from the main road, Drumconner boasts beautiful gardens. The home competes in the 'Bournemouth in Bloom' contest and often does very well: the home hasn't placed outside the top two for the last six years. There is an activities coordinator at the home who organises visits from entertainers and exercise.

Registered places: 36
Guide weekly rate: £575–£705
Specialist care: Nursing
Medical services: Podiatry, dentist, optician
Qualified staff: Meets standard

Home details

Location: Rural area, 2.5 miles from Upton
Communal areas: Lounge, dining room, conservatory, patio
Accessibility: *Floors:* 3 • *Access:* Lift • *Wheelchair access:* Good
Smoking: x
Pets: ✓
Routines: Flexible

Room details

Single: 34
Shared: 4
En suite: Undisclosed
Facilities: TV point

Door lock: x
Lockable place: ✓

Services provided

Beauty services: Hairdressing
Mobile library: x
Religious services: x
Transport: x
Activities: *Coordinator.* ✓ • *Examples*: Themed days • *Outings:* x
Meetings: ✓

Forest Hill House Nursing Home

Manager: Julie Dove
Owner: Royal Bay Care Homes Ltd
Contact: Rushall Lane, Corfe Mullen,
Wimborne, Dorset, BH21 3RT
) 01202 631741
@ foresthilloffice@aol.com

Forest Hill House is set in a rural area with spacious wooded grounds. Many rooms of the home have views of the grounds. A conservatory leads out onto a patio area with a pond, raised flowerbeds and seating. The activities coordinator organises events centred on memorable days, such as the Queen's birthday, sporting events or seasons. A summer fête is also an annual occurrence.

Friary House

Manager: Peter Fry
Owner: Michael Fry
Contact: 26 Carlton Road North, Weymouth, Dorset, DT4 7PY

☎ 01305 782574
@ enquiries@kfcare.co.uk
🖱 www.kfcare.co.uk

Situated in a quiet residential area of Weymouth, Friary House is one of two homes owned by Michael Fry. His son is currently the home's manager. Set in grounds that are surrounded by hedges and trees, Friary House is near local shops. All the food is home cooked and it includes lots of fresh local produce. There is a variable choice of food and residents are welcome to eat in their room if they prefer. There is an activities coordinator at the home and outings occur regularly.

Registered places: 16
Guide weekly rate: £375–£450
Specialist care: Respite
Medical services: Podiatry, occupational therapy, physiotherapy
Qualified staff: Exceeds standard: 75% at NVQ level 2

Home details
Location: Residential area, 1 mile from Weymouth centre
Communal areas: Lounge, dining room, garden
Accessibility: *Floors:* 3 • *Access:* Lift • *Wheelchair access:* Good
Smoking: ✕
Pets: ✕
Routines: Flexible

Room details
Single: 16
Shared: 0
En suite: 16
Facilities: None

Door lock: ✓
Lockable place: ✓

Services provided
Beauty services: Hairdressing, manicures
Mobile library: ✕
Religious services: ✕
Transport: ✕
Activities: *Coordinator.* ✓ • *Examples:* Bingo, games • *Outings:* ✓
Meetings: ✕

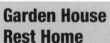

Garden House Rest Home

Manager: Gillian Houghton
Owner: Garden House Rest Home Ltd
Contact: Priestlands, Sherborne, Dorset, DT9 4HN

☎ 01935 813188

Garden House is located in Sherborne town, six miles from Yeovil. There is a regular programme of activities, including weekly bingo, daily crosswords and various outings arranged. Residents also enjoy visiting school children and entertainers. A good working relationship has been formed with the local GP. There is good contact with the local community and staff encourage residents to remain active.

Registered places: 15
Guide weekly rate: Undisclosed
Specialist care: Respite
Medical services: Podiatry, optician
Qualified staff: Exceeds standard: 70% at NVQ Level 2

Home details
Location: Residential area, in Sherborne
Communal areas: Lounge, dining room, conservatory, patio and garden
Accessibility: *Floors:* 1 • *Wheelchair access:* Good
Smoking: ✕
Pets: ✓
Routines: Flexible

Room details
Single: 15
Shared: 0
En suite: 15
Facilities: TV point

Door lock: ✓
Lockable place: ✓

Services provided
Beauty services: Hairdressing
Mobile library: ✕
Religious services: Communion service
Transport: ✕
Activities: *Coordinator.* ✕ • *Examples:* Bingo, daily crosswords, quizzes • *Outings:* ✓
Meetings: ✕

Registered places: 26
Guide weekly rate: £323–£495
Specialist care: Dementia, respite
Medical services: Podiatry, dentist, optician
Qualified staff: Exceeds standard: 66% at NVQ level 2

Home details
Location: Residential area, 1 mile from Weymouth
Communal areas: 2 lounges, dining room, patio and garden
Accessibility: *Floors:* 2 • *Access:* Lift and stair lift
Wheelchair access: Good
Smoking: In designated area
Pets: At manager's discretion
Routines: Flexible

Room details
Single: 24
Shared: 1
En suite: 25
Facilities: TV point, telephone point

Door lock: ✓
Lockable place: ✓

Services provided
Beauty services: Hairdressing
Mobile library: ✗
Religious services: Monthly Anglican Communion service,
monthly Baptist service
Transport: ✗
Activities: *Coordinator:* ✓ • *Examples*: Bingo, quizzes,
visiting entertainers • *Outings:* ✗
Meetings: ✗

Goldcrest

Manager: Linda Smith
Owner: Rajendrasen and Angela Purusram
Contact: 183 Dorchester Road,
Weymouth, Dorset, DT4 7LF
☎ 01305 830400
@ goldcrestcare@btconnect.com
🖥 www.goldcrestresthome.com

Goldcrest is located on the main Dorchester to Weymouth road, a short walk from local shops and a pub. It is around a 15-minute walk to the town, approximately one mile away. The home has two lounges for residents to relax in, as well as a garden with a patio area they can enjoy in the summer. The home arranges an Anglican Communion service once a month in addition to a Baptist service once a month. The home also has an activities coordinator who arranges quizzes as well as performances from visiting entertainers as part of the activities programme.

Registered places: 11
Guide weekly rate: £440–£450
Specialist care: None
Medical services: Podiatry, optician, physiotherapy
Qualified staff: Fails standard

Home details
Location: Residential area, in Dorchester
Communal areas: Lounge, dining room, conservatory,
patio and garden
Accessibility: *Floors:* 2 • *Access:* Lift • *Wheelchair access:* Good
Smoking: ✗
Pets: At manager's discretion
Routines: Flexible

Room details
Single: 11
Shared: 0
En suite: 6
Facilities: TV point, telephone point

Door lock: ✓
Lockable place: ✓

Services provided
Beauty services: Hairdressing
Mobile library: ✓
Religious services: Monthly Communion service
Transport: Car
Activities: *Coordinator:* ✗ • *Examples*: Coffee mornings, games,
music to movement • *Outings:* ✓
Meetings: ✓

Grassington House

Manager: Marion Franklin
Owner: Marion Franklin
Contact: 50 Prince of Wales Road,
Dorchester, Dorset, DT1 1PP
☎ 01305 267968
@ Neill1@onetel.com

A Victorian property set in a residential area of Dorchester, Grassington House has enclosed gardens that feature flower borders and shrubs along with a paved terrace. There is also ample communal space for the 11 residents, including a lounge, dining room and conservatory. There is no activities coordinator at the home, but staff run coffee morning, games and exercise for residents. They also take them on occasional outings.

Greenbushes Nursing Home

Manager: Beverly Welch
Owner: Dorchester Care Ltd
Contact: 10 Weymouth Avenue,
Dorchester, Dorset, DT1 2EN
☎ 01305 262192
@ greenbushes@bmlhealthcare.co.uk
🖰 www.bmlhealthcare.co.uk

Greenbushes Nursing Home is set in a detached house on the southern edge of Dorchester, within walking distance to the town centre. The house is made up partially of the traditional building and well as a new extension, housing 10 rooms. It is surrounded by lawned gardens with flowerbeds. There is a bus stop right outside the home, with services into town. A dedicated activities coordinator organises local outings and visiting entertainers.

Registered places: 42
Guide weekly rate: £550–£700
Specialist care: Nursing
Medical services: Podiatry, optician, physiotherapy
Qualified staff: Meets standard

Home details
Location: Residential area, in Dorchester
Communal areas: Lounge, dining room, conservatory
Accessibility: *Floors:* 2 • *Access:* Lift • *Wheelchair access:* Good
Smoking: ✗
Pets: ✗
Routines: Flexible

Room details
Single: 32
Shared: 5   **Door lock:** ✓
En suite: 17   **Lockable place:** ✓
Facilities: None

Services provided
Beauty services: Hairdressing
Mobile library: ✗
Religious services: ✗
Transport: ✗
Activities: *Coordinator:* ✓ • *Examples:* Visiting entertainers
     Outings: ✓
Meetings: ✓

Hillsdon Private Nursing Home

Manager: Alison Thomas
Owner: Baselink Care Ltd
Contact: 37 Springfield Road,
Lower Parkstone, Poole, Dorset, BH14 0LG
☎ 01202 742753
@ graham.thomas@
     baselinegroup.org.uk
🖰 www.hillsdonnursing.co.uk

A detached building that is situated close to the centre of Poole, Hillsdon Private Nursing Home is 10 minutes' walk away from the local shops and is serviced by local buses. With large windows in the bedrooms to let in the sun, Hillsdon also has a decked area in the garden where residents may pass the time outside and work on a sensory garden is expected to be completed shortly. There are regular resident and relative meetings every six months and with pets welcome in the home, Hillsdon also has a cat living on site.

Registered places: 21
Guide weekly rate: £525–£675
Specialist care: Nursing, respite
Medical services: Podiatry, dentist, optician, physiotherapy
Qualified staff: Exceeds standard: 64% at NVQ level 2

Home details
Location: Residential area, 1.5 miles from Poole
Communal areas: Lounge, dining room, garden
Accessibility: *Floors:* 2 • *Access:* Lift • *Wheelchair access:* Good
Smoking: ✗
Pets: ✓
Routines: Flexible

Room details
Single: 13
Shared: 4   **Door lock:** ✓
En suite: 5   **Lockable place:** ✓
Facilities: TV point, telephone point

Services provided
Beauty services: Hairdressing
Mobile library: Library facilities
Religious services: Monthly Communion service
Transport: ✗
Activities: *Coordinator:* ✗ • *Examples:* Gentle exercise, singalongs
     Outings: ✗
Meetings: ✓

Registered places: 13
Guide weekly rate: £400–£460
Specialist care: Day care, respite
Medical services: Podiatry, dentist, optician, physiotherapy
Qualified staff: Meets standard

Home details

Location: Village location, 1 mile from Bridport
Communal areas: Lounge, dining room, garden
Accessibility: *Floors:* 2 • *Access:* Stair lift
    Wheelchair access: Limited
Smoking: ✗
Pets: At manager's discretion
Routines: Flexible

Room details

Single: 11
Shared: 1   Door lock: ✗
En suite: 5   Lockable place: ✗
Facilities: TV point, telephone point

Services provided

Beauty services: Hairdressing
Mobile library: ✗
Religious services: Monthly Anglican Communion service
Transport: Car
Activities: *Coordinator:* ✗ • *Examples:* Games, theme days
    Outings: ✓
Meetings: ✓

The Homestead

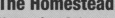

Manager: Susan Butler
Owner: Adrian and Susan Butler
Contact: 101 West Bay Road,
Bridport, Dorset, DT6 4AY
☏ 01308 423338
@ adrianbutler@hstead.eclipse.co.uk

The Homestead is a Georgian building located mid-way between Bridport and West Bay, approximately one mile from both. Susan and Adrian Butler, the owners, live in a private flat on the second floor. With a rear sloped garden that contains a vegetable patch, the home also has an attractive 'sensory' garden at the front with a seating area. Situated half a mile from the sea and 20 minutes' walk from the nearest shop, residents are well equipped for an independent lifestyle. The Homestead is a pet-friendly home and currently has a cat.

Registered places: 12
Guide weekly rate: Undisclosed
Specialist care: Nursing
Medical services: Podiatry
Qualified staff: Meets standard

Home details

Location: Residential area, 2 miles from Christchurch
Communal areas: Lounge, garden
Accessibility: *Floors:* 2 • *Access:* Lift • *Wheelchair access:* Good
Smoking: ✗
Pets: ✓
Routines: Flexible

Room details

Single: 4
Shared: 4   Door lock: ✓
En suite: 0   Lockable place: ✓
Facilities: None

Services provided

Beauty services: Hairdressing, manicures
Mobile library: ✗
Religious services: ✗
Transport: ✗
Activities: *Coordinator:* ✗ • *Examples:* Scrabble • *Outings:* ✗
Meetings: ✗

Kelso

Manager: Angela Ackrill
Owner: Kenneth and Angela Ackrill
Contact: 10 Clifton Road, Southbourne,
Bournemouth, Dorset, BH6 3PA
☏ 01202 432655

Kelso is situated near the seafront in a residential area of Southbourne. An emphasis is put on the residents' health needs and they are treated with dignity by the staff. The environment surrounding the property is well maintained. Residents are encouraged by staff to personalise their rooms with pictures, mementos and small items of furniture.

Kingsley Court

Manager: Becky Chapman
Owner: Michael Fry
Contact: 28 Dorchester Road, Weymouth, Dorset, DT4 7JU

) 01305 782343
@ kingsleycourt28@aol.com
🖰 www.kfcare.co.uk

Part of a family-run business, Kingsley Court is a detached home located on the Dorchester Road five minutes from both the beach and local shops. Well located for residents wishing to retain their independence, the home is also a five-minute bus ride from the town. Although the home generally has good wheelchair access, three of the home's bedrooms are only accessible to those able to walk. The home has secluded gardens and is visited regularly by Pets As Therapy.

Registered places: 18
Guide weekly rate: £450–£600
Specialist care: Respite
Medical services: Podiatry, dentist, optician, physiotherapy
Qualified staff: Fails standard

Home details
Location: Residential area, in Weymouth
Communal areas: Lounge, dining room, garden
Accessibility: *Floors:* 2 • *Access:* Stair lift • *Wheelchair access:* Good
Smoking: ✗
Pets: At manager's discretion
Routines: Flexible

Room details
Single: 14
Shared: 2
En suite: 16
Facilities: TV point, telephone point

Door lock: ✓
Lockable place: ✓

Services provided
Beauty services: Hairdressing, manicures
Mobile library: ✓
Religious services: ✗
Transport: ✗
Activities: *Coordinator.* ✓ • *Examples:* Visiting entertainers
 Outings: ✓
Meetings: ✗

Knyveton Hall Rest Home

Manager: Elaine Coggins
Owner: Alan Coggins Ltd
Contact: 34 Knyveton Road, East Cliff, Bournemouth, Dorset, BH1 3QR

) 0202 557671

Knyveton Hall lies between Bournemouth and Boscombe – 100 yards from Boscmobe Gardens and a short five-minute drive from the seafront. A family-run home where the proprietors live on the premises, the building began life as a school before becoming a hotel and then a care home. Bedrooms in Knyveton Hall exceed minimum sizing standards. The home offers two or three outings a year and has a comprehensive activities programme.

Registered places: 39
Guide weekly rate: £325–£425
Specialist care: Day care, respite
Medical services: Podiatry, dentist, optician
Qualified staff: Undisclosed

Home details
Location: Residential area, 2 miles from Bournemouth centre
Communal areas: 3 lounges, dining room, garden
Accessibility: *Floors:* 4 • *Access:* Lift • *Wheelchair access:* Good
Smoking: In designated area
Pets: At manager's discretion
Routines: Flexible

Room details
Single: 35
Shared: 2
En suite: 37
Facilities: TV, telephone point

Door lock: ✓
Lockable place: ✓

Services provided
Beauty services: Hairdressing, manicures
Mobile library: ✓
Religious services: Weekly Anglican and Catholic visits
Transport: Car
Activities: *Coordinator.* ✗ • *Examples:* Arts and crafts, games, visiting entertainers • *Outings:* ✓
Meetings: ✗

Registered places: 24
Guide weekly rate: From £500
Specialist care: None
Medical services: Podiatry, dentist, occupational therapy, optician
Qualified staff: Fails standard: 40% at NVQ level 2

Home details
Location: Village location, 0.5 miles from Blandford
Communal areas: Lounge, dining room, conservatory,
    patio and garden
Accessibility: *Floors:* 2 • *Access:* Lift • *Wheelchair access:* Good
Smoking: ×
Pets: ×
Routines: Flexible

Room details
Single: 20
Shared: 2   Door lock: ✓
En suite: 21   Lockable place: ✓
Facilities: TV, telephone point

Services provided
Beauty services: Hairdressing
Mobile library: ✓
Religious services: Monthly Communion service
Transport: ×
Activities: *Coordinator.* ✓ • *Examples:* Bingo, games • *Outings:* ✓
Meetings: ✓

Larks Leas

Manager: Andrea Falconer
Owner: Castle Farm Care Ltd
Contact: Milldown Road,
Blandford, Dorset, DT11 7DE
) 01258 452777
@ admin@larksleas.co.uk
🖰 www.larksleas.co.uk

A detached property located on a main road, only half a mile from Blandford, Larks Leas is a modern building with an attractive garden that features paving and colourful flowers. There is also a conservatory so the garden can be enjoyed on cold days as well. The home offers occupational therapy as well as other support services. It also has an activities coordinator who facilitates the social atmosphere and organises games. It has a happy atmosphere with good caring, has a home feeling rather that of an institution.

Registered places: 55
Guide weekly rate: £330–£600
Specialist care: Emergency admissions, respite
Medical services: Podiatry, dentist, optician, physiotherapy
Qualified staff: Undisclosed

Home details
Location: Residential area, 2 miles from Poole centre
Communal areas: 5 lounges, 4 dining rooms, patio and garden
Accessibility: *Floors:* 2 • *Access:* Lift • *Wheelchair access:* Good
Smoking: In designated area
Pets: At manager's discretion
Routines: Flexible

Room details
Single: 53
Shared: 1   Door lock: ✓
En suite: 54   Lockable place: ✓
Facilities: TV point, telephone point

Services provided
Beauty services: Hairdressing
Mobile library: ✓
Religious services: Monthly nondenominational Communion service
Transport: ×
Activities: *Coordinator.* ✓ • *Examples:* Bingo, exercise to music
    Outings: ✓
Meetings: ✓

The Laurels and Pine Lodge

Manager: Shona Sydenham
Owner: Jocelyn Evans
Contact: 33–37 Foxholes Road,
Oakdale, Poole, Dorset, BH15 3NA
) 01202 743202
@ thelaurels33@aol.com

Comprised of two houses and situated in a residential area of Poole, The Laurels and Pine Lodge are five minutes' walk away from the local newsagents and are situated on a bus route. Residents can enjoy a variety of activities, including games and a Pimm's afternoon in the summer. Regular outings are organised throughout the year. There is ample choice of communal areas, including five lounge areas, four dining rooms and a patio area.

The Laurels Retirement Home

Manager: Tarina Price
Owner: Richard and Elizabeth Kitchen
Contact: 195 Barrack Road, Christchurch, Dorset, BH23 2AR
) 01202 470179
@ info@laurels.uk.net

The Laurels Retirement Home is an older-style property, with a more recent extension, situated on one of the main roads into Christchurch town centre. The home has a lounge and dining room, which also has seated area that looks onto the patio. To the rear of the property is a private patio area, which also has seating where residents can entertain visitors.

Registered places: 20
Guide weekly rate: £345–£550
Specialist care: Dementia
Medical services: Podiatry, dentist, optician
Qualified staff: Exceeds standard: 85% at NVQ level 2

Home details
Location: Residential area, 1 mile from Christchurch centre
Communal areas: Lounge, dining room, patio and garden
Accessibility: *Floors:* 2 • *Access:* Stair lift
   Wheelchair access: Limited
Smoking: x
Pets: ✓
Routines: Flexible

Room details
Single: 12
Shared: 4
En suite: 3
Facilities: TV

Door lock: ✓
Lockable place: ✓

Services provided
Beauty services: Hairdressing, manicures
Mobile library: x
Religious services: x
Transport: x
Activities: *Coordinator:* x • *Examples:* Arts and crafts, exercises, visiting entertainers • *Outings:* x
Meetings: x

Linkfield Court

Manager: Yolanda Farrell
Owner: Linkfield Court Ltd
Contact: 19 Knyveton Road, East Cliff, Bournemouth, Dorset, BH1 3QG
) 01202 558301
@ Linkfieldcourt@btinternet.com

Linkfield Court is a former hotel, retaining many of its original features. It is set in three quarters of an acre of gardens, 10 minutes' walk from the beach. On a main bus route and five minutes from the train station and a supermarket, residents here are well equipped for an independent lifestyle. As well as holding regular resident and relatives meetings, Linkfield Court also belongs to the care aware scheme – an advocacy service offered to the families of residents. A self-contained independent living area is also available within the main building for one non-permanent resident over the age of 40.

Registered places: 29
Guide weekly rate: £269–£650
Specialist care: Day care, respite
Medical services: Podiatry, dentist, optician, physiotherapy
Qualified staff: Undisclosed

Home details
Location: Residential area, 1 mile from Bournemouth
Communal areas: 2 lounge/dining rooms, patio and garden
Accessibility: *Floors:* 2 • *Access:* Lift • *Wheelchair access:* Good
Smoking: In designated area
Pets: At manager's discretion
Routines: Flexible

Room details
Single: 23
Shared: 3
En suite: 11
Facilities: TV point, telephone point

Door lock: ✓
Lockable place: ✓

Services provided
Beauty services: Hairdressing
Mobile library: ✓
Religious services: Monthly Anglican visits
Transport: x
Activities: *Coordinator:* x • *Examples:* Bingo, mobility exercises • *Outings:* ✓
Meetings: ✓

Registered places: 17
Guide weekly rate: £475–£650
Specialist care: Emergency admissions, respite
Medical services: Podiatry, dentist, optician
Qualified staff: Fails standard

Home details
Location: Residential area, 2 miles from Bournemouth centre
Communal areas: Lounge, dining room, garden
Accessibility: *Floors:* 2 • *Access:* Lift • *Wheelchair access:* Good
Smoking: ✗
Pets: At manager's discretion
Routines: Flexible

Room details
Single: 15
Shared: 1
En suite: 13
Facilities: TV point, telephone point

Door lock: ✓
Lockable place: ✓

Services provided
Beauty services: Hairdressing
Mobile library: ✓
Religious services: ✗
Transport: Car
Activities: *Coordinator:* ✗ • *Examples:* Bingo, exercise class, musical entertainment • *Outings:* ✓
Meetings: ✓

Long Close

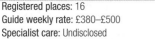

Manager: Christine Barrow
Owner: Keith London-Webb
Contact: 23 Forest Road,
Branksome Park, Poole,
Dorset, BH13 6DQ
☎ 01202 765090
@ long_close@btconnect.com

In a quiet residential area of Branksome Park, Long Close is set in woodland; approximately 15 minutes' walk from the nearest shop in Westbourne and close to the beach. Appealing to those with a horticultural interest, the home has attractive secluded gardens. As well as for outings, the home's own car can be used to take residents out on an individual basis

---

Registered places: 16
Guide weekly rate: £380–£500
Specialist care: Undisclosed
Medical services: Podiatry, dentist, optician
Qualified staff: Fails standard

Home details
Location: Residential area, 1 mile from Sherborne
Communal areas: Lounge, dining room, patio and garden
Accessibility: *Floors:* 2 • *Access:* Stair lift • *Wheelchair access:* Good
Smoking: ✗
Pets: ✓
Routines: Flexible

Room details
Single: 16
Shared: 0
En suite: 13
Facilities: None

Door lock: ✗
Lockable place: ✓

Services provided
Beauty services: Hairdressing
Mobile library: ✓ Religious services: ✗
Transport: ✗
Activities: *Coordinator:* ✗ • *Examples:* Arts and crafts, music for health • *Outings:* ✗
Meetings: ✓

Ludbourne Hall

Manager: Denise Read
Owner: Scosa Ltd
Contact: South Street, Sherborne,
Dorset, DT9 3LT
☎ 01935 816382

An older property which has features dating back to the 18th-century, Ludbourne Hall is situated close to local amenities. The home is within easy access of the town's facilities including the railway station, gardens and Abbey. Plans and risk assessments are in place for each resident and contain detailed guidance so that staff can meet identified needs.

Lytchetts

Manager: Alison Borries
Owner: Carl and Alison Borries
Contact: 4 Chalky Road,
Broadmayne, Dorset, DT2 8PJ
) 01305 853524

Lytchetts is a detached property in a residential area of Broadmayne village, situated in the heart of the Dorset and 10 minutes' walk from local amenities such as a shop and pub. The main communal area provides views of the plants and wildlife in the garden and some bedrooms have patio doors which lead directly into it. The home operates a flexible visiting policy and residents may invite guests to stay for meals free of charge. There are also facilities available for the resident to make their guest light refreshments.

Registered places: 12
Guide weekly rate: £560
Specialist care: Day care, respite
Medical services: Podiatry, dentist, optician
Qualified staff: Meets standard

Home details
Location: Village location, 4 miles from Dorchester
Communal areas: Lounge/dining room, garden
Accessibility: *Floors:* 1 • *Wheelchair access:* Good
Smoking: In designated area
Pets: At manager's discretion
Routines: Flexible

Room details
Single: 12
Shared: 0
En suite: 12
Facilities: TV point, telephone point
Door lock: ✓
Lockable place: ✓

Services provided
Beauty services: Hairdressing, reflexology
Mobile library: Library facilities
Religious services: Monthly Communion service
Transport: Car
Activities: *Coordinator:* x • *Examples:* Arts and crafts, games, musical entertainment • *Outings:* ✓
Meetings: ✓

The Malthouse

Manager: Susan Bracher
Owner: Nicola Lewis
Contact: Bay Road, Gillingham, Dorset, SP8 4EW
) 01747 822667
@ care@malthouserh.co.uk
⌂ www.malthouserh.co.uk

A 17th-century building that has been greatly extended, The Malthouse is situated on the outskirts of Gillingham and can be found down a quiet lane. Approximately 10 minutes' walk from the nearest shop, the home has spacious gardens with a courtyard area, raised flowerbeds and bird Avery. In addition to the registered bedrooms, there are three ground-floor apartments and five 'lodges' that have been built in the grounds of the home.

Registered places: 33
Guide weekly rate: £585–£720
Specialist care: Day care, emergency admissions, respite
Medical services: Podiatry, dentist, optician
Qualified staff: Undisclosed

Home details
Location: Village location, 0.5 miles from Gillingham centre
Communal areas: 2 lounges, lounge/dining room, dining room, patio and garden
Accessibility: *Floors:* 3 • *Access:* Lift • *Wheelchair access:* Good
Smoking: In designated area
Pets: At manager's discretion
Routines: Flexible

Room details
Single: 27
Shared: 3
En suite: 29
Facilities: TV point, telephone point
Door lock: ✓
Lockable place: x

Services provided
Beauty services: Hairdressing, aromatherapy, manicures
Mobile library: ✓
Religious services: Fortnightly Anglican Communion service
Transport: People carrier
Activities: *Coordinator:* ✓ • *Examples:* Games, reminiscence *Outings:* ✓
Meetings: x

Registered places: 48
Guide weekly rate: Undisclosed
Specialist care: Nursing, respite
Medical services: None
Qualified staff: Undisclosed

Home details

Location: Residential area, 1.5 miles from Gillingham
Communal areas: Lounge, dining room, garden
Accessibility: *Floors:* 2 • *Access:* Lift • *Wheelchair access:* Good
Smoking: x
Pets: ✓
Routines: Flexible

Room details

Single: 48
Shared: 0 | Door lock: ✓
En suite: 48 | Lockable place: ✓
Facilities: TV, telephone

Services provided

Beauty services: Hairdressing, aromatherapy
Mobile library: ✓
Religious services: Monthly Communion service
Transport: x
Activities: *Coordinator.* ✓ • *Examples:* Arts and crafts, singalongs, quizzes, visiting entertainers • *Outings:* ✓
Meetings: ✓

The Mellowes

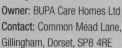

Manager: Jane Jones
Owner: BUPA Care Homes Ltd
Contact: Common Mead Lane, Gillingham, Dorset, SP8 4RE
) 01747 826677
@ bupacarehomes.co.uk

The Mellowes is located one and a half miles from the town of Gillingham and is serviced by a bus route. The home has 48 places for residential and nursing and respite care. The home has its own activities coordinator who arranges games, quizzes and visiting entertainers. There are also outings arranged to garden centres, the pub and the cinema. The residents have a flexible daily routine with set meal times. The home also has its own palliative care coordinator and prides itself on its standard of palliative care. The home has a monthly Communion service and offers the services of a hairdresser and a mobile library.

Registered places: 20
Guide weekly rate: From £480
Specialist care: Respite
Medical services: Podiatry, dentist, occupational therapy, optician
Qualified staff: Undisclosed

Home details

Location: Residential area, 1 mile from Wimborne
Communal areas: 2 lounges, dining room, garden
Accessibility: *Floors:* 2 • *Access:* Lift • *Wheelchair access:* Limited
Smoking: x
Pets: At manager's discretion
Routines: Flexible

Room details

Single: 20
Shared: 0 | Door lock: ✓
En suite: 20 | Lockable place: ✓
Facilities: TV point, telephone point

Services provided

Beauty services: Hairdressing, massage
Mobile library: ✓
Religious services: Monthly nondenominational Communion service
Transport: x
Activities: *Coordinator.* ✓ • *Examples:* Creative group, exercise
    Outings: ✓
Meetings: ✓

Mile Oak Rest Home

Manager: Lisa Sutton
Owner: Mile Oak Ltd
Contact: 2 The Acorns Wimborne Road, West Wimborne, Dorset BH21 2EU
) 01202 885225
@ mileoak@onetel.net

Set in over half an acre of garden and partly bordered by a stream which runs into the River Stour, Mile Oak Rest Home is so named by the oak tree which greets residents as they enter the home. Situated in a quiet residential area, the home lies opposite a garage and shop. With large windows which feature throughout the home and let in much light, one of the lounges in the home is a quiet sun lounge. The gardens are a particular feature with mature trees and shrubs as well as a pond. The home prides itself on its homely atmosphere, and currently has two cats.

Millbrook House

Manager: Sharon Chalke
Owner: Millbrook House Ltd
Contact: Child Okeford, Blandford, Dorset, DT11 8EY
☎ 01258 860330

A Georgian house that has been extended, Millbrook House is located seven miles from the town centre of Blandford. There is a bus service to the town. Pets are allowed in the home and there are designated smoking areas. There are three floors with three lifts and good wheelchair access. The home offers a manicure service every week and a mobile library visits every six weeks. The home arranges activities such as games, visiting entertainers and quizzes and organises outings to the seaside and to the theatre.

Registered places: 33
Guide weekly rate: £525–£620
Specialist care: None
Medical services: Podiatry, dentist, optician, physiotherapy
Qualified staff: Exceeds standard: 60% at NVQ Level 2

Home details
Location: Village location, 7 miles from Blandford
Communal areas: 3 lounges, 2 dining rooms, hairdressing salon, conservatory, garden
Accessibility: *Floors:* 3 • *Access:* 3 lifts • *Wheelchair access:* Good
Smoking: In designated area
Pets: ✓
Routines: Flexible

Room details
Single: 25
Shared: 4
En suite: 29
Facilities: TV, telephone
Door lock: ✓
Lockable place: ✓

Services provided
Beauty services: Hairdressing, manicures
Mobile library: ✓
Religious services: Weekly church service
Transport: ✓
Activities: *Coordinator.* ✗ • *Examples:* Arts and crafts, games, visiting entertainers • *Outings:* ✓
Meetings: ✗

Milton Lodge Residential Care Home

Manager: Beverley McNulty
Owner: Clive and Sheila Burden
Contact: 32 Milton Road, Bournemouth, Dorset, BH8 8LP
☎ 01202 556873

Situated in a residential area in Charminster, two minutes' walk from amenities such as shops, a post office and cafés, Milton Lodge is set back from the road with attractive, enclosed gardens. Also positioned five minutes' drive from the beach, the home is located close to a bus route with regular services. Although outings are mostly restricted to summer, the home holds a summer party each year and residents enjoy frequent visits from Pets As Therapy. Residents benefit from weekly meetings called 'get-togethers' where they may informally discuss aspects of their care.

Registered places: 18
Guide weekly rate: £490–£550
Specialist care: Dementia
Medical services: Podiatry, dentist, optician, physiotherapy
Qualified staff: Exceeds standard: 66% at NVQ level 2

Home details
Location: Residential area, 1.5 miles from Bournemouth centre
Communal areas: Lounge, dining room, conservatory, garden
Accessibility: *Floors:* 2 • *Access:* Stair lift • *Wheelchair access:* Good
Smoking: ✗
Pets: At manager's discretion
Routines: Flexible

Room details
Single: 16
Shared: 1
En suite: 1
Facilities: TV point, telephone point
Door lock: ✓
Lockable place: ✗

Services provided
Beauty services: Hairdressing
Mobile library: ✓
Religious services: Monthly Catholic Communion service, weekly Anglican service
Transport: ✗
Activities: *Coordinator.* ✗ • *Examples:* Bingo, exercise, reminiscence *Outings:* ✗
Meetings: ✓

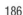

Registered places: 22
Guide weekly rate: £500–£640
Specialist care: Day care, respite
Medical services: Podiatry, dentist, optician
Qualified staff: Exceeds standard: 63% at NVQ level 2

Home details

Location: Residential area, in Dorchester
Communal areas: 2 lounges, dining room, garden
Accessibility: *Floors:* 2 • *Access:* Lift • *Wheelchair access:* Good
Smoking: ×
Pets: ×
Routines: Flexible

Room details

Single: 22
Shared: 0   Door lock: ✓
En suite: 15   Lockable place: ✓
Facilities: TV point, telephone point

Services provided

Beauty services: Hairdressing, massage
Mobile library: ✓
Religious services: Monthly Communion service
Transport: Car
Activities: *Coordinator.* ×• *Examples:* Arts and crafts, bingo, yoga
    Outings: ✓
Meetings: ✓

Montrose Residential Care Home

Manager: Sara Hallett
Owner: Mrs Taylor
Contact: 40 Prince of Wales Road, Dorchester, Dorset, DT1 1PW
☎ 01305 262274
@ montroseresidential@ukonline.co.uk
🖰 www.montroseresidential.co.uk

Montrose Residential Care Home is an attractive building situated 10 minutes' walk from Dorchester town centre. The proprietor's private accommodation is on the third floor, and their daughter manages the home. As well as a recently installed suggestions box, a questionnaire is submitted to residents and relatives every three months. Outside there is a large patio with raised flowerbeds while a wide path leads to an attractive lawned area with pergola and stone birdbath. Families of residents are able to stay for meals free of charge.

Registered places: 40
Guide weekly rate: £675–£725
Specialist care: Nursing, respite
Medical services: Podiatry, dentist, occupational therapy, optician, speech therapy
Qualified staff: Meets standard

Home details

Location: Residential area, 4.5 miles from Bournemouth centre
Communal areas: Lounge, dining room, 2 conservatories, garden
Accessibility:*Floors:* 2 • *Access:* Lift • *Wheelchair access:* Good
Smoking: ×
Pets: ×
Routines: Structured

Room details

Single: 40
Shared: 0   Door lock: ✓
En suite: 40   Lockable place: ✓
Facilities: TV point, telephone point

Services provided

Beauty services: Hairdressing, aromatherapy, massage
Mobile library: ✓
Religious services: Monthly Anglican Communion service, Catholic Mass
Transport: ×
Activities: *Coordinator.* ✓ • *Examples:* Bingo, exercise • *Outings:* ✓
Meetings: ✓

Muscliff

Manager: Dedrey Charles
Owner: Muscliff Medical Ltd
Contact: 5 Tolpuddle Gardens, Muscliff, Bournemouth, Dorset, BH9 3RE
☎ 01202 516999

Owned by Muscliff Medical Ltd – a group of four doctors and a pharmacist– Muscliff is a purpose-built home which is currently undergoing renovation work. The home produces a newsletter monthly, containing details of upcoming activities and birthdays. The accessible landscaped garden boasts a fishpond and patio areas. Services provide include massage and aromatherapy as well as hairdressing. Monthly Anglican and Catholic services take place as well as regular activities.

Nazareth Lodge

Manager: Ann Ambrose
Owner: Susan Trimble
Contact: Penny Street,
Sturminster Newton, Dorset, DT10 1DE
) 01258 472511
@ Nazareth.lodge@tiscali.co.uk

A purpose-built home set in its own gardens, Nazareth Lodge is located in the small town of Sturminster Newton, close to local amenities including shops and a church. There are two lounges in the home, one of which is used as a meeting room for residents to greet guests in a more private space. There is no activities coordinator at the home, but staff organise games and beauty therapy for residents.

Registered places: 22
Guide weekly rate: Undisclosed
Specialist care: Day care, respite
Medical services: Podiatry, physiotherapy
Qualified staff: Fails standard

Home details
Location: Village location, 9 miles from Blandford
Communal areas: 2 lounges, dining room, conservatory, garden
Accessibility: *Floors:* 2 • *Access:* Lift • *Wheelchair access:* Good
Smoking: ✗
Pets: ✓
Routines: Flexible

Room details
Single: 20
Shared: 2
En suite: 11
Facilities: TV point, telephone point
Door lock: ✓
Lockable place: ✗

Services provided
Beauty services: Hairdressing, hydrotherapy, manicures
Mobile library: ✓
Religious services: Monthly Anglican Communion service
Transport: ✗
Activities: *Coordinator:* ✗ • *Examples:* Games • *Outings:* ✗
Meetings: ✗

Oakdene

Manager: Linda Harmer
Owner: Dorset Health Care Ltd
Contact: Ringwood Road,
Three Legged Cross, Wimborne,
Dorset, BH21 6RB
) 01202 813722
@ info@oakdenecare.co.uk
⌂ www.oakdenecare.co.uk

A purpose-built care home, Oakdene is situated within walking distance of Three Legged Cross village shops. The home has landscaped gardens with raised flowerbeds and a terrace area. An activities coordinator organises in-house activities such as arts and crafts and visits from entertainers and Pets As Therapy. A mobile library also visits frequently.

Registered places: 45
Guide weekly rate: £475–£730
Specialist care: Nursing
Medical services: Podiatry, optician, physiotherapy
Qualified staff: Fails standard

Home details
Location: Village location, 2 miles from West Moors
Communal areas: 2 lounges, dining room, conservatory, garden
Accessibility: *Floors:* 2 • *Access:* Lift • *Wheelchair access:* Good
Smoking: ✗
Pets: ✓
Routines: Flexible

Room details
Single: 43
Shared: 1
En suite: 44
Facilities: TV point, telephone point
Door lock: ✓
Lockable place: ✗

Services provided
Beauty services: Hairdressing
Mobile library: ✓
Religious services: ✗
Transport: ✗
Activities: *Coordinator:* ✓ • *Examples:* Arts and crafts, musical entertainment • *Outings:* ✓
Meetings: ✗

Registered places: 28
Guide weekly rate: £450–£650
Specialist care: Respite
Medical services: Podiatry, dentist, occupational therapy, optician
Qualified staff: Meets standard

Home details
Location: Village location, in Stalbridge
Communal areas: 3 lounges, dining room, patio and garden
Accessibility: *Floors:* 3 • *Access:* Lift • *Wheelchair access:* Good
Smoking: ✗
Pets: At manager's discretion
Routines: Flexible

Room details
Single: 28
Shared: 0 | Door lock: ✓
En suite: 11 | Lockable place: ✓
Facilities: TV, telephone point

Services provided
Beauty services: Hairdressing
Mobile library: ✗
Religious services: Monthly Communion service
Transport: Minibus
Activities: *Coordinator:* ✓ • *Examples:* Exercise, skittles, quizzes
   Outings: ✓
Meetings: ✗

The Old Rectory

Manager: Kelly Henshall
Owner: Mr and Mrs Wagner-Brouwer
Contact: High Street, Stalbridge,
Dorset, DT10 2LL
) 01963 362624
@ kelly.henshall@yahoo.co.uk
🖰 www.theoldrectory.co.uk

A 17th-century Queen Anne building in the heart of the small, thriving town of Stalbridge, The Old Rectory is within level walking distance of less than five minutes from shops, a post office and a pub. With views of the Dorset countryside, the home also has secure walled gardens. A bus service offers routes to other nearby towns such as Blandford and Yeovil while the home's minibus assists less-mobile residents with frequent outings. Meals are available for guests on request at no extra charge, and a questionnaire is given out every six months to ensure a good service.

Registered places: 35
Guide weekly rate: Undisclosed
Specialist care: Day care, respite
Medical services: Podiatry, hygienist, optician, physiotherapy
Qualified staff: Meets standard

Home details
Location: Rural area, 8 miles from Yeovil
Communal areas: Lounge, 2 dining rooms, garden
Accessibility: *Floors:* 2 • *Access:* Stair lift • *Wheelchair access:* Good
Smoking: In designated area
Pets: At manager's discretion
Routines: Flexible

Room details
Single: 31
Shared: 2 | Door lock: ✓
En suite: 33 | Lockable place: ✓
Facilities: TV, telephone point

Services provided
Beauty services: Hairdressing, aromatherapy, reflexology
Mobile library: ✓
Religious services: Monthly Anglican Communion service
Transport: Car
Activities: *Coordinator:* ✓ • *Examples:* Arts and crafts, talks
   Outings: ✓
Meetings: ✓

The Old Vicarage

Manager: Natalie Foy
Owner: Tovic Ltd
Contact: Leigh, Sherborne,
Dorset, DT9 6HL
) 01935 873033
@ natalie@tovic.com
🖰 www.theoldvicarage-leigh.co.uk

The Old Vicarage is a well-established home set in spacious grounds. It is on a regular bus route to Yeovil and its amenities including shops and a cinema. As well as a comprehensive activities programme, The Old Vicarage has a shop trolley which visits residents weekly. In 2004 the home was the first in Dorset to be awarded the Investors in People award. The Old Vicarage is also the first care home in the country to be working towards accreditation as a Practice Development Unit with Bournemouth University.

Park Lodge

Manager: Ann and David Taylor
Owner: Ann and David Taylor
Contact: 18 Ridgeway, Broadstone,
Poole, Dorset, BH18 8EA
) 01202 694232

Park Lodge is located in Broadstone, on a bus route and within a quarter of a mile of local amenities including a shopping centre and library. It is also close to Broadstone Golf Club. There are two lounges for the 17 residents to choose from and a conservatory area, providing ample communal space. There is an Anglican service at the home where Communion is given every six weeks.

Registered places: 17
Guide weekly rate: £440–£450
Specialist care: None
Medical services: Podiatry
Qualified staff: Fails standard

Home details
Location: Residential area, in Broadstone
Communal areas: 2 lounges, dining room, conservatory, garden
Accessibility: *Floors:* 2 • *Access:* Lift • *Wheelchair access:* Good
Smoking: ✗
Pets: ✗
Routines: Structured

Room details
Single: 17
Shared: 0   **Door lock:** ✓
En suite: 11   **Lockable place:** ✓
Facilities: TV point, telephone point

Services provided
Beauty services: Hairdressing
Mobile library: ✗
Religious services: Anglican Communion service every 6 weeks
Transport: ✗
Activities: *Coordinator:* ✗ • *Examples:* Bingo, exercise sessions, scrabble • *Outings:* ✗
Meetings: ✓

Queensmount

Manager: Elizabeth Shacklady
Owner: BUPA Care Homes Ltd
Contact: 18 Queens Park West Drive,
Bournemouth, Dorset, BH8 9DA
) 01202 391144
@ QueensmountALL@BUPA.com
⌐ www.bupacarehomes.co.uk

Queensmount is in a peaceful setting close to the centre of Bournemouth and the seafront. Purpose-built, it offers spacious accommodation. There are four lounges and there is a licensed bar where residents may enjoy a pre-dinner drink. There are patio areas and an ornamental fountain to enjoy on a sunny afternoon. Local places of interest such as the owl sanctuary, the New Forest and Bournemouth itself may be enjoyed on organised trips or with friends and family.

Registered places: 52
Guide weekly rate: Undisclosed
Specialist care: Nursing, palliative care, respite, terminal care
Medical services: Podiatry, occupational therapy, physiotherapy
Qualified staff: Undisclosed

Home details
Location: Residential area, 2.5 miles from Bournemouth centre
Communal areas: 4 lounges, dining room, hairdressing salon, bar, kitchenette, patio and garden
Accessibility: *Floors:* 3 • *Access:* Lift • *Wheelchair access:* Good
Smoking: ✗
Pets: ✓
Routines: Flexible

Room details
Single: 44
Shared: 10   **Door lock:** ✓
En suite: 47   **Lockable place:** ✗
Facilities: TV point, telephone point

Services provided
Beauty services: Hairdressing, aromatherapy
Mobile library: ✓
Religious services: ✓
Transport: ✓
Activities: *Coordinator:* ✓ • *Examples:* Bingo, exercises • *Outings:* ✓
Meetings: ✓

Registered places: 39
Guide weekly rate: £600
Specialist care: Nursing
Medical services: Podiatry, optician
Qualified staff: Meets standard

Home details

Location: Residential area, in Sherborne
Communal areas: 2 lounges, dining room, conservatory, garden
Accessibility:*Floors:* 2 • *Access:* Lift • *Wheelchair access:* Good
Smoking: ✗
Pets: ✓
Routines: Flexible

Room details

Single: 29
Shared: 5
En suite: 31
Facilities: TV point, telephone point

Door lock: ✓
Lockable place: ✓

Services provided

Beauty services: Hairdressing, aromatherapy
Mobile library: ✓
Religious services: Weekly Catholic Communion service,
   monthly Anglican Communion service
Transport: ✗
Activities: *Coordinator.* ✓ • *Examples:* Exercise sessions,
   flower arranging, gardening • *Outings:* ✓
Meetings: ✓

Riverside

Manager: Judith Maidment
Owner: Riverside Nursing Home Ltd
Contact: Westbury, Sherborne,
Dorset, DT9 3QZ
☎ 01935 812046
@ riversidehouse@tiscali.co.uk

Overlooking the playing fields of Sherborne School, Riverside is within walking distance of the town centre though for less mobile residents a weekly trolley shop enables individuals to purchase confectionary, toiletries and stationary. The home offers individual shopping trips to parks and to the town's shops, coffee shops and the market which takes place on Thursdays and Saturdays. As well as a comprehensive activities programme, residents with an interest in gardening may use the home's greenhouse. Many residents are keen on gardening and the house organises annual competitions.

Registered places: 35
Guide weekly rate: £450–£485
Specialist care: Emergency admissions, respite
Medical services: Podiatry, dentist, occupational therapy, optician
Qualified staff: Meets standard

Home details

Location: Residential area, 2 miles from Bournemouth centre
Communal areas: Lounge, dining room, 2 conservatories, garden
Accessibility: *Floors:* 3 • *Access:* Lift and stair lift
   Wheelchair access: Limited
Smoking: ✗
Pets: At manager's discretion
Routines: Flexible

Room details

Single: 33
Shared: 1
En suite: 25
Facilities: TV point, telephone point

Door lock: ✓
Lockable place: ✓

Services provided

Beauty services: Hairdressing, aromatherapy
Mobile library: ✗
Religious services: Monthly Anglican service
Transport: Car
Activities: *Coordinator:* ✓ • *Examples:* Craft sessions, exercises,
   singalongs • *Outings:* ✓
Meetings: ✓

Shalden Grange

Manager: Janine May
Owner: Amrik and Kuldeep Benepal
Contact: 1–3 Watkin Road,
Boscombe, Bournemouth,
Dorset, BH5 1HP
☎ 01202 301918

A modern building that consists of two older properties joined together, Shalden Grange is situated in a residential area 10 minutes' walk from Boscombe's main shopping area and five minutes from the sea. With its location equipping residents well with the promise of independent living, the home is decorated in a homely fashion with residents enjoying a varied activities programme. As well as having visits from Pets As Therapy, Shalden Grange is also currently home to a pet budgie.

Southmead

Manager: Penelope Fletcher
Owner: Penelope Fletcher
Contact: 159 York Road,
Broadstone, Poole, Dorset, BH18 8ES
☎ 01202 694726
@ robert@southmead.co.uk
🖰 www.southmead.co.uk

Situated in a quiet, residential area of Broadstone, Southmead is a family-run home located on a bus route. The home has a lounge, a dining room, a garden with a patio area and a conservatory. There is a TV and a telephone in each of the rooms and a lockable place for valuables is available on request. The home has an activities coordinator who arranges daily activities such as bingo and visiting entertainers, as well as outings to the local garden centre. The home has its own cats but pets are not permitted for residents. The home arranges for a mobile library to visit and there is monthly Communion.

Registered places: 16
Guide weekly rate: £475
Specialist care: None
Medical services: Podiatry, dentist, optician, physiotherapy
Qualified staff: Exceeds standard

Home details
Location: Residential area, 3.5 miles from Poole centre
Communal areas: Lounge, dining room, conservatory, patio and garden
Accessibility: *Floors:* 2 • *Access:* Stair lift • *Wheelchair access:* Good
Smoking: ✗
Pets: ✗
Routines: Flexible

Room details
Single: 10
Shared: 3
En suite: 3
Facilities: TV, telephone

Door lock: ✓
Lockable place: ✓

Services provided
Beauty services: Hairdressing
Mobile library: ✓
Religious services: Weekly Communion service
Transport: ✓
Activities: *Coordinator:* ✓ • *Examples:* Bingo, dominoes, musical entertainment • *Outings:* ✓
Meetings: ✓

Southwood Lodge

Manager: Toni Bailey
Owner: Lesley Wilson
Contact: 36–40 Southwood Avenue,
Southbourne, Bournemouth,
Dorset, BH6 3QB
☎ 01202 422213

Located in a residential area in Boscombe, close to Bournemouth centre, Southwood Lodge benefits from its seaside location and residents often enjoy taking walks along the cliff tops. Southwood Lodge is also a short walk from local amenities including shops and a post office. There is an activities coordinator at the home and a hairdresser and beautician visit. The home has a designated room to watch a video in peace and quiet.

Registered places: 32
Guide weekly rate: £350–£550
Specialist care: Respite
Medical services: Podiatry, dentist, optician
Qualified staff: Meets standard

Home details
Location: Residential area, 3 miles from Bournemouth centre
Communal areas: Lounge, dining room, video room, garden
Accessibility: *Floors:* 3 • *Access:* Stair lift • *Wheelchair access:* Good
Smoking: ✗
Pets: At manager's discretion
Routines: Flexible

Room details
Single: 32
Shared: 0
En suite: 32
Facilities: TV point, telephone point

Door lock: ✓
Lockable place: ✓

Services provided
Beauty services: Hairdressing, beautician
Mobile library: ✓
Religious services: Monthly Anglican Communion service
Transport: ✗
Activities: *Coordinator:* ✓ • *Examples:* Bingo, games, visiting entertainers • *Outings:* ✗
Meetings: ✗

Registered places: 10
Guide weekly rate: £445
Specialist care: Day care, emergency admissions, respite
Medical services: Podiatry, dentist, optician, physiotherapy
Qualified staff: Fails standard

Home details

Location: Residential area, 2 miles from Bournemouth centre
Communal areas: Lounge, dining room, patio and garden
Accessibility: *Floors:* 2 • *Access:* Lift • *Wheelchair access:* Good
Smoking: In designated area
Pets: At manager's discretion
Routines: Flexible

Room details

Single: 10
Shared: 0
En suite: 1
Facilities: TV point, telephone point

Door lock: ✓
Lockable place: ✓

Services provided

Beauty services: Hairdressing
Mobile library: ✓
Religious services: Monthly Catholic visits
Transport: ✗
Activities: *Coordinator:* ✗ • *Examples:* Arts and crafts, bingo
   Outings: ✓
Meetings: ✗

St Bridget's Residential Home

Manager: Denise Simpson
Owner: Anthony Howell
Contact: 42 Stirling Road, Talbot Woods, Bournemouth, Dorset, BH3 7JH
☎ 01202 515969

A converted 1930s house, St Bridget's Residential Home is a small home located in a quiet residential area. A 15-minute walk from Winton, active residents may enjoy a stroll up to the town's local facilities. Priding itself on its homely atmosphere, St Bridget's encourages those with an interest in gardening to utilise the home's facilities. There is a cat called Thomas that lives at the home. Other notable features are St Bridget's coloured windows.

Registered places: 21
Guide weekly rate: £600–£650
Specialist care: Day care, respite
Medical services: Podiatry, dentist, optician, physiotherapy
Qualified staff: Meets standard

Home details

Location: Residential area, 0.5 miles from Shaftesbury centre
Communal areas: Lounge, dining room, garden room, garden
Accessibility: *Floors:* 2 • *Access:* 2 lifts • *Wheelchair access:* Good
Smoking: ✗
Pets: ✓
Routines: Flexible

Room details

Single: 21
Shared: 0
En suite: 21
Facilities: TV, telephone

Door lock: ✓
Lockable place: ✓

Services provided

Beauty services: Hairdressing, aromatherapy, manicures
Mobile library: ✓
Religious services: Monthly
Transport: ✗
Activities: *Coordinator:* ✓ • *Examples:* Daily crossword, visiting
   entertainers • *Outings:* ✓
Meetings: ✓

St Denis Lodge

Manager: Patricia Butler
Owner: St Denis Lodge Ltd
Contact: Salisbury Road, Shaftesbury, Dorset, SP7 8BS
☎ 01747 854596
@ Beverley@stdenislodge.ffnet.co.uk
🖱 www.stdenislodge.co.uk

St Denis is a large Georgian property set in its own grounds. The home is privately owned and is maintained as a country house hotel. There are 21 single rooms all with en suite facilities and some with views overlooking the garden. The home is suitable for those with low to moderate needs, who wish to retain a degree of independence, but is also accessible to those with physical frailty. An activities coordinator arranges a variety of activities for the residents such as exercise sessions twice a week, National Trust slide shows and outings once a month on a bus trip.

St James' Park Nursing Home

Manager: Helen Holden
Owner: BUPA Care Homes Ltd
Contact: Higher Street, Bradpole,
Bridport, Dorset, DT6 3EU
) 01308 421174
@ StJamesParkEveryone@BUPA.com
♨ www.bupacarehomes.co.uk

St James' Park is situated in the centre of the village of Bradpole. The original house was a 19th-century country residence. It is surrounded by landscaped gardens and a patio, overlooking the Dorset countryside. The accommodation includes a lounge, library and restaurant-style dining room in the conservatory, and there is full lift access to the upper floors. Many bedrooms have views over the grounds and beyond, and most have en suite facilities. Daily activities are offered, and personal interests are encouraged. St James' Park also offers care to older people with physical disabilities.

Registered places: 46
Guide weekly rate: Undisclosed
Specialist care: Nursing, physical disability, respite
Medical services: Podiatry, physiotherapy
Qualified staff: Undisclosed

Home details
Location: Village location, 1 mile from Bridport
Communal areas: 2 lounges, conservatory/dining room, kitchenette, library, garden
Accessibility: *Floors:* 3 • *Access:* Lift • *Wheelchair access:* Good
Smoking: ✗
Pets: ✗
Routines: Flexible

Room details
Single: 29
Shared: 7
En suite: 32
Facilities: TV point, telephone point
Door lock: ✓
Lockable place: ✗

Services provided
Beauty services: Hairdressing, aromatherapy
Mobile library: ✓
Religious services: ✓
Transport: ✓
Activities: *Coordinator.* ✓ • *Examples:* Bingo, exercises • *Outings:* ✓
Meetings: ✓

Staddon Lodge

Manager: Sheena Davis
Owner: David and Sheena Davis
Contact 25 Nelson Road, Branksome,
Poole, Dorset, BH12 1ER
) 01202 764269

An older-style Edwardian property located in a residential area, Staddon Lodge is positioned five minutes' walk from Westbourne shopping area and the Bournemouth upper gardens. A family-run home, one of the home's proprietors, Mrs Davis, also doubles as the home's manager while one member of staff lives on the premises. The home's gardens include a summerhouse, providing a pleasant place to sit in hot weather.

Registered places: 12
Guide weekly rate: £350–£585
Specialist care: Day care, emergency admissions, respite
Medical services: Podiatry, dentist, optician
Qualified staff: Exceeds standard: 70% at NVQ level 2

Home details
Location: Residential area, 1.5 miles from Bournemouth centre
Communal areas: Lounge, dining room, garden
Accessibility: *Floors:* 2 • *Access:* None • *Wheelchair access:* None
Smoking: ✗
Pets: At manager's discretion
Routines: Flexible

Room details
Single: 12
Shared: 0
En suite: 8
Facilities: TV point, telephone point
Door lock: ✓
Lockable place: ✓

Services provided
Beauty services: Hairdressing
Mobile library: Library facilities
Religious services: Monthly nondenominational Communion service
Transport: Car
Activities: *Coordinator.* ✗ • *Examples:* Games, musical entertainment
Outings: ✓
Meetings: ✗

Registered places: 36
Guide weekly rate: Undisclosed
Specialist care: Respite
Medical services: Podiatry, dentist, optician, physiotherapy
Qualified staff: Meets standard

Home details

Location: Rural area, 6 miles from Dorchester
Communal areas: Lounge, 2 dining room, conservatory, library, swimming pool, garden
Accessibility: *Floors:* 3 • *Access:* Lift • *Wheelchair access:* Good
Smoking: In designated area
Pets: At manager's discretion
Routines: Flexible

Room details

Single: 24
Shared: 6
En suite: 30
Facilities: TV point, telephone point

Door lock: ✓
Lockable place: ✓

Services provided

Beauty services: Hairdressing, aromatherapy
Mobile library: ✓
Religious services: Monthly Communion service
Transport: Car
Activities: *Coordinator:* ✓ • *Examples:* Games, visiting entertainers
  Outings: ✓
Meetings: ✓

Steepleton Manor

Manager: Vacant
Owner: Altogether Care LLP
Contact: Winterbourne Steepleton, Dorchester, Dorset, DT2 9LG
) 01305 889316
⌂ www.steepletonmanor.co.uk

A large Grade II listed Victorian manor house, Steepleton Manor is located in a rural area and set in six and a half acres of grounds. With a river running alongside the property and a Victorian walled garden, its grounds are attractive and varied. While some rooms have dedicated private bathrooms instead of an en suite, the home's extensive facilities also include an outdoor heated swimming pool. The home is located eight miles from Weymouth, and six miles from Dorchester.

Registered places: 12
Guide weekly rate: £380–£450
Specialist care: None
Medical services: Podiatry, dentist, optician
Qualified staff: Meets standard

Home details

Location: Residential area, in Wimbourne
Communal areas: Lounge, dining room, garden
Accessibility: *Floors:* 2 • *Access:* None • *Wheelchair access:* None
Smoking: ✗
Pets: ✓
Routines: Flexible

Room details

Single: 8
Shared: 2
En suite: 10
Facilities: TV point

Door lock: ✓
Lockable place: ✓

Services provided

Beauty services: Hairdressing
Mobile library: ✓
Religious services: Monthly nondenominational Communion service
Transport: Minibus
Activities: *Coordinator:* ✗ • *Examples:* One-to-one sessions
  Outings: ✓
Meetings: ✗

Stoneleigh House

Manager: Helen Edbrooke
Owner: Helen Edbrooke
Contact: 2 Rowlands Hill, Wimborne, Dorset, BH21 1AN
) 01202 884908
@ Helen@stoneleighhouse.com
⌂ www.stoneleighhouse.com

An older property, situated 200 yards from the nearest shop, Stoneleigh House is close to Wimborne's amenities which include a community centre, shops and pubs. The owner doubles as the manager and lives on the second floor. A dog also lives on the premises. With mature gardens, individuals with an interest in horticulture may take pleasure in gardening a small patch of the gardens while weekly outings ensure residents are never bored. Although the home does not have structured and regular residents meetings, the home is small enough that people are able to discuss issues openly.

Stratfield Lodge Residential Home

Manager: Ernest Pickering
Owner: Stratfield Lodge Ltd
Contact: 63 Wellington Road, Bournemouth, Dorset, BH8 8JL

) 01202 553596
@ ernestpickering@aol.com

Stratfield Lodge is a small family-owned home which caters to individuals with a learning disability as well as offering care to the elderly. The home is located one mile from Bournemouth and there is a bus service to the town centre. There are 14 single rooms most of which have en suite facilities. The home has a lounge, a dining room, a garden and a patio area. The home has its own transport and arranges for a mobile library to visit. Pets are allowed but smoking is not permitted. The home arranges daily activities for the residents.

Registered places: 14
Guide weekly rate: Undisclosed
Specialist care: Learning disability, respite
Medical services: Dentist, optician
Qualified staff: Meets standard

Home details
Location: Residential area, 1 mile from Bournemouth
Communal areas: Lounge, dining room, patio and garden
Accessibility: *Floors:* 2 • *Access:* Lift • *Wheelchair access:* Good
Smoking: ✗
Pets: ✓
Routines: Undisclosed

Room details
Single: 14
Shared: 0
En suite: Undisclosed
Facilities: TV, telephone

Door lock: ✓
Lockable place: ✓

Services provided
Beauty services: Hairdressing, manicures
Mobile library: ✓
Transport: ✓
Activities: *Coordinator:* ✗ • *Examples:* Bingo, games • *Outings:* ✓
Meetings: ✗

Summerhill Residential Home

Manager: Mrs Farrar
Owner: Mr and Mrs Farrar
Contact: 46 Glenwood Road, West Moors, Ferndown, Dorset, BH22 0ER

) 01202 870935

Summerhill Residential Home is located in a quiet, residential area of West Moors within walking distance of the local shops. It is also located on bus routes which run to both Poole and Bournemouth. The home has 15 single rooms all of which have en suite facilities. There is also a call system in each room. The home has a large lounge, a dining room and a conservatory. The garden is accessible for all the residents. The home has its own transport and takes residents on outings to local gardens and shopping.

Registered places: 15
Guide weekly rate: £430–£500
Specialist care: Respite
Medical services: Podiatry
Qualified staff: Meets standard

Home details
Location: Residential area, in West Moors
Communal areas: Lounge, dining room, conservatory, garden
Accessibility: *Floors:* 2 • *Access:* Lift • *Wheelchair access:* Good
Smoking: ✗
Pets: ✗
Routines: Structured

Room details
Single: 15
Shared: 0
En suite: 15
Facilities: None

Door lock: ✗
Lockable place: ✗

Services provided
Beauty services: Hairdressing
Mobile library: ✓
Religious services: Weekly Catholic visits
Transport: ✓
Activities: *Coordinator:* ✗ • *Examples:* Games, visiting entertainers
Outings: ✓
Meetings: ✗

Registered places: 18
Guide weekly rate: From £475
Specialist care: None
Medical services: Podiatry, dentist, optician
Qualified staff: Undisclosed

Home details

Location: Rural area, 2 miles from Lyme Regis
Communal areas: Lounge, dining room, patio and garden
Accessibility: *Floors:* 2 • *Access:* Stair lift
   Wheelchair access: Limited
Smoking: x
Pets: x
Routines: Flexible

Room details

Single: 17
Shared: 6
En suite: 2
Facilities: Telephone

Door lock: ✓
Lockable place: x

Services provided

Beauty services: Hairdressing
Mobile library: x
Religious services: Communion service every 3 weeks
Transport: x
Activities:*Coordinator.* x • *Examples:* Exercise sessions,
   videos, visiting entertainers • *Outings:* x
Meetings: x

Thistlegate House

Manager: Vacant
Owner: John Corney and June Webb
Contact: Axminster Road, Charmouth,
Dorset, DT6 6BY
) 01297 560569

Thistlegate is a Grade II listed Georgian building which stands in four acres of grounds. The home is situated near the coast, two miles from Lyme Regis. The landscaped grounds offer views over Lyme Bay and there is a seating area for residents to enjoy. There are a variety of activities arranged for the residents including exercise sessions and visiting entertainers. The residents have a flexible daily routine and may have their meals in their room if they wish. The home has two floors with a stair lift but there is limited access for wheelchair users.

Registered places: 17
Guide weekly rate: Undisclosed
Specialist care: Dementia, mental disorder, respite
Medical services: Podiatry, optician
Qualified staff: Fails standard

Home details

Location: Residential area, 2 miles from West Moors
Communal areas: Lounge, dining room, garden
Accessibility: *Floors:* 2 • *Access:* Lift • *Wheelchair access:* Good
Smoking: In designated area
Pets: At manager's discretion
Routines: Flexible

Room details

Single: 17
Shared: 0
En suite: 17
Facilities: TV point, telephone point

Door lock: ✓
Lockable place: ✓

Services provided

Beauty services: Hairdressing
Mobile library: ✓
Religious services: x
Transport: Car
Activities: *Coordinator.* x • *Examples:* Arts and crafts • *Outings:* x
Meetings: x

Thornfield Care Home

Manager: Mohammad Poordil
Owner: Sindamanee and
Mohammad Poordil
Contact: 434 Ringwood Road,
Ferndown, Dorset, BH22 9AY
) 01202 861845
@ poordil@yahoo.co.uk

Thornfield Care Home is an extended family home that is located on a main road between West Moors and Ferndown. The home is close to public transport and local amenities. As well as providing care for the elderly, the home provides specialist care for those with dementia and mental disorders. There is no activities coordinator at the home but relevant activities are organised by the staff.

Two Cedars

Manager: Jean Williams
Owner: John and Jean Williams
Contact: 81 Dunyeats Road, Broadstone, Poole, Dorset, BH18 8AF
) 01202 694942

Two Cedars was built in 1908 but has been extended so as to accommodate 17 individuals. Situated near the town that include shops, a post office and bus services, it is set back from the road in mature gardens. The home is very involved in the local community. Students and dogs visit regularly and there are many outings into Broadstone and to schools when they hold events.

Registered places: 17
Guide weekly rate: £500
Specialist care: Respite
Medical services: Podiatry, physiotherapy
Qualified staff: Undisclosed

Home details
Location: Residential area, in Broadstone
Communal areas: Lounge, dining room, patio and garden
Accessibility: *Floors:* 2 • *Access:* Lift • *Wheelchair access:* Good
Smoking: x
Pets: x
Routines: Flexible

Room details
Single: 17
Shared: 0
En suite: 17
Facilities: TV, telephone.

Door lock: ✓
Lockable place: x

Services provided
Beauty services: Hairdressing
Mobile library: x
Religious services: Monthly Communion service
Transport: x
Activities: *Coordinator:* x • *Examples:* Classical music, games
  Outings: ✓
Meetings: ✓

Whitecliffe House

Manager: Julie Schooling
Owner: Colten Care Ltd
Contact: 30–40 Whitecliffe Mill Street, Blandford, Dorset, DT11 7BQ
) 01258 450011
@ whitecliffehouse@coltencare.co.uk
⌂ www.coltencare.co.uk

Located five minutes' walk from Blandford town centre, Whitecliffe House is in a central location. An older-style building that was purpose-built, it is a red-bricked building that lies in a courtyard setting. A mobile library visits frequently and the home has its own minibus so residents can go on outings. The activities coordinator also organises in-house activities such as music therapy and visits from local entertainers.

Registered places: 28
Guide weekly rate: £680–£780
Specialist care: Nursing
Medical services: Podiatry, dentist, optician
Qualified staff: Fails standard

Home details
Location: Residential area, in Blandford
Communal areas: Lounge, dining room
Accessibility: *Floors:* 3 • *Access:* Lift • *Wheelchair access:* Good
Smoking: x
Pets: At manager's discretion
Routines: Flexible

Room details
Single: 28
Shared: 0
En suite: 0
Facilities: None

Door lock: ✓
Lockable place: ✓

Services provided
Beauty services: Hairdressing
Mobile Library: ✓
Religious services: x
Transport: Minibus
Activities: *Coordinator:* ✓ • *Examples:* Music therapy,
  visiting entertainers • *Outings:* ✓
Meetings: x

Registered places: 28
Guide weekly rate: £690
Specialist care: Nursing, emergency admissions, respite
Medical services: Podiatry, dentist, optician, physiotherapy
Qualified staff: Meets standard

Home details

Location: Village location, 2 miles from Wimborne town
Communal areas: 2 lounges, dining room, garden
Accessibility: *Floors:* 2 • *Access:* Lift • *Wheelchair access:* Good
Smoking: ✗
Pets: ✗
Routines: Flexible

Room details

Single: 24
Shared: 2   Door lock: ✓
En suite: 23   Lockable place: ✓
Facilities: TV point, telephone point

Services provided

Beauty services: Hairdressing
Mobile library: ✗
Religious services: Monthly Anglican service
Transport: ✗
Activities: *Coordinator.* ✓ • *Examples*: Bingo, visiting entertainers
    Outings: ✓
Meetings: ✗

The Wimborne

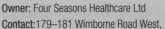

Manager: Helene Dunbar
Owner: Four Seasons Healthcare Ltd
Contact: 179–181 Wimborne Road West,
Stapehill, Wimborne, Dorset, BH21 2DJ
☎ 01202 877614
@ the.wimborne@fshc.co.uk
🖱 www.fshc.co.uk

A purpose-built home easily accessed by the A31. The Wimborne is an attractive and spacious home within walking distance of local amenities and on a bus route. Although the home does not allow residents to bring in pets, they are welcome to visit. As well as current visits from Pets As Therapy, The Wimborne currently has a dog which, owned by a staff member, does not stay overnight. The home has a shop trolley which goes round the home twice a week, and also has an organ.

Registered places: 31
Guide weekly rate: £595–£725
Specialist care: Emergency admissions, respite
Medical services: Podiatry, dentist, optician
Qualified staff: Meets standard

Home details

Location: Village location, 2 miles from Dorchester
Communal areas: 2 lounges, 2 dining rooms, conservatory, garden
Accessibility: *Floors:* 3 • *Access:* Lift • *Wheelchair access:* Good
Smoking: ✗
Pets: ✗
Routines: Flexible

Room details

Single: 23
Shared: 5   Door lock: ✓
En suite: 28   Lockable place: ✓
Facilities: TV point, telephone point

Services provided

Beauty services: Hairdressing
Mobile library: ✓
Religious services: Monthly Anglican Communion service
Transport: Minibus
Activities: *Coordinator.* ✓ • *Examples*: Discussions, quizzes, visiting
    entertainers • *Outings:* ✓
Meetings: ✓

Wolfeton Manor

Manager: Pauline Stevenson
Owner: Wolfeton Manor Healthcare Ltd
Contact: East Hill, Charminster,
Dorchester, Dorset, DT2 9QL
☎ 01305 262340
@ info@wolfetonmanor.co.uk
🖱 www.wolfetonmanor.co.uk

Built in the 19th-century as a private residence for Dorchester's Town Clerk, Wolfeton Manor sits in a tranquil setting 10 minutes from the local shop and on a bus route to Dorchester, Yeovil and Weymouth. Set in two and a half acres of garden, it is situated on a hill overlooking the Cerne and Frome Rivers with attractive gardens that feature wooded paths and an extensively stocked pond. There is a piano in the lounge for residents' use. Wolfeton Manor also has five assisted living suites for the more able resident.

Woodside Lodge

Manager: Natasha Ketchen
Owner: Woodside Lodge Ltd
Contact: 160 Burley Road,
Bransgore, Christchurch, Dorset
BH23 8DB

) 01425 673030
@ chotoblossom@aol.com

Set in a semi-rural location a few miles from Christchurch, Woodside Lodge is a modern home situated 10 minutes' walk from the local shops and on a bus route which passes right outside the home. With a huge garden complete with bird tables and spectacular views of the surrounding scenery, the home is also close to lots of natural wildlife. Residents with an interest in gardening are encouraged to exercise their passion on the grounds and may meet foxes and pheasants.

Registered places: 21
Guide weekly rate: £585–£600
Specialist care: Dementia, emergency admissions, mental disorder, respite
Medical services: Podiatry, dentist, optician, physiotherapy
Qualified staff: Exceeds standard: 100% at NVQ level 2

Home details
Location: Village location, 5 miles from Christchurch
Communal areas: 2 lounges, dining room, patio and garden
Accessibility: *Floors:* 2 • *Access:* Lift • *Wheelchair access:* Good
Smoking: ✗
Pets: At manager's discretion
Routines: Flexible

Room details
Single: 17
Shared: 2
En suite: 12
Facilities: TV point, telephone point

Door lock: ✓
Lockable place: ✓

Services provided
Beauty services: Hairdressing, manicures, reflexology
Mobile library: ✓
Religious services: Monthly nondenominational Communion service
Transport: ✗
Activities: *Coordinator:* ✗ • *Examples:* Knitting, painting, visiting entertainers • *Outings:* ✓
Meetings: ✗

Registered places: 47
Guide weekly rate: Undisclosed
Specialist care: Nursing, palliative care, respite, terminal care
Medical services: Podiatry, physiotherapy
Qualified staff: Undisclosed

Home details
Location: Residential area, in Cirencester
Communal areas: 3 lounges, dining room, bar, hairdressing salon, kitchenette, patio and garden
Accessibility: *Floors:* 3 • *Access:* Lift and stair lift
Wheelchair access: Good
Smoking: In designated area
Pets: ✓
Routines: Flexible

Room details
Single: 38
Shared: 6
En suite: 44
Facilities: TV point, telephone point

Door lock: ✓
Lockable place: ✗

Services provided
Beauty services: Hairdressing, aromatherapy
Mobile library: ✓
Religious services: Monthly Communion service
Transport: ✓
Activities: *Coordinator.* ✓ • *Examples* Games, one-to-one sessions, quizzes • *Outings:* ✓
Meetings: ✓

Ashley House Nursing Home

Manager: Ann Alden
Owner: BUPA Care Homes Ltd
Contact: 118 Trafalgar Road, Cirencester, Gloucestershire, GL7 2ED
) 01285 650671
@ AshleyHouseALL@BUPA.com
🖳 www.bupacarehomes.co.uk

Ashley House is conveniently situated within the historic Roman town of Cirencester, and is within easy reach of local shops, amenities and the Abbey grounds. Purpose-built in traditional Cotswold stone, the home is set around a sheltered courtyard garden. The home has number of lounges, and a licensed bar is available where residents may enjoy a pre-dinner drink. The activities coordinator ensures there is always something going on, including games of bridge and scrabble, art workshops and musical entertainment. Outings are organised to near-by attractions like the Cirencester Polo Club, the Abbey Grounds and the charming Cotswold countryside.

Registered places: 64
Guide weekly rate: £650–£820
Specialist care: Nursing, dementia, physical disability
Medical services: Podiatry
Qualified staff: Meets standard

Home details
Location: Rural area, 4.5 miles from Cheltenham
Communal areas: Lounge, dining room, garden
Accessibility: *Floors:* 2 • *Access:* Lifts • *Wheelchair access:* Good
Smoking: In designated area
Pets: ✓
Routines: Flexible

Room details
Single: 56
Shared: 4
En suite: 60
Facilities: TV

Door lock: ✓
Lockable place: ✓

Services provided
Beauty services: Hairdressing, aromatherapy
Activities: Coordinators: ✓ • *Examples*: Arts and crafts, visiting entertainers • *Outings:* ✓
Meetings: ✗

Badgeworth Court Care Centre

Manager: Teresa Berry
Owner: Barchester Healthcare Ltd
Contact: Badgeworth, Cheltenham, Gloucestershire GL51 4UL
) 01452 715015
@ www.barchester.com/oulton

Badgeworth Court is a Grade II listed building set in 18 acres of formal gardens. The home is divided into four sections, each caring for a diversity of needs – from the elderly and frail to dementia patients. There are three activities coordinators at the home to cater for every resident's needs. Events include Chinese New Year celebrations, a Burn's Night and Valentine's Day. '*The Badgeworth Times*' is produced for residents and visitors to keep up-to-date with news and events at the home. There are also outings on offer for the residents.

Barrington Lodge Nursing Home

Manager: Tracy Gardner
Owner: BUPA Care Homes Ltd
Contact: 138 Cirencester Road,
Charlton Kings, Cheltenham,
Gloucestershire, GL538 DS
📞 01242 263434
@ BarringtonLodgeALL@BUPA.com
🖱 www.bupacarehomes.co.uk

Originally a large private house, Barrington Lodge has been extended and converted. It is situated in a peaceful residential area of Charlton Kings, close to local shops and on a bus route to nearby Cheltenham. There are attractive landscaped gardens and a patio to enjoy on a sunny afternoon. All the bedrooms have garden views, and all have en suite facilities. Daily activities include arts and crafts, gardening, games and quizzes and trips to local places of interest. Barrington Lodge also offers care to people with Parkinson's disease and those who have had a stroke.

Registered places: 46
Guide weekly rate: Undisclosed
Specialist care: Nursing, palliative care, respite, terminal care
Medical services: Podiatry, physiotherapy, occupational therapy
Qualified staff: Undisclosed

Home details
Location: Residential area, 2 miles from Cheltenham
Communal areas: Lounge, dining room, hairdressing salon, conservatory, patio and garden
Accessibility: *Floors:* 3 • *Access:* Lift and stair lift
Wheelchair access: Good
Smoking: In designated area
Pets: ✓
Routines: Flexible

Room details
Single: 37
Shared: 0
En suite: 37
Facilities: TV point, telephone point

Door lock: ✓
Lockable place: ✗

Services provided
Beauty services: Hairdressing, aromatherapy
Mobile library: ✓
Religious services: Monthly Communion service
Transport: ✓
Activities: *Coordinator:* ✓ • *Examples:* Arts and crafts, gardening, quizzes • *Outings:* ✓
Meetings: ✓

Bay Tree Court Care Home

Manager: Natalie Bonner
Owner: European Healthcare Group Plc
Contact: High Street, Prestbury,
Cheltenham, Gloucestershire, GL52 3AU
📞 01242 236000
@ baytreecourt@ehguk.com

An modern building situated on the outskirts of Cheltenham, Bay Tree Court is a purpose-built home that provides nursing and residential care on two separate floors. With an attractive courtyard and spacious conservatory, there are many places in which to relax. Offering a flexible daily routine with two meal sittings for the main lunchtime meal, the involvement of relatives in the home's day-to-day running is also encouraged with relatives meetings taking place every three months. Although Bay Tree Court does not allow pets to live in the home, they are welcome to visit.

Registered places: 59
Guide weekly rate: From £610
Specialist care: Nursing, emergency admissions, palliative care, respite
Medical services: Podiatry, dentist, optician
Qualified staff: Undisclosed

Home details
Location: Residential area, 3 miles from Cheltenham centre
Communal areas: 4 lounges, 2 dining rooms, 2 conservatories, hairdressing salon, courtyard and garden
Accessibility: *Floors:* 2 • *Access:* Lift • *Wheelchair access:* Good
Smoking: ✗
Pets: At manager's discretion
Routines: Flexible

Room details
Single: 59
Shared: 0
En suite: 59
Facilities: TV point, telephone point

Door lock: ✗
Lockable place: ✗

Services provided
Beauty services: Hairdressing, aromatherapy, reflexology
Mobile library: ✗
Transport: Minibus and car
Religious services: ✗
Activities: *Coordinator:* ✓ • *Examples:* Bingo, current affairs discussions, painting • *Outings:* ✓
Meetings: ✓

Registered places: 55
Guide weekly rate: £660–£720
Specialist care: Nursing
Medical services: Podiatry, dentist
Qualified staff: Undisclosed

Home details

Location: Residential area, 0.5 miles from Thornbury
Communal areas: 2 lounges, 2 dining rooms, hairdressing salon,
   conservatory, patio and garden
Accessibility: *Floors:* 2 • *Access:* Lift • *Wheelchair access:* Good
Smoking: ✕
Pets: At manager's discretion
Routines: Flexible

Room details

Single: 49
Shared: 3
En suite: 52
Facilities: TV, telephone point

Door lock: ✕
Lockable place: ✕

Services provided

Beauty services: Hairdressing
Mobile library: ✕
Religious services: ✕
Transport: ✕
Activities: *Coordinator.* ✓ • *Examples*: Exercise classes
   Outings: ✓
Meetings: ✕

Beech House

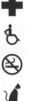

Manager: Judith Peachey
Owner: Beechcare Ltd
Contact: 11 Prowse Close, Thornbury,
South Gloucestershire, BS35 1EG
☎ 01454 412266
@ beechhousecare@aol.com

A purpose-built home in a quiet area, Beech House is approximately half a mile from Thornbury. Beech House is home to two cats and other pets would be permitted at the manager's discretion. The surrounding garden is of a high standard, and houses a gazebo, which is enjoyed by the residents. Residents are provided variety of meals, and various activities are always available, such as exercise classes. There are also outings on offer.

Registered places: 26
Guide weekly rate: £435–£485
Specialist care: Respite
Medical services: Podiatry, dentist
Qualified staff: Meets standard

Home details

Location: Residential area, 2 miles from Cheltenham
Communal areas: 2 lounges, dining room, conservatory, garden
Accessibility: *Floors:* 2 • *Access:* Lift • *Wheelchair access:* Good
Smoking: ✕
Pets: ✓
Routines: Flexible

Room details

Single: 26
Shared: 0
En suite: 26
Facilities: None

Door lock: ✓
Lockable place: ✓

Services provided

Beauty services: Hairdressing
Mobile library: ✕
Religious services: ✕
Transport: ✕
Activities: *Coordinator.* ✕ • *Examples*: Bingo, one-to-one sessions
   Outings: ✕
Meetings: ✕

Bredon View

Manager: Katrina Mitchell
Owner: CTCH Ltd
Contact: 24–26 Libertus Road,
Cheltenham, Gloucestershire, GL51 7EL
☎ 01242 525087

Situated in a residential area close to the railway station, Bredon View is a care home converted from two semi-detached older properties. The home has landscaped gardens and a conservatory. The food is satisfactory but there is a wide degree of choice as well. The home offers a safe system for the protection of personal belongings for residents. There are one-to-one sessions available as well as group activities such as bingo.

Bridge House Residential Home

Manager: Rachel Parnell
Owner: Bridge House Ltd
Contact: 31 Rectory Road,
Frampton Cotterell,
South Gloucestershire, BS36 2BN
) 01454 772888
@ bridgehouseoh@btconnect.com

Bridge House is a family-run home situated close to the River Frome in a residential area. The home is close to small village amenities and is on the bus route to Bristol and Yate. The home is run on Christian principles, with regular prayer sessions and services. It is also close to a number of churches. A model railway runs through the grounds of Bridge House and on bank holidays the home holds open days. The home arranges outings for the residents as well as regular activities such as crafts and quizzes.

Registered places: 16
Guide weekly rate: £440
Specialist care: Day care
Medical services: Podiatry
Qualified staff: Undisclosed

Home details
Location: Village location, 9 miles from Bristol
Communal areas: Lounge, dining room, conservatory, garden
Accessibility: *Floors:* 2 • *Access:* Lift • *Wheelchair access:* Good
Smoking: ×
Pets: ×
Routines: Structured

Room details
Single: 16
Shared: 0
En suite: 0
Facilities: TV point, telephone point

Door lock: ✓
Lockable place: ✓

Services provided
Beauty services: Hairdressing, aromatherapy
Mobile Library: ✓
Religious services: Daily prayer service, weekly Communion service
Transport: ×
Activities: *Coordinator:* × • *Examples:* Arts and crafts, quizzes, visiting entertainers • *Outings:* ✓
Meetings: ×

Broadleas Residential Care Home

Manager: Katherine Halstead
Owner: ACER Care Homes Ltd
Contact: 9 Eldorado Road, Cheltenham,
Gloucestershire, GL50 2PU
) 01242 256095

In a quiet residential area of Cheltenham, Broadleas Residential Care Home is located close to the railway station and nearby shops. With a small lawn at the front of the house and allocated parking at either side of the home, the Broadlea's rear gardens are tended, in part, by a resident who lives at the home. The home arranges outings for the residents as well as internal activities such as performances by visiting entertainers.

Registered places: 20
Guide weekly rate: £375–£500
Specialist care: Respite
Medical services: Podiatry, dentist, optician
Qualified staff: Fails standard

Home details
Location: Residential area, 1 mile from Cheltenham
Communal areas: Lounge, dining room, garden
Accessibility: *Floors:* 4 • *Access:* Lift • *Wheelchair access:* Limited
Smoking: ×
Pets: ×
Routines: Flexible

Room details
Single: 20
Shared: 0
En suite: 20
Facilities: None

Door lock: ×
Lockable place: ✓

Services provided
Beauty services: Hairdressing
Mobile library: ×
Religious services: ×
Transport: ×
Activities: *Coordinator:* × • *Examples:* Music and movement, visiting entertainers • *Outings:* ✓
Meetings: ×

Registered places: 12
Guide weekly rate: £380–£400
Specialist care: Mental disorder, respite
Medical services: Podiatry, dentist, optician
Qualified staff: Undisclosed

Home details

Location: Village location, 13 miles from Stroud
Communal areas: Lounge, dining room, garden
Accessibility: *Floors:* 2 • *Access:* Stair lift • *Wheelchair access:* Good
Smoking: In designated area
Pets: At manager's discretion
Routines: Flexible

Room details

Single: 12
Shared: 0
En suite: 9
Door lock: ✗
Lockable place: ✓
Facilities: TV point, telephone point

Services provided

Beauty services: Hairdressing
Mobile library: ✓
Religious services: Monthly Communion service
Transport: ✗
Activities: *Coordinator:* ✗ • *Examples:* Bingo, games, quizzes
Outings: ✗
Meetings: ✗

Canonbury Residential Home

Manager: Michaela Hayden
Owner: Oliveira Care Ltd
Contact: 19 Canonbury Street, Berkeley, Gloucestershire, GL13 9BE
) 01453 810292

An attractive 17th-century Grade II listed building set in the heart of Berkeley, Canonbury Residential Home was once a farm. It is ideally situated next to local shops, a post office and bank. Retaining much of its personal history, Canonbury Residential Home has a courtyard and terrace as well as a water feature in its garden. Small and homely, the home's lounge has an open fire and the manager encourages residents to discuss their views on the home openly, after quizzes or one-to-one with staff.

Registered places: 45
Guide weekly rate: £450–£558
Specialist care: Nursing, dementia, physical disability
Medical services: Podiatry
Qualified staff: Fails standard

Home details

Location: Rural area, 20 miles from Bristol
Communal areas: Lounge, dining room, library, hairdressing salon, patio and garden
Accessibility: *Floors:* 3 • *Access:* Lift and 2 stair lifts
Wheelchair access: Good
Smoking: ✗
Pets: ✓
Routines: Flexible

Room details

Single: 27
Shared: 8
En suite: 14
Door lock: ✓
Lockable place: ✓
Facilities: TV

Services provided

Beauty services: Hairdressing
Mobile library: ✗
Religious services: ✗
Transport: ✗
Activities: *Coordinator:* ✓ • *Examples:* Music and movement, visiting entertainers • *Outings:* ✓
Meetings: ✗

Castleford House Nursing Home

Manager: Madeleine Parsons
Owner: Milkwood Care Ltd
Contact: Castleford Hill, Tutshill, Nr Chepstow, Gloucestershire, NP16 7LE
) 01291 629929

Castleford House is situated on the Gloucestershire/Gwent border and overlooks the town of Chepstow and the River Severn. The home is a red-bricked building spread on three floors, each with a mezzanine level. A large reception area provides a pleasant welcoming area, and there is also a lounge, dining room and library which acts as a quiet lounge. There is a patio to the rear of the property and a walled garden with flowerbeds. An activities coordinator works several days a week and organises special events, music and movement and visiting entertainment, which are all displayed on a notice board.

Chargrove Lawn

Manager: Katie Allen
Owner: CTCH Ltd
Contact: Shurdington Road,
Cheltenham, Gloucestershire, GL51 5XA
☎ 01242 862686
@ enquiries@ctch.co.uk
🖰 www.ctch.co.uk

Set in a semi-rural location, Chargrove Lawn is an adapted property that is lies one mile from local shops and three miles from Cheltenham. The home offers views over fields to Leckhampton Hill. The home won a 'Cheltenham in Bloom' award for its garden displays for three years in a row. The home publishes a monthly newsletter to keep residents up to date with birthdays, activities and so on. There is a residents meeting every six weeks.

Registered places: 26
Guide weekly rate: £462–£513
Specialist care: Day care
Medical services: Podiatry, hygienist, optician, physiotherapy
Qualified staff: Meets standard

Home details
Location: Residential area, 3 miles from Cheltenham
Communal areas: 2 lounges, conservatory, dining room, hairdressing salon, library, patio and garden
Accessibility: Floors: 2 • Access: Lift • Wheelchair access: Good
Smoking: In designated area
Pets: At manager's discretion
Routines: Flexible

Room details
Single: 26
Shared: 0
En suite: 26
Facilities: TV point, telephone point

Door lock: ✓
Lockable place: ✓

Services provided
Beauty services: Hairdressing
Mobile library: ✓
Religious services: ✗
Transport: Minibus
Activities: Coordinator: ✗ • Examples: Games, one-to-one sessions
  Outings: ✓
Meetings: ✓

Charnwood House

Manager: Melanie Holland
Owner: Apsley Park Ltd
Contact: 49 Barnwood Road,
Gloucester, GL2 0SD
☎ 01452 523478
@ mel_holland123@yahoo.co.uk

Charnwood House is located in a residential area, seven miles from Gloucester. The home has a lounge and a conservatory, which is used as a dining room. The home arranges Communion from a Catholic priest and there are also visits from clergy of other denominations. The home employs an activities coordinator who arranges coffee mornings and musical entertainment. There are also outings on offer, including boat trips.

Registered places: 35
Guide weekly rate: £390–£850
Specialist care: Nursing, respite
Medical services: Podiatry, dentist, optician
Qualified staff: Meets standard

Home details
Location: Residential area, 7 miles from Gloucester
Communal areas: Lounge, dining room, conservatory, garden
Accessibility: Floors: 3 • Access: Lift and stair lift
  Wheelchair access: Good
Smoking: In designated area
Pets: ✗
Routines: Flexible

Room details
Single: Undisclosed
Shared: Undisclosed
En suite: Undisclosed
Facilities: TV

Door lock: ✗
Lockable place: ✓

Services provided
Beauty services: Hairdressing
Mobile library: ✗
Religious services: Catholic Communion
Transport: ✓
Activities: Coordinator: ✓ • Exmaples: Coffee mornings, musical entertainment • Outings: ✓
Meetings: ✓

Registered places: 16
Guide weekly rate: £390–£530
Specialist care: None
Medical services: Podiatry, optician, physiotherapy
Qualified staff: Meets standard

Home details
Location: Rural area, 5.6 miles from Stroud
Communal areas: 2 lounges, dining room, garden
Accessibility: *Floors:* 3 • *Access:* Lift • *Wheelchair access:* Good
Smoking: ✗
Pets: ✓
Routines: Flexible

Room details
Single: 14
Shared: 1
En suite: 12
Facilities: TV point

Door lock: ✓
Lockable place: ✓

Services provided
Beauty services: Hairdressing
Mobile library: ✗
Religious services: Weekly Catholic visits,
    monthly Communion service
Transport: ✗
Activities: *Coordinator:* ✗ • *Examples:* Food tasting sessions,
    musical entertainment • *Outings:* ✗
Meetings: ✗

Church Court Care Centre

Manager: Rita Poole
Owner: Blanchworth Care
Contact: Church Street, Stroud,
Gloucestershire, GL5 1JL
✆ 0845 3455785

Church Court Care centre is situated next door to an Anglican church, approximately six miles from Stroud. Church Court is a Grade II listed building dating back to the 17th-century. The home is part of Blanchworth Care. Residents benefit from a range of activities on offer in the home and there are close links with the local church which some residents are involved in. There are weekly visits from a Catholic priest and a monthly Communion service.

Registered places: 33
Guide weekly rate: £385–£510
Specialist care: Physical disability, respite
Medical services: Podiatry, dentist, optician
Qualified staff: Undisclosed

Home details
Location: Residential area, 7 miles from Bristol
Communal areas: Dining room, garden
Accessibility: *Floors:* 2 • *Access:* Lift • *Wheelchair access:* Good
Smoking: ✗
Pets: At manager's discretion
Routines: Flexible

Room details
Single: 32
Shared: 1
En suite: 33
Facilities: TV

Door lock: ✓
Lockable place: ✓

Services provided
Beauty services: None
Mobile library: ✗
Religious services: ✗
Transport: Minibus
Activities: *Coordinator:* ✗ • *Examples:* Bingo, card making, quizzes
    Outings: ✗
Meetings: ✓

Cleeve Lodge

Manager: Marie Rochester
Owner: Shields Care Ltd
Contact: Cleeve Lodge Close, Downend,
South Gloucestershire, BS16 6AQ
✆ 0117 970 2273
@ cleevelodge@shieldscare.com
🖱 www.shieldscare.com

Cleeve Lodge is a listed building dating back to the 18th century. The home is situated in a residential area, seven miles from Bristol. The home supports and encourages the residents to maintain independence in order to enhance their quality of life. The home has its own minibus for transportation and offers residents a variety of activities including quizzes and bingo.

Collingwood

Manager: Wendy Pullin
Owner: Frances Bailey
Contact: 78a Bath Road, Longwell Green, South Gloucestershire, BS30 9DG
) 0117 9324527

Situated in a cul-de-sac in the residential area of Longwell Green, Collingwood resides near local amenities and is six and a half miles from Bristol. Well served by public transport, a bus stop is also nearby. There is a welcoming environment at Collingwood, which offers a good standard of accommodation. The home traditionally has a low staff turnover, which indicates that there is continuity of care to the people who live in the home. The home takes the residents on outings and arranges other activities such as bingo and performances by visiting entertainers.

Registered places: 21
Guide weekly rate: Undisclosed
Specialist care: None
Medical services: Undisclosed
Qualified staff: Undisclosed

Home details
Location: Residential area, 6.5 miles from Bristol
Communal areas: 2 lounges, dining room, garden
Accessibility: *Floors:* 2 • *Access:* Lift • *Wheelchair access:* Good
Smoking: x
Pets: x
Routines: Flexible

Room details
Single: 21
Shared: 0
En suite: 21
Facilities: None

Door lock: x
Lockable place: x

Services provided
Beauty services: Hairdressing
Mobile library: x
Religious services: x
Transport: x
Activities: *Coordinator:* x • *Examples:* Bingo, visiting entertainers
Outings: ✓
Meetings: Undisclosed

The Court

Manager: Angela Dilley
Owner: Blanchworth Care
Contact: Culverhay, Wotton-under-Edge, Gloucestershire, GL12 7LS
) 08453 455791

This Grade II listed building is a specially adapted Georgian mansion set in one acre of walled gardens. Positioned close to the Cotswold town of Wotten-under-Edge residents are within easy walking distance of shops, banks and a post office. The home has two large lounges and a garden for residents to relax in and the home arranges activities such as baking to amuse the residents. There is a monthly Communion service in the home and there is a hairdressing service on offer.

Registered places: 13
Guide weekly rate: £550
Specialist care: None
Medical services: None
Qualified staff: Undisclosed

Home details
Location: Residential area, 0.2 miles from Wotton-under-Edge
Communal areas: 2 lounges, dining room, garden
Accessibility: *Floors:* 2 • *Access:* Stair lift • *Wheelchair access:* Good
Smoking: x
Pets: x
Routines: Flexible

Room details
Single: 10
Shared: 2
En suite: 12
Facilities: TV, telephone

Door lock: ✓
Lockable place: ✓

Services provided
Beauty services: Hairdressing
Mobile library: x
Religious services: Monthly Communion service
Transport: x
Activities: *Coordinator:* x • *Examples:* Baking • *Outings:* x
Meetings: x

Registered places: 13
Guide weekly rate: £313–£390
Specialist care: None
Medical services: Podiatry, physiotherapy, optician
Qualified staff: Exceeds standard: 60% at NVQ level 2

Home details

Location: Residential area, 2 miles from Cheltenham
Communal areas: Dining room, garden
Accessibility: *Floors:* 2 • *Access:* Lift • *Wheelchair access:* Good
Smoking: ✗
Pets: ✓
Routines: Flexible

Room details

Single: 13
Shared: 9
En suite: 8
Facilities: TV

Door lock: ✓
Lockable place: ✓

Services provided

Beauty services: None
Mobile library: ✗
Religious services: ✗
Transport: ✗
Activities: *Coordinator.* ✗ • *Examples:* Bingo • *Outings:* ✓
Meetings: ✗

Darley Dale

Manager: John O'Connor
Owner: Mary O'Connor
Contact: 24–26 Libertus Road,
Cheltenham, Gloucestershire, GL51 7EL
☎ 01242 513389

Darley Dale is a Victorian house that has been extended to provide personal care for 13 elderly people. There is a ramp providing access to the garden area, which has seating and outdoor heating. The home always make family and friends feel welcome. The home provides a homely and relaxed environment for residents, and a good standard of home-cooked food is provided, with consideration to individual likes and dislikes.

Registered places: 13
Guide weekly rate: Undisclosed
Specialist care: Respite
Medical services: Podiatry, dentist, optician
Qualified staff: Exceeds standard: 100% at NVQ level 2

Home details

Location: Residential area, 8 miles from Bristol
Communal areas: Lounge, conservatory, dining room, garden
Accessibility: *Floors:* 2 • *Access:* Lift • *Wheelchair access:* Good
Smoking: In designated area
Pets: ✗
Routines: Flexible

Room details

Single: 13
Shared: 0
En suite: 3
Facilities: TV point, telephone point

Door lock: ✓
Lockable place: ✓

Services provided

Beauty services: Hairdressing
Mobile library: ✓
Religious services: Fortnightly
Transport: ✗
Activities: *Coordinator.* ✗ • *Examples:* Bingo, games, musical entertainment • *Outings:* ✓
Meetings: ✓

Edgemont House

Manager: Linda Abrahams
Owner: Linda Abrahams
Contact: 20 West Street, Oldland Common,
South Gloucestershire,
BS30 9QS
☎ 0117 9325558

Set in a residential area near a main road, residents at Edgemont House are in easy reach of bus services to Kingswood, two miles away and Bristol, eight miles away. The home's garden boasts a fishpond and patio areas. There is also a conservatory in the home. There are residents meetings every six months and a religious service takes place once a fortnight. The home also arranges outings and activities such as bingo and games.

Edgemont View

Manager: Helen Hopson
Owner: Linda Abrahams
Contact: 160 High Street, Oldland Common, South Gloucestershire, BS30 9TA
) 0117 9077380

Located in Oldland Common close to its sister home, Edgemont View is situated near several facilities, including a pub and a number of shops. The home has a dedicated activities coordinator who arranges a variety of activities for the residents, such as games and performances by visiting entertainers. The home also offers residents the opportunity to go on outings in the local area. There is a garden and two conservatories at the home for residents to relax and socialise in.

Registered places: 21
Guide weekly rate: £580
Specialist care: Nursing, respite
Medical services: Podiatry, dentist, optician
Qualified staff: Meets standard

Home details
Location: Residential area, 8 miles from Bristol
Communal areas: Lounge, dining room, 2 conservatories, garden
Accessibility: *Floors:* 2 • *Access:* None • *Wheelchair access:* Limited
Smoking: ×
Pets: ×
Routines: Flexible

Room details
Single: 15
Shared: 3
En suite: 1
Facilities: None

Door lock: ✓
Lockable place: ✓

Services provided
Beauty services: Hairdressing
Mobile library: × Religious services: ×
Transport: ×
Activities: *Coordinator.* ✓ • *Examples:* Games, singalongs, visiting entertainers • *Outings:* ✓
Meetings: ×

Elm Grove Nursing Home

Manager: Ann Carter
Owner: BUPA Care Homes Ltd
Contact: 42 Somerford Road, Cirencester, Gloucestershire, GL7 1TX
) 01285 653057
@ ElmGroveALL@BUPA.com
⌂ www.bupacarehomes.co.uk

Originally a large private house, Elm Grove has been converted to meet the needs of elderly residents. Within the grounds is Chestnut Lodge, a separate house providing residential care. Elm Grove is situated in a pleasant residential area on the outskirts of Cirencester, within walking distance of local shops and on a bus route. Sherry and wine are served with meals in the dining room overlooking the gardens. Daily activities are offered, including musical entertainment, games and quizzes, and trips to local places of interest. Elm Grove also offers care to older people with physical disabilities.

Registered places: 60
Guide weekly rate: Undisclosed
Specialist care: Nursing, dementia, palliative care, physical disability, respite, terminal care
Medical services: Podiatry, physiotherapy
Qualified staff: Undisclosed

Home details
Location: Residential area, 0.5 miles from Cirencester centre
Communal areas: 2 lounges, 2 dining rooms, hairdressing salon, patio and garden
Accessibility: *Floors:* 2 • *Access:* Lift • *Wheelchair access:* Good
Smoking: ×
Pets: ✓
Routines: Flexible

Room details
Single: 58
Shared: 0
En suite: 49
Facilities: TV point, telephone point

Door lock: ✓
Lockable place: ×

Services provided
Beauty services: Hairdressing
Mobile library: ✓
Religious services: ✓
Transport: ✓
Activities: *Coordinator.* ✓ • *Examples:* Games, musical entertainment, quizzes • *Outings:* ✓
Meetings: ✓

Registered places: 16
Guide weekly rate: £400–£450
Specialist care: Mental disorder, respite
Medical services: Podiatry, dentist, optician
Qualified staff: Fails standard

Home details

Location: Residential area, 7.3 miles from Gloucester
Communal areas: Lounge, dining room, conservatory, garden
Accessibility: *Floors:* 2 • *Access:* Stair lift • *Wheelchair access:* Good
Smoking: ×
Pets: ×
Routines: Flexible

Room details

Single: 14
Shared: 1
En suite: 1
Facilities: TV

Door lock: ×
Lockable place: ×

Services provided

Beauty services: Hairdressing
Mobile library: × Religious services: Weekly Catholic service
Transport: ×
Activities: *Coordinator:* × • *Examples:* Bingo, parties, sherry evenings
  Outings: ×
Meetings: ×

Elmbridge Residential Home

Manager: Caroline O'Grady
Owner: Caroline O'Grady
Contact: 21 Embridge Road, Longlevens, Gloucester GL2 0NY
) 01452 524147

Elmbridge Residential Home is a traditional old-style house set back from the road and conveniently placed near such local amenities as shops and a post office With brightly lit and attractively decorated rooms, Elmbridge also has attractive and secluded gardens with flower borders and fruit trees. A hairdresser comes twice a week and there are regular make up and nail care sessions. The home hosts parties for special occasions and one resident celebrated her 69th wedding anniversary with her husband at Elmbridge. Staff are keen to walk with residents around the garden or to the local shops.

Registered places: 31
Guide weekly rate: £390–£630
Specialist care: Nursing, day care, respite
Medical services: Podiatry, hygienist, optician, physiotherapy
Qualified staff: Fails standard

Home details

Location: Village location, 2 miles from Coleford
Communal areas: Lounge, lounge/dining room, conservatory,
  patio and garden
Accessibility: *Floors:* 4 • *Access:* Lift • *Wheelchair access:* Good
Smoking: ×
Pets: ×
Routines: Structured

Room details

Single: 31
Shared: 0
En suite: 31
Facilities: None

Door lock: ×
Lockable place: ✓

Services provided

Beauty services: Hairdressing
Mobile library: ×
Religious services: ×
Transport: Minibus
Activities: *Coordinator:* × • *Examples:* Bingo, darts, musical
  entertainment • *Outings:* ✓
Meetings: ✓

The Elms

Manager: Vacant
Owner: Brickjet Ltd
Contact: Staunton, Coleford, Gloucestershire, GL16 8NX
) 08453 455793

A purpose-built home situated alongside the main road between Coleford and Monmouth, The Elms is found two miles from Coleford. The home has large gardens and a conservatory for residents to enjoy the sunshine. The Elms has many outings for residents, borrowing a minibus from another nursing home. As well as these outings there are activities throughout the week for the residents, such as darts and musical entertainment. The home also has visits from a Pets As Therapy dog although it does not allow pets to stay in the house.

Faith House

Manager: Toni Stevens
Owner: Toni and Gary Stevens
Contact: Station Road, Severn Beach,
South Gloucestershire, BS35 4PL
) 01454 632611
@ wlsnest04@btinternet.com

A small home that consists of a bungalow with first floor extension, Faith House is situated in Severn Beach close to the seafront and approximately 100 yards from the train station. The home has Christian roots, but is not run as a Christian home: residents of all faiths are welcome. The home holds a church service once a month. Residents often eat their meals in the home's kitchen. There are visits from a mobile library and the home arranges outings for the residents.

Registered places: 8
Guide weekly rate: £450–£470
Specialist care: Day care, respite
Medical services: Podiatry
Qualified staff: Exceeds standard: 75% at NVQ level 2

Home details
Location: Residential area, 17.5 miles from Bristol
Communal areas: Lounge/dining room, garden
Accessibility: *Floors:* 2 • *Access:* None • *Wheelchair access:* Limited
Smoking: ×
Pets: At manager's discretion
Routines: Flexible

Room details
Single: 8
Shared: 0
En suite: 6
Facilities: TV point, telephone point

Door lock: ✓
Lockable place: ✓

Services provided
Beauty services: Hairdressing
Mobile library: ✓
Religious services: Monthly church service
Transport: ×
Activities: *Coordinator.* × • *Examples:* Board games, scrabble
   Outings: ✓
Meetings: ×

Firgrove House

Manager: Lorraine Beer
Owner: Kenneth and Jennifer Roberts
Contact: Station Road, Yate,
South Gloucestershire, BS37 4AH
) 01454 310636

Made up of the Main House and smaller Coach House, Firgrove House is situated a five-minute walk from the town centre. The home is located in a residential area, approximately 12 miles from Bristol. The gardens at the home have recently been landscaped and there is a conservatory. The home has been awarded a five-star food hygiene award. There are regular residents meetings and an Anglican Communion service once a month. The home arranges outings for the residents and regular activities such as bingo and reminiscence sessions.

Registered places: 20
Guide weekly rate: £435
Specialist care: Dementia, respite
Medical services: Podiatry, optician, physiotherapy
Qualified staff: Meets standard

Home details
Location: Residential area, 12 miles from Bristol
Communal areas: Lounge, dining room, conservatory, garden
Accessibility: *Floors:* 3 • *Access:* Stair lift • *Wheelchair access:* Good
Smoking: In designated area
Pets: ✓
Routines: Flexible

Room details
Single: 16
Shared: 2
En suite: 5
Facilities: TV point, telephone point

Door lock: ✓
Lockable place: ✓

Services provided
Beauty services: Hairdressing
Mobile library: ✓
Religious services: Monthly Anglican Communion service
Transport: ×
Activities: *Coordinator.* × • *Examples:* Bingo, gentle exercises,
   reminiscence • *Outings:* ✓
Meetings: ✓

Registered places: 20
Guide weekly rate: £425–£625
Specialist care: Day care, respite
Medical services: Podiatry, dentist, optician
Qualified staff: Exceeds standard: 85% at NVQ level 2

Home details

Location: Residential area, 5 miles from Bristol
Communal areas: 2 lounges, dining room, library, garden
Accessibility: *Floors:* 2 • *Access:* Lift • *Wheelchair access:* Good
Smoking: ✗
Pets: At manager's discretion
Routines: Flexible

Room details

Single: 20
Shared: 0
En suite: 20
Facilities: TV point, telephone point

Door lock: ✓
Lockable place: ✓

Services provided

Beauty services: Hairdressing, aromatherapy
Mobile library: Library facilities
Religious services: Weekly service, monthly Anglican
　Communion service
Transport: Car
Activities: *Coordinator:* ✓ • *Examples:* Bingo, films, visiting
　entertainers • *Outings:* ✓
Meetings: ✓

Gables Residential Care Home Ltd

Manager: Ann Aubrey
Owner: Gables Residential Care Home Ltd
Contact: 1a Sydenham Way, Hanham
Green, South Gloucestershire, BS15 3TG
📞 0117 914 0799
@ Annaubrey1960@yahoo.co.uk

Situated in a rural suburb close to a pub, post office and shops, Gables Residential Care Home is located five miles from Bristol. The home has two lounges and a garden for residents to enjoy, as well as its own library facilities. There are residents meetings held every quarter to allow residents to voice any issues they may have. The home has its own car and often takes the residents on outings. There are daily activities such as film showing and there are regular religious services.

Registered places: 53
Guide weekly rate: £635–£970
Specialist care: Nursing, physical disability, respite
Medical services: Podiatry, optician, physiotherapy
Qualified staff: Meets standard

Home details

Location: Rural area, 10 miles from Bristol
Communal areas: 4 lounges, dining room, garden
Accessibility: *Floors:* 3 • *Access:* Lift • *Wheelchair access:* Good
Smoking: ✗
Pets: ✗
Routines: Flexible

Room details

Single: 41
Shared: 6
En suite: 42
Facilities: TV, telephone

Door lock: ✗
Lockable place: ✓

Services provided

Beauty services: Hairdressing, manicures
Mobile library: ✗
Religious services: Weekly Anglican service, monthly Communion
　service
Transport: Minibus
Activities: *Coordinator:* ✓ • *Examples:* Arts and crafts, keep fit,
　visiting entertainers • *Outings:* ✓
Meetings: ✗

Glebe House

Manager: Jacqueline Brown
Owner: Avonedge Ltd
Contact: 5 Sundays Hill,
Lower Almondsbury,
South Gloucestershire, BS32 4DS
📞 01454 616116
@ glebenursinghome@btconnect.com
🖱 www.bristolcarehomes.co.uk

Set in landscaped gardens in a quiet area next to a church and pub, Glebe House is a converted vicarage, built at the turn of the century, which has been extended. The home is located in a rural area, 10 miles from Bristol. Although residents are not allowed to keep pets in the home, they are welcome to visit. The home also has a mobile shop. The home has an Anglican Communion service once a month and a service once a week. There is a minibus at the home and outings are on offer to the residents.

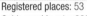

The Grange

Manager: Sam William
Owner: CTCH Ltd
Contact: Grange Road,Northway,
Tewkesbury, Gloucestershire, GL20 8HQ
) 01684 850111

A purpose-built home situated in a residential area of Tewkesbury, eight miles from the town centre. The Grange has a conservatory to relax in and enjoy the sunshine. The home is close to local facilities, which include a shopping precinct and pub. Outings on offer to the residents can be trips to a safari park and the seaside. Activities include a popular 'knitter-natter' club, which (as the name suggests) involves knitting and chatting. A visiting beautician offers hairdressing and manicures.

Registered places: 69
Guide weekly rate: £451–£520
Specialist care: Nursing
Medical services: Podiatry, hygienist, optician, physiotherapy
Qualified staff: Exceeds standard: 70% at NVQ level 2

Home details

Location: Residential area, 8 miles from Tewkesbury
Communal areas: 8 lounges, 4 dining rooms, conservatory, patio and garden
Accessibility: *Floors:* 3 • *Access:* Lift • *Wheelchair access:* Good
Smoking: ✗
Pets: ✗
Routines: Flexible

Room details

Single: 64
Shared: 5
En suite: 69
Facilities: TV

Door lock: ✓
Lockable place: ✓

Services provided

Beauty services: Hairdressing, beautician
Mobile library: ✓
Religious services: Anglican Communion service
Transport: ✗
Activities: *Coordinator.* ✓ • *Examples:* Bingo, quizzes • *Outings:* ✓
Meetings: ✗

Hampton House

Manager: Rosalind Elliott
Owner: Curtis Homes Ltd
Contact: 94 Leckhampton Road,
Cheltenham, Gloucestershire, GL53 0BN
) 01242 520527
@ roz@hamptonhousecare.co.uk
www.hamptonhousecare.co.uk

A detached period property that has been carefully refurbished over the years, Hampton House is situated in a pleasant residential area of Leckhampton five minutes' walk from the local shops. This area is also easily accessed by public transport, with buses to local areas and Cheltenham. Complete with a pond, the gardens are extensive and enclosed by shrub borders and can also be enjoyed from both the comfort of the patio and conservatory.

Registered places: 21
Guide weekly rate: £480–£540
Specialist care: Day care, respite
Medical services: Podiatry, dentist, optician, physiotherapy
Qualified staff: Undisclosed

Home details

Location: Residential area, 0.75 miles from Cheltenham
Communal areas: 2 lounges, dining room, conservatory, garden
Accessibility: *Floors:* 2 • *Access:* Lift • *Wheelchair access:* Good
Smoking: ✗
Pets: At manager's discretion
Routines: Flexible

Room details

Single: 21
Shared: 0
En suite: 16
Facilities: TV point, telephone point

Door lock: ✓
Lockable place: ✓

Services provided

Beauty services: Hairdressing
Mobile library: ✓
Religious services: Monthly nondenominational Communion service
Transport: ✗
Activities: *Coordinator.* ✓ • *Examples:* Bingo, sherry parties, visiting entertainers • *Outings:* ✓
Meetings: ✗

Registered places: 21
Guide weekly rate: £475
Specialist care: Day care, respite
Medical services: Podiatry, dentist, optician, physiotherapy
Qualified staff: Meets standard

Home details

Location: Residential area, 6 miles from Bristol
Communal areas: Lounge, dining room, patio and garden
Accessibility: *Floors:* 3 • *Access:* Lift • *Wheelchair access:* Good
Smoking: In designated area
Pets: At manager's discretion
Routines: Flexible

Room details

Single: 21
Shared: 0
En suite: Undisclosed
Facilities: TV, telephone point

Door lock: ✓
Lockable place: ✓

Services provided

Beauty services: Hairdressing, aromatherapy, manicures
Mobile library: ✓
Religious services: ✓
Transport: ✓
Activities: *Coordinator:* ✓ • *Examples:* Arts and crafts, games, visiting entertainers • *Outings:* ✓
Meetings: ✓

Harefield Hall

Manager: Susan Evans
Owner: Banff Securities Ltd
Contact: 171 Bath Road, Willsbridge, South Gloucestershire, BS30 9DD
☏ 0117 9323245

Situated in its own large grounds between Longwell Green and Willsbridge, Harefield Hall is near to a post office and local shops and is six miles from the town centre. There is a bus service which stops just outside the home. The home has a large garden with a seating area, as well as a lounge and a dining room. The home's activities coordinator arranges activities for both the morning and the afternoon, such as arts and crafts, visiting entertainers and bingo. The home has its own transport and organises outings to Bath for the residents.

Registered places: 30
Guide weekly rate: £505–£535
Specialist care: Nursing, day care, respite
Medical services: Podiatry, dentist, optician, physiotherapy
Qualified staff: Meets standard

Home details

Location: Residential area, 0.4 miles from Chipping Sodbury
Communal areas: 2 Lounges, 2 dining rooms, patio
Accessibility: *Floors:* 2 • *Access:* Lift • *Wheelchair access:* Good
Smoking: ✗
Pets: ✗
Routines: Flexible

Room details

Single: 14
Shared: 8
En suite: 0
Facilities: TV

Door lock: ✗
Lockable place: ✗

Services provided

Beauty services: Hairdressing, aromatherapy
Mobile library: ✗
Religious services: Monthly Communion service
Transport: ✗
Activities: *Coordinator:* ✓ • *Examples:* Arts and crafts, bingo *Outings:* ✓
Meetings: ✓

The Heathers Nursing Home

Manager: Roger Tippings
Owner: Hitan Patel
Contact: Bowling Hill, Chipping Sodbury, South Gloucestershire, BS37 6AX
☏ 01454 312726
@ theheathers@
   acaciacare.wanadoo.co.uk

A Grade II listed Georgian manor house situated in Chipping Sodbury, The Heathers has excellent access to shops and other amenities. The home has a large patio instead of a garden. The dedicated activities coordinator organises arts and crafts, quizzes, bingo and outings such as visits to the zoo. Residents also get regular exercise. The home arranges a Communion service to take place once a month.

Hunters Care Centre

Manager: Sue Stannard
Owner: Barchester Healthcare Ltd
Contact: Cherry Tree Lane,
Cirencester, Gloucestershire, GL7 5DT

☏ 01285 653707
@ hunters@barchester.com
🖰 www.barchester.com/hunters

Attractively located on the outskirts of Cirencester, Hunters Care Centre is situated close to the luscious Cotswold countryside while still retaining good links to the A417. A purpose-built home, Hunters Care Centre provides a specialist dementia programme that is aimed at promoting freedom and life skills in a secure environment. As well as their own fully licensed bar, Hunters Care Centre also has an enclosed garden and a number of spacious lounges — some of which may provide privacy to residents meeting with relatives. The home is close to local amenities.

Number of registered beds: 89
Guide weekly rate: Undisclosed
Specialist care: Nursing, dementia
Medical services: Podiatry, dentistry, physiotherapy, occupational therapy, optician
Qualified staff: Undisclosed

Home details
Location: Rural area, 2 miles from Cirencester
Communal areas: 4 lounges, dining room, bar, garden
Accessibility: *Floors:* 2 • *Access:* Lift • *Wheelchair access:* Good
Smoking: ✗
Pets: ✗
Routines: Flexible

Room details
Single: Undisclosed
Shared: Undisclosed
En suite: 89
Facilities: TV, telephone

Door lock: ✗
Lockable place: ✗

Services provided
Beauty services: Hairdressing
Mobile library: ✗
Religious services: ✗
Transport: Minibus
Activities: *Coordinator.* ✓ • *Examples:* Coffee mornings, crosswords
Outings: ✗
Meetings: Undisclosed

Hyperion House

Manager: Katie Boyce
Owner: Diva Care Ltd
Contact: London Street, Fairford,
Gloucestershire, GL7 4AH

☏ 01285 712349
@ info@divacare.co.uk
🖰 www.divacare.co.uk

Hyperion House's vast and luscious grounds are situated comfortably close to the centre of Fairford and its surrounding community. Originally a hotel, the building was converted in 1985. Whilst necessary alterations have ensured residents can live freely and comfortably, the home's bar ensures that its service industry roots have not been forgotten! Although the home does not have its own transport, for those requiring trips out to the shops or for outpatient visits, transport can be arranged.

Registered places: 45
Guide weekly rate: £425–£750
Specialist care: Nursing, day care, respite
Medical services: Podiatry, dentist, optician
Qualified staff: Undisclosed

Home details
Location: Rural area, 0.2 miles from Fairford
Communal areas: Lounge, dining room, conservatory, bar, patio and garden
Accessibility: *Floors:* 2 • *Access:* Lift • *Wheelchair access:* Good
Smoking: ✗
Pets: At manager's discretion
Routines: Flexible

Room details
Single: 9
Shared: 16
En suit: 25
Facilities: TV point, telephone point

Door lock: ✓
Lockable place: ✓

Services provided
Beauty services: Hairdressing
Mobile library: ✗
Religious services: Monthly Communion service
Transport: ✗
Activities: *Coordinator.* ✗ • *Examples:* Bingo, quizzes, socials
Outings: ✓
Meetings: ✗

Registered places: 30
Guide weekly rate: Undisclosed
Specialist care: Dementia
Medical services: Podiatry, dentist, optician, physiotherapy
Qualified staff: Exceeds standard: 75% at NVQ level 2

Home details

Location: Residential area, 5 miles from Bristol
Communal areas: 3 lounges, dining room/conservatory,
   2 quiet rooms, garden
Accessibility: *Floors:* 3 • *Access:* Lift and stair lift
   Wheelchair access: Good
Smoking: In designated area
Pets: At manager's discretion
Routines: Flexible

Room details

Single: 28
Shared: 1
En suite: 24
Facilities: TV point

Door lock: ✓
Lockable place: ✓

Services provided

Beauty services: Hairdressing
Mobile library: ✓ Religious services: ✓
Transport: ✓
Activities: Coordinators: ✓• *Examples*: Coffee mornings, painting
   Outings: ✓
Meetings: ✓

Kenver House

Manager: Nicola Johnson
Owner: Twaleb Seehootoorah
Contact: 56 Hill Street, Kingswood,
South Gloucestershire, BS15 4EX
⟫ 0117 9674236

Kenver House has good access to local facilities and is a short walk to the main shopping complex of Kingswood. The home has three lounges, one of which is a quiet lounge where movies are shown. There is also a garden with a paved area which is regularly tended by a gardener. A greenhouse has recently been built to allow residents to grow vegetables. The home offers a range of activities to the residents including coffee mornings to discuss the news and outings to the shops. There are also regular meetings with the residents and their relatives.

Registered places: 33
Guide weekly rate: £560–£675
Specialist care: Nursing, physical disability, respite
Medical services: Podiatry, hygienist, optician, physiotherapy
Qualified staff: Exceeds standard: 64% at NVQ level 2

Home details

Location: Residential area, 0.3 miles from Tetbury
Communal areas: 2 lounges, dining room, conservatory,
   patio and garden
Accessibility: *Floors:* 4 • *Access:* Lift • *Wheelchair access:* Good
Smoking: ✗
Pets: ✗
Routines: Flexible

Room details

Single: 13
Shared: 10
En suite: Undisclosed
Facilities: Telephone

Door lock: ✗
Lockable place: ✗

Services provided

Beauty services: Hairdressing
Mobile library: ✗
Religious services: Monthly Communion service
Transport: ✗
Activities: *Coordinator.* ✓ • *Examples*: Visiting entertainers
   Outings: ✓
Meetings: ✓

Kingsley House Nursing Home

Manager: Barbara Harpwood
Owner: The Cotswold Nursing Home
Company Ltd
Contact: Gumstool Hill, Tetbury,
Gloucestershire, GL8 8DG
⟫ 01666 503333
@ Kingsleyhouse.nursinghome@
   virgin.net

An adapted 18th-century building, Kingsley House is in the centre of the town, opposite a pub and a short walk away from the shops and other amenities. The home has a conservatory and patio-garden for residents to enjoy. The home prides itself on the level of care they offer to their residents, and certain projects that they are involved in. These include the 'End of life care' initiative in association with Southampton Hospital, and being part of research studies. Snacks are available on request throughout the night.

Kingswood Care Centre

Manager: Pat Sheppard
Owner: Southern Cross Healthcare Ltd
Contact: Wotton Road, Kingswood,
Nr Wotton-under-Edge,
Gloucestershire, GL12 8RA

☎ 01453 844647
@ kingswood@schealthcare.co.uk
🖰 www.schealthcare.co.uk

An extended listed building that is situated close to its sister home Highgrove, Kings Lodge is located approximately 17 miles from Kingswood. The home is situated a 15-minute walk from the local village. There is a communal safe in the office for valuables. The home has its own activities coordinator. There are organised outings once a year to the seaside in the minibus. The home organises regular religious services and there also is a hairdressing service.

Registered places: 44
Guide weekly rate: Undisclosed
Specialist care: Nursing, respite
Medical services: Podiatry, dentist, optician, physiotherapy
Qualified staff: Meets standard

Home details
Location: Village location, 16.5 miles from Kingswood
Communal areas: Lounges, dining room, patio and garden
Accessibility: *Floors:* 2 • *Access:* 2 lifts • *Wheelchair access:* Good
Smoking: In designated area
Pets: ✗
Routines: Flexible

Room details
Single: 36
Shared: 4
En suite: 44
Facilities: Telephone

Door lock: ✓
Lockable place: ✗

Services provided
Beauty services: Hairdressing
Mobile library: ✗
Religious services: ✓
Transport: ✓
Activities: *Coordinator.* ✓ • *Examples:* Bingo • *Outings:* ✓
Meetings: ✓

Kingswood Court

Manager: Aubrey Sibiya
Owner: Four Seasons Healthcare Ltd
Contact: Soundwell Road, Kingswood,
South Gloucestershire, BS15 1PN

☎ 0117 9603722

Kingswood Court is a purpose-built home located in Kingswood, under a mile from the city of Bristol. The home has a mobile shop where residents can purchase items. The home holds a Baptist service once a fortnight and there is a residents meeting which takes place every quarter. The home has a gardening group residents can join and residents are also offered the chance to go on outings. The home also has visits from a mobile library.

Registered places: 66
Guide weekly rate: £600–£650
Specialist care: Nursing
Medical services: Podiatry, optician
Qualified staff: Undisclosed

Home details
Location: Residential area, 0.7 miles from Kingswood
Communal areas: 3 lounge, dining room, garden
Accessibility: *Floors:* 3 • *Access:* Lift • *Wheelchair access:* Good
Smoking: In designated area
Pets: At manager's discretion
Routines: Flexible

Room details
Single: 60
Shared: 3
En suite: Undisclosed
Facilities: TV point, telephone point

Door lock: ✗
Lockable place: ✓

Services provided
Beauty services: Hairdressing
Mobile library: ✓
Religious services: Fortnightly Baptist service
Transport: ✗
Activities: *Coordinator.* ✗ • *Examples:* Gardening group • *Outings:* ✓
Meetings: ✓

Registered places: 22
Guide weekly rate: £349–£450
Specialist care: Respite
Medical services: Podiatry
Qualified staff: Meets standard

Home details
Location: Rural area, 5.5 miles from Cheltenham
Communal areas: 2 lounges, dining room, garden
Accessibility: *Floors:* 2 • *Access:* Lift • *Wheelchair access:* Good
Smoking: ✗
Pets: ✗
Routines: Flexible

Room details
Single: 22
Shared: 0
En suite: 3
Facilities: None

Door lock: ✓
Lockable place: ✓

Services provided
Beauty services: Hairdressing
Mobile library: ✓
Religious services: ✗
Transport: Minibus
Activities: *Coordinator.* ✗ • *Examples:* Singalongs • *Outings:* ✓
Meetings: ✓

Knightsbridge Lodge

Manager: Carol Coates
Owner: Ann and David Easdown
Contact: Knightsbridge Green, Cheltenham, Gloucestershire, GL51 9TA
☎ 01242 680168

Situated near the hamlet of Knightsbridge, Knightsbridge Lodge was originally a Victorian Toll House. The home is located in a rural area, five and a half miles from Cheltenham. Residents are served a good standard of varied and nutritious food, using fresh produce when possible. The home has its own minibus and often takes residents on outings in the local area. There are regular residents meetings and a mobile library comes to the home. The home has two lounges for residents to relax in as well as a garden.

Registered places: 29
Guide weekly rate: Undisclosed
Specialist care: Respite
Medical services: Podiatry, optician
Qualified staff: Fails standard

Home details
Location: Residential area, 5 miles from Gloucester
Communal areas: Lounge, lounge/dining room, garden
Accessibility: *Floors:* 3 • *Access:* Lift • *Wheelchair access:* Good
Smoking: In designated area
Pets: ✓
Routines: Structured

Room details
Single: 29
Shared: 0
En suite: 0
Facilities: TV point, telephone point

Door lock: ✓
Lockable place: ✓

Services provided
Beauty services: Hairdressing
Mobile library: ✗
Religious services: Monthly Communion service
Transport: ✗
Activities: *Coordinator.* ✗ • *Examples:* Bingo, visiting entertainers
   Outings: ✗
Meetings: ✓

The Knoll

Manager: Theresa Johnson
Owner: Alder Meadows Ltd
Contact: 335a Stroud Road, Gloucester GL4 0BD
☎ 01452 526146

A large house that has been extended, The Knoll stands in its own grounds with views over the city and towards May Hill in the Forest of Dean. The home lies five miles from Gloucester. There are regular residents meetings and the home arranges for a Communion service to take place once a month. There are activities available in the home such as bingo and the home also organises performances from visiting entertainers.

The Laurels

Manager: Patricia McCreery
Owner: Patricia McCreery
Contact: Main Road, Huntley,
Gloucestershire, GL19 3EA
) 01452 831484

This small care home, housing eight residents, is situated six miles from the city of Gloucester in the village of Huntley. There is a small private garden to the rear of the home. The size of the home gives staff the opportunity to cater well for every individual's unique needs, particularly with special dietary needs. There is a mobile library which comes to the home and there are regular residents meetings held to discuss any issues the residents may have.

Registered places: 8
Guide weekly rate: £390–£425
Specialist care: Undisclosed
Medical services: Podiatry, dentist, optician
Qualified staff: Fails standard

Home details
Location: Village location, 6 miles from Gloucester
Communal areas: Lounge/dining room, garden
Accessibility: *Floors:* 1 • *Wheelchair access:* Good
Smoking: ✗
Pets: ✗
Routines: Flexible

Room details
Single: 8
Shared: 0
En suite: 5
Facilities: None

Door lock: ✓
Lockable place: ✓

Services provided
Beauty services: Hairdressing
Mobile library: ✓
Religious services: ✗
Transport: ✗
Activities: *Coordinator.* ✗ • *Examples*: Bingo, cards • *Outings:* ✗
Meetings: ✓

Littlecroft Residential Home

Manager: Mark Hewlett
Owner: Quality Care Homes Ltd
Contact: 44 Barry Road,
Oldland Common,
South Gloucestershire, BS30 6QY
) 0117 9324204

A converted property situated in Oldland Common, Littlecroft Residential Home is close to a local shop. Littlecroft is seven and a half miles away from Bristol in a residential area, within walking distance of a local garden centre. The home arranges for an Anglican Communion service to take place every month and there is a residents meeting every three months. The home arranges outings for the residents as well as internal activities such as crafts and bingo.

Registered places: 17
Guide weekly rate: £392–£525
Specialist care: Respite
Medical services: Podiatry, dentist, optician
Qualified staff: Exceeds standard: 60% at NVQ level 2

Home details
Location: Residential area, 7.5 miles from Bristol
Communal areas: 2 lounges, dining room, garden
Accessibility: *Floors:* 2 • *Access:* Lift • *Wheelchair access:* Limited
Smoking: ✗
Pets: At manager's discretion
Routines: Structured

Room details
Single: 17
Shared: 0
En suite: 10
Facilities: TV point, telephone point

Door lock: ✓
Lockable place: ✓

Services provided
Beauty services: Hairdressing
Mobile library: ✓
Religious services: Monthly Anglican Communion service
Transport: ✗
Activities: *Coordinator.* ✗ • *Examples*: Arts and crafts, bingo *Outings:*
✓
Meetings: ✓

Registered places: 67
Guide weekly rate: £750–£895
Specialist care: Nursing, dementia, mental disorder,
    physical disability, respite
Medical services: Undisclosed
Qualified staff: Fails standard

Home details
Location: Rural area, 1.3 miles from Stonehouse
Communal areas: Lounge, dining room, garden
Accessibility: *Floors:* 3 • *Access:* Lift • *Wheelchair access:* Good
Smoking: x
Pets: x
Routines: Flexible

Room details
Single: 60
Shared: 7
En suite: 60
Door lock: x
Lockable place: x
Facilities: TV point, telephone point

Services provided
Beauty services: Hairdressing
Mobile library: x
Religious services: x
Transport: Minibus
Activities: *Coordinator.* ✓ • *Examples:* Arts and crafts, computer
    classes, visiting entertainers • *Outings:* ✓
Meetings: Undisclosed

Moreton Hill Care Centre

Manager: Charlotte Tily
Owner: Barchester Healthcare Ltd
Contact: Standish, Stonehouse,
Gloucestershire, GL10 3BZ
) 01453 826000
@ sue.stannard@barchester.com
⌂ www.barchester.com

A renovated farmhouse that is set on a hill, permitting views of the Cotswold countryside, Moreton Hill Care Centre is a former winner of the Care Home Design Award. The home provides a variable programme of activities and substantial work has been done in providing individual memory box displays for residents with dementia. The home has also invested in air conditioning to maintain appropriate medication storage temperatures.

Registered places: 20
Guide weekly rate: From £350
Specialist care: Dementia
Medical services: Podiatry, hygienist, optician, physiotherapy
Qualified staff: Exceeds standard: 80% at NVQ level 2

Home details
Location: Village location, 0.6 miles from Longhope
Communal areas: 2 lounges, dining room, conservatory,
    patio and garden
Accessibility:*Floors:* 2 • *Access:* Lift • *Wheelchair access:* Good
Smoking: x
Pets: x
Routines: Structured

Room details
Single: 20
Shared: 0
En suite: 20
Door lock: ✓
Lockable place: ✓
Facilities: TV, telephone

Services provided
Beauty services: Hairdressing
Mobile Library: ✓
Religious services: Weekly Catholic visits, monthly Anglican
    Communion service
Transport: Car
Activities: *Coordinator.* ✓ • *Examples:* Arts and crafts, exercise,
    reminiscing • *Outings:* ✓
Meetings: x

The Old Rectory

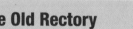

Manager: Rosemarie Halifax
Owner: Eric Hardy
Contact: School Lane, Church Road,
Longhope, Gloucestershire, GL17 0LJ
) 01452 831135
@ oldrectory123@btconnect.com

A Georgian building set in its own grounds, The Old Rectory is in a small village, 10 minutes away from buses and other amenities. While 19 residents are accommodated in the main building, there is an additional lodge available for a more independent resident. This includes a kitchenette, lounge and spare bedroom for a carer to sleep in at night. The dining room has views out towards the countryside and there is a lovely sun lounge to appreciate the view and the garden, which has a water feature.

Parton House

Manager: Margaret Littler
Owner: CTCH Ltd
Contact: Parton Road, Churchdown,
Gloucester GL3 2JE
☏ 01452 856779

An older-style property that has been recently extended, Parton House is set in its own large grounds in a semi-rural location. The home lies around six and a half miles from the centre of Gloucester. The home has its own small cinema where residents watch films and the rooms in the new extension receive Sky TV. The home has its own minibus and organises a Communion service to take place once a month. There are regular residents meetings and a mobile library comes to the home.

Registered places: 36
Guide weekly rate: £451–£565
Specialist care: Respite
Medical services: Podiatry, dentist, optician, physiotherapy
Qualified staff: Exceeds standard: 75% at NVQ level 2

Home details
Location: Residential area, 6.5 miles from Gloucester
Communal areas: 2 lounges, dining room, hairdressing salon, garden
Accessibility: *Floors:* 2 • *Access:* Lift • *Wheelchair access:* Good
Smoking: In designated area
Pets: At manager's discretion
Routines: Flexible

Room details
Single: 36
Shared: 0
En suite: 36
Facilities: TV point, telephone point

Door lock: ✓
Lockable place: ✓

Services provided
Beauty services: Hairdressing
Mobile library: ✓
Religious services: Monthly Communion service
Transport: Minibus
Activities: *Coordinator.* ✓ • *Examples:* Arts and crafts, games, film showings • *Outings:* ✗
Meetings: ✓

Queensbridge House

Manager: June Stanton
Owner: Queensbridge Care Ltd
Contact: 63 Queens Road, Cheltenham,
Gloucestershire, GL50 2NF
☏ 01242 519690

Close to Cheltenham train station and on a bus route, Queensbridge House is a detached house, which overlooks a nature reserve. The home is found in a residential area, approximately one and a half miles from Cheltenham town centre. The home has an enclosed garden that can be enjoyed during the summer months. The home also has four lounges for residents to relax in. There is a residents meeting every six months and the home organises a Communion service to take place on a monthly basis.

Registered places: 27
Guide weekly rate: £425–£750
Specialist care: Dementia, physical disability
Medical services: Podiatry, hygienist, optician, physiotherapy
Qualified staff: Exceeds standard

Home details
Location: Residential area, 1.6 miles from Cheltenham
Communal areas: 4 lounges, dining room, conservatory, 2 gardens
Accessibility: Floors: 2 • Access: Lift • Wheelchair access: Good
Smoking: In designated area
Pets: ✗
Routines: Structured

Room details
Single: 25
Shared: 1
En suite: 23
Facilities: TV point, telephone point

Door lock: ✓
Lockable place: ✓

Services provided
Beauty services: Hairdressing, manicures
Mobile library: ✓
Religious services: Monthly Communion service
Transport: Cars
Activities: *Coordinator.* ✓ • *Examples:* Armchair exercises, games *Outings:* ✗
Meetings: ✓

Registered places: 26
Guide weekly rate: Undisclosed
Specialist care: Day care, respite
Medical services: Podiatry, dentist, optician
Qualified staff: Undisclosed

Home details

Location: Residential area, 1 mile from Gloucester
Communal areas: 2 lounges, 2 dining rooms, conservatory, garden
Accessibility: *Floors:* 2 • *Access:* None • *Wheelchair access:* Limited
Smoking: In designated area
Pets: At manager's discretion
Routines: Flexible

Room details

Single: 26
Shared: 0
En suite: 23
Facilities: TV point, telephone point

Door lock: ✓
Lockable place: ✓

Services provided

Beauty services: Hairdressing
Mobile library: ✗
Religious services: ✗
Transport: Minibus
Activities: *Coordinator.* ✗ • *Examples:* Games, music and movement, sherry mornings • *Outings:* ✓
Meetings: ✓

Redlands Acre

Manager: Chris Whittington
Owner: CTCH Ltd
Contact: 35 Tewkesbury Road, Longford, Gloucester GL2 9BD
☎ 01452 507248
🖰 www.ctch.co.uk

Situated on a main route into Gloucester, Redlands Acre has a bus stop outside the home, providing easy access to the city centre, one mile away. The home provides residential care for 26 residents and is set on two floors. There is no lift or stair lift, so the resident must be able-bodied. There are also eight attached bungalows at the rear of the property which provide sheltered accommodation. The home has its own minibus and residents are taken on a variety of outings such as sightseeing and shopping. The home also arranges internal activities such as music and movement and sherry mornings.

Registered places: 13
Guide weekly rate: £475
Specialist care: Day care, physical disability, respite
Medical services: Podiatry, dentist, optician, physiotherapy
Qualified staff: Exceeds standard: 75% at NVQ level 2

Home details

Location: Residential area, 0.2 miles from Stonehouse
Communal areas: Lounge, dining room, summerhouse, conservatory, garden
Accessibility: *Floors:* 2 • *Access:* Lift • *Wheelchair access:* Good
Smoking: ✗
Pets: At manager's discretion
Routines: Structured

Room details

Single: 9
Shared: 2
En suite: 11
Facilities: TV, telephone

Door lock: ✓
Lockable place: ✓

Services provided

Beauty services: Hairdressing, manicures
Mobile library: ✗
Religious services: Weekly Communion service
Transport: ✓
Activities: *Coordinator.* ✗ • *Examples:* Bingo, crosswords
Outings: ✗
Meetings: ✓

Regency Retirement Home

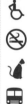

Manager: Margaret Buckingham
Owner: Trevor and Margaret Buckingham
Contact: 52 Regent Street, Stonehouse, Gloucestershire, GL10 2AD
☎ 01453 823139

The Regency Retirement Home is located a two-minute walk from the town centre of Stonehouse. The home has a lounge, a dining room and a summerhouse in the garden. The residents have a daily routine which includes crosswords twice a week, a daily walk and manicures once a week. The Regency Retirement Home offers a personalised service to its small number of residents and holds regular residents meetings. The home has its own transport and a weekly religious service.

St Jude's Residential Home For The Elderly

Manager: Winifred Morgan
Owner: Paul Morgan
Contact: Front Street, Nympsfield,
Nr Stonehouse, Gloucestershire,
GL10 3TY
) 01453 860682

St Jude's is a small, family-run care home set in the village of Nympsfield. The home has a list of planned outings and activities each year, which includes two monthly exercise classes – Chi Gong and 'balance'. The home has also purchased an allotment where residents are welcome to participate in gardening. The home does not have a lift, so it is essential that residents on the second floor must be mobile. The home is found five miles from Stonehouse.

Registered places: 10
Guide weekly rate: From £400
Specialist care: Respite
Medical services: Podiatry
Qualified staff: Undisclosed

Home details
Location: Village location, 5 miles from Stonehouse
Communal areas: Lounge, dining room
Accessibility: *Floors:* 2 • *Access:* None • *Wheelchair access:* Limited
Smoking: In designated area
Pets: ✓
Routines: Flexible

Room details
Single: 8
Shared: 1
En suite: Undisclosed
Facilities: None

Door lock: ✓
Lockable place: ✓

Services provided
Beauty services: Hairdressing
Mobile library: ✗
Religious services: ✗
Transport: ✗
Activities: *Coordinator:* ✗ • *Examples:* Exercise classes • *Outings:* ✗
Meetings: ✗

St Paul's Residential Home

Manager: Mobina Sayani
Owner: Mobina Sayani
Contact: 127–131 Stroud Road,
Gloucester GL1 5JL
) 01452 505485

St Paul's Residential Home comprises three older houses that have been joined and adapted. An extension is being built to enlarge the capacity of the home. It is situated a 10-minute walk from Gloucester city. There is a portable telephone in the home which residents can use. Pets are allowed to visit the home but smoking is not permitted. The residents have regular meetings and the home arranges regular religious services. The home currently has two lounges, a dining room, a garden and a conservatory although this may change with the extension.

Registered places: 21
Guide weekly rate: Undisclosed
Specialist care: Respite
Medical services: Podiatry, dentist, optician
Qualified staff: Meets standard

Home details
Location: Residential area, 4.7 miles from Gloucester
Communal areas: 2 lounges, dining room, conservatory, garden
Accessibility: *Floors:* 2 • *Access:* Lift • *Wheelchair access:* Good
Smoking: ✗
Pets: ✓
Routines: Flexible

Room details
Single: 19
Shared: 1
En suite: Undisclosed
Facilities: TV

Door lock: ✓
Lockable place: ✗

Services provided
Beauty services: Hairdressing
Mobile library: ✗
Religious services: ✓
Transport: ✗
Activities: *Coordinator:* ✓ • *Examples:* Bingo, music, board games
Outings: ✗
Meetings: ✓

Registered places: 48
Guide weekly rate: £521–£650
Specialist care: Nursing, emergency admissions
Medical services: Podiatry, dentist, optician
Qualified staff: Undisclosed

Home details
Location: Residential area, 0.5 miles from Yate
Communal areas: 2 lounges, 2 dining rooms, garden
Accessibility: *Floors:* 2 • *Access:* Lift • *Wheelchair access:* Good
Smoking: In designated area
Pets: ✗
Routines: Flexible

Room details
Single: 36
Shared: 6
En suite: 0
Facilities: None

Door lock: ✓
Lockable place: ✓

Services provided
Beauty services: Hairdressing
Mobile library: ✓
Religious services: Fortnightly Anglican and Baptist services
Transport: ✗
Activities: *Coordinator.* ✓ • *Examples:* Bingo, gardening, musical entertainment • *Outings:* ✗
Meetings: ✓

Stanshawes

Manager: Jeen Davis
Owner: Four Seasons Healthcare Ltd
Contact: 11 Stanshawes Drive, Yate, South Gloucestershire, BS37 4ET
☎ 01454 850005
@ stanshawes@fshc.co.uk
🖰 www.fshc.co.uk

Stanshawes is a purpose-built home in a residential location. It is situated a gentle half-mile walk from the town of Yate. Yate town centre has over 100 shops and a number of parks that are all within easy access of the home. The home has an activities coordinator who arranges group activities, such as a gardening club and bingo, as well as one-to-one sessions. The home also arranges fortnightly religious services for either Anglican or Baptist denominations.

Registered places: 21
Guide weekly rate: £460–£560
Specialist care: Respite
Medical services: Podiatry
Qualified staff: Exceeds standard: 60% at NVQ level 2

Home details
Location: Residential area, 0.5 miles from Nailsworth
Communal areas: 2 lounges, 2 dining rooms, patio and garden
Accessibility: *Floors:* 3 • *Access:* Lift • *Wheelchair access:* Good
Smoking: In designated area
Pets: ✓
Routines: Flexible

Room details
Single: 21
Shared: 0
En suite: 21
Facilities: TV point, telephone point

Door lock: ✓
Lockable place: ✓

Services provided
Beauty services: Hairdressing, manicures
Mobile library: Local library brings books
Religious services: ✓
Transport: ✗
Activities: *Coordinator.* ✓ • *Examples:* Board games, exercise sessions, films • *Outings:* ✓
Meetings: ✓

The Steppes Residential Home

Manager: Joanne Smith
Owner: The Steppes Care Ltd
Contact: Cossack Square, Nailsworth, Gloucester GL6 0DB
☎ 01453 832406
@ steppescare@aol.com

The Steppes is an older property that has been extended over time and accommodates 21 residents. The Steppes is a family-run and family-orientated home which is situated in the centre of town, half a mile from Nailsworth. The home has two lounges, two dining rooms and a garden with a stream running through it. There is an activities coordinator who arranges exercise sessions and games, as well as outings to areas interest. The home is located near the local library and books are brought to the home for residents to enjoy.

Stinchcombe Manor

Manager: Joanne Howells
Owner: Blanchworth Care
Contact: Stinchcombe, Nr Dursley,
Gloucestershire, GL11 6BQ
) 08453 455783

Situated in Stinchcombe village, Stinchcombe Manor is a large house that resides in its own grounds, 20 miles from Gloucester. The home has two lounges and a garden with a patio area for residents to enjoy. There is also a path for residents to walk on with views of the surrounding area. The home arranges a monthly Communion service and there are regular residents meetings. The activities coordinator arranges a varied programme for the residents, which includes armchair aerobics and gardening. There are also outings on offer for the residents.

Registered places: 36
Guide weekly rate: £390–£654
Specialist care: Nursing, respite
Medical services: Podiatry
Qualified staff: Fails standard

Home details
Location: Village location, 20 miles from Gloucester
Communal areas: 2 lounges, dining room, patio and garden
Accessibility: *Floors:* 2 • *Access:* 2 lifts and stair lift
   Wheelchair access: Good
Smoking: ×
Pets: ×
Routines: Flexible

Room details
Single: 20
Shared: 8
En suite: 18
Facilities: TV, telephone

Door lock: ✓
Lockable place: ×

Services provided
Beauty services: Hairdressing
Mobile library: ✓
Religious services: Monthly Communion service
Transport: ×
Activities: *Coordinator.* ✓ • *Examples:* Armchair aerobics, cheese tasting, gardening • *Outings:* ✓
Meetings: ✓

Tewkesbury Nursing Home

Manager: Jenifer King
Owner: Tewkesbury Nursing Home Ltd
Contact: The Oxhey, Bushley,
Nr Tewkesbury, Gloucestershire, GL20 6HP
) 01684 850311
@ tewkesbury@majesticare.co.uk
www.majesticare.co.uk

A single-storey building set in the countryside with comfortable rooms for relaxing and socialising, Tewkesbury Nursing Home is accessible and friendly. The activities coordinator spends one-to-one time with residents, making them feel welcomed and valued. There is a courtyard with raised flowerbeds and many rooms have views of the surrounding countryside. The home produces a newsletter twice a month. There is no smoking within the house, but there is a designated smoking area. The home is situated in a rural area, 12 miles from Tewkesbury.

Registered places: 59
Guide weekly rate: From £600
Specialist care: Nursing, dementia, physical disability
Medical services: Podiatry, dentist, optician
Qualified staff: Fails standard: 44% at NVQ level 2

Home details
Location: Rural area, 12 miles from Tewkesbury
Communal areas: 3 lounges, 2 dining rooms, conservatory, patio and garden
Accessibility: *Floors:* 1 • *Wheelchair access:* Good
Smoking: In designated area
Pets: At manager's discretion
Routines: Flexible

Room details
Single: 48
Shared: 4
En suite: 28
Facilities: TV point

Door lock: ✓
Lockable place: ✓

Services provided
Beauty services: Hairdressing, aromatherapy, manicures
Mobile library: ✓
Religious services: ×
Transport: ×
Activities: *Coordinator.* ✓ • *Examples:* Bingo, music and movement, one-to-one sessions • *Outings:* ✓
Meetings: ×

Registered places: 58
Guide weekly rate: £392–£630
Specialist care: Nursing, dementia
Medical services: Podiatry, hygienist, optician, physiotherapy
Qualified staff: Fails standard: 40% at NVQ level 2

Home details

Location: Village location, 7.5 miles from Bristol
Communal areas: 4 lounges, 3 dining rooms, conservatory, garden
Accessibility: *Floors:* 2 • *Access:* Lift and stair lift
   Wheelchair access: Good
Smoking: ×
Pets: ×
Routines: Structured

Room details

Single: 56
Shared: 1
En suite: Undisclosed
Facilities: Telephone point

Door lock: ✓
Lockable place: ✓

Services provided

Beauty services: Hairdressing
Mobile library: ×
Religious services: Monthly Anglican visits
Transport: ×
Activities: *Coordinator.* ✓ • *Examples:* Gentle exercise,
   Outings: ✓
Meetings: ×

Warmley House Care Home

Manager: Janet Goodfellow
Owner: Lunan House Ltd
Contact: Tower Road North,Warmley,
South Gloucestershire,
BS30 8XN
☎ 0117 9674872

A Grade II listed building that is split into two sections and includes a purpose-built nursing wing, Warmley House Care Home offers care until end of life. Its beautiful setting sets the tone for a relaxing experience, with gentle exercise and many services provided. Residents are provided with a variety of food as well as a wide range of social activities both in the home and externally. There are monthly visits from an Anglican minister.

Registered places: 45
Guide weekly rate: £480–£600
Specialist care: Nursing
Medical services: Podiatry, dentist, occupational therapy, optician,
   physiotherapy
Qualified staff: Undisclosed

Home details

Location: Village location, 4 miles from Chipping Sodbury
Communal areas: 3 lounges, 3 dining rooms, patio and garden
Accessibility:*Floors:* 2 • *Access:* Lift • *Wheelchair access:* Good
Smoking: ×
Pets: ✓
Routines: Flexible

Room details

Single: 39
Shared: 3
En suite: Undisclosed
Facilities: None

Door lock: ×
Lockable place: ✓

Services provided

Beauty services: Hairdressing
Mobile library: ×
Religious services: ×
Transport: ×
Activities: *Coordinator.* ✓ • *Examples:* Arts and crafts, baking
   Outings: ✓
Meetings: ×

Wickwar Nursing and Residential Home

Manager: Amanda Waldron
Owner: Ashbourne Ltd
Contact: Castle House, Sodbury Road,
Wickwar, South Gloucestershire,
GL12 8NR
☎ 01454 294426
@ wickwar@ashbourne.co.uk
🖰 www.schealthcare.co.uk

A converted property located on the Sodbury Road, Wickwar Nursing and Residential Home benefits from its close proximity to a bus stop where there is a bus service up to three times a day. Close to village facilities, Chipping Sodbury is four miles away and the home has a mobile shop. The activities coordinator in the home puts together a varied programme which includes baking and bingo. There are also regular outings on offer.

Willow Cottage

Manager: Pauline Rodman
Owner: Jennifer and David Roberts
Contact: 127 Station Road, Yate, South Gloucestershire, BS37 5AL

) 01454 318738

@ willowcottage@dsl.pitex.com

Situated close to Firgrove House, Willow Cottage is located in the centre of Yate opposite the main shopping centre. The home has two lounges for residents to relax in, as well as a conservatory and a garden. The home arranges group activities for the residents such as armchair exercises and bingo, in addition to individual sessions. There is a residents meeting every six weeks and there are regular outings on offer.

Registered places: 34
Guide weekly rate: £430–£550
Specialist care: Nursing
Medical services: Podiatry, optician, physiotherapy
Qualified staff: Exceeds standard: 80% at NVQ level 2

Home details
Location: Residential area, 0.3 miles from Yate
Communal areas: 2 lounges, dining room, conservatory, garden
Accessibility: *Floors:* 3 • *Access:* Lift • *Wheelchair access:* Good
Smoking: ×
Pets: ×
Routines: Flexible

Room details
Single: 28
Shared: 3
En suite: 2
Facilities: TV point, telephone point

Door lock: ×
Lockable place: ×

Services provided
Beauty services: Hairdressing
Mobile library: ✓
Religious services: Monthly Communion service
Transport: ×
Activities: *Coordinator:* × • *Examples:* Armchair exercises, art therapy, bingo • *Outings:* ✓
Meetings: ✓

Winslow House

Manager: Jean Walker
Owner: Winslow House Ltd
Contact: Springhill, Nailsworth Gloucestershire, GL6 0LS

) 01453 832269

A converted Victorian property situated close to the facilities of Nailsworth, which are within walking distance of the home. Winslow House also permits its residents attractive views of the surrounding countryside. There are monthly visits to the home by Anglican and Catholic clergy and the home has its own car to take residents on outings. There is a mobile library which comes to the home and there are regular residents meetings.

Registered places: 35
Guide weekly rate: £450–£850
Specialist care: Undisclosed
Medical services: Podiatry, hygienist, optician, physiotherapy
Qualified staff: Exceeds standard: 68% at NVQ level 2

Home details
Location: Residential area, 0.7 miles from Nailsworth
Communal areas: Lounge, lounge/dining room, dining room, conservatory, patio and garden
Accessibility: *Floors:* 4 • *Access:* Lift • *Wheelchair access:* Good
Smoking: ×
Pets: ✓
Routines: Structured

Room details
Single: Undisclosed
Shared: Undisclosed
En suite: 35
Facilities: TV, telephone

Door lock: ✓
Lockable place: ✓

Services provided
Beauty services: Hairdressing, manicures
Mobile Library: ✓
Religious services: Monthly Anglican and Catholic visits
Transport: Car
Activities: *Coordinator:* ✓ • *Examples:* Bingo • *Outings:* ✓
Meetings: ✓

Registered places: 18
Guide weekly rate: £349–£485
Specialist care: Day care, respite
Medical services: Podiatry, dentist, optician
Qualified staff: Undisclosed

Home details

Location: Residential area, 0.7 miles from Cheltenham
Communal areas: 2 lounges, 2 dining rooms, garden
Accessibility: *Floors:* 3 • *Access:* Stair lifts
   Wheelchair access: Good
Smoking: In designated area
Pets: At manager's discretion
Routines: Flexible

Room details

Single: 18
Shared: 0   Door lock: ✓
En suite: 18   Lockable place: ✓
Facilities: TV point, telephone point

Services provided

Beauty services: Hairdressing
Mobile library: ✗
Religious services: ✗
Transport: Minibus
Activities: *Coordinator:* ✗ • *Examples:* Games, movement and music
   Outings: ✓
Meetings: ✓

Winstonian House

Manager: Sally Hobson
Owner: CTCH Ltd
Contact: 42 All Saints Road,
Cheltenham, Gloucestershire,
GL52 2EZ
☎ 01242 577927
🖰 www.ctch.co.uk

Winstonian House comprises three terrace houses, including an end of terrace house, that have been converted into one property. The home is located in the All Saints area of Cheltenham. The home has connecting lounges, two dining rooms and al garden where residents can sit. The home has its own minibus and residents are taken shopping and to local sights. The home welcomes visitors to the home, and encourages them to get involved in the life of the home. Residents are encouraged to participate socially in the home, and several good community contacts are in place.

Registered places: 40
Guide weekly rate: £635–£750
Specialist care: Nursing, physical disability
Medical services: Podiatry, hygienist, optician, physiotherapy
Qualified staff: Meets standard

Home details

Location: Rural location, 1.7 miles from Winterbourne
Communal areas: 2 lounges, dining room, 2 conservatories,
   patio and garden
Accessibility: *Floors:* • 2 *Access:* Lift • *Wheelchair access:* Good
Smoking: ✗
Pets: ✗
Routines: Structured

Room details

Single: 36
Shared: 2   Door lock: ✓
En suite: 11   Lockable place: ✓
Facilities: TV, telephone point

Services provided

Beauty services: Hairdressing, manicures
Mobile Library: ✓
Religious services: Monthly Anglican Communion service
Transport: ✗
Activities: *Coordinator:* ✓ • *Examples:* Music and movement
   Outings: ✗
Meetings: ✗

Woodlands Manor

Manager: Cheryl Lawrence
Owner: Woodlands Manor
Care Home Ltd
Contact: Ruffet Road, Kendleshire,
South Gloucestershire, BS36 1AN
☎ 01454 250593

In a rural location almost two miles from Winterbourne, Woodlands Manor provides care for 40 residents. There is a bus stop at end of the drive and easy access to the motorway. Woodlands Manor is set in its own grounds. The carers have a good, established reputation and try to make the house a home. Downend also makes an effort to send out a quarterly newsletter.

Woodstock Nursing Home

Manager: Millie Barnes
Owner: Millie and John Barnes
Contact: 35 North Upton Lane, Barnwood, Gloucester GL4 3TD
☎ 01452 616291

Situated in a residential area of Barnwood close to a small parade of shops, Woodstock Nursing Home is a large home set in its own grounds and overlooking attractive, enclosed gardens. These encompass a flat grassy area surrounded by a circular paved walkway. With three lounges in total, one is dedicated to quiet while another is used for group activities. Outings are arranged monthly with in-house entertainment provided by visiting professionals.

Registered places: 29
Guide weekly rate: Undisclosed
Specialist care: Nursing, dementia, physical disability
Medical services: Podiatry, dentist, optician, physiotherapy
Qualified staff: Undisclosed

Home details
Location: Residential area, 2 miles from Gloucester centre
Communal areas: 3 lounges, dining room, garden
Accessibility: *Floors:* 3 • *Access:* Lift • *Wheelchair access:* Good
Smoking: ✗
Pets: ✗
Routines: Flexible

Room details
Single: 29
Shared: 0
En suite: 29
Facilities: TV point, telephone point

Door lock: ✓
Lockable place: ✓

Services provided
Beauty services: Hairdressing
Mobile library: ✗
Religious services: Monthly Anglican Communion service
Transport: ✗
Activities: *Coordinator.* ✓ • *Examples:* One-to-one sessions
    Outings: ✓
Meetings: ✗

Wotton Rise Nursing Home

Manager: Diana Martinez
Owner: Mr and Mrs Martinez
Contact: 140 London Road, Gloucester GL1 3PL
☎ 01452 303073

Wotton Rise is situated a mile from the city centre of Gloucester and provides care for 27 residents. The home can also care for two patients with physical disability. The laid back approach to the social and recreational needs gives the residents freedom to choose. The home has a daily activities programme including board games and in the summer the home organises outings to the church fête and for walks in the park. Pets would be allowed in the home and there are regular residents meetings.

Registered places: 27
Guide weekly rate: £530
Specialist care: Nursing, physical disability, respite
Medical services: None
Qualified staff: Exceeds standard: 100% at NVQ level 2

Home details
Location: Residential area, 1 mile from Gloucester
Communal areas: Lounge, dining room, conservatory, garden
Accessibility: *Floors:* 2 • *Access:* Lift • *Wheelchair access:* Good
Smoking: ✗
Pets: At manager's discretion
Routines: Flexible

Room details
Single: 21
Shared: 3
En suite: 9
Facilities: TV, telephone point

Door lock: ✓
Lockable place: ✓

Services provided
Beauty services: Hairdressing, manicures
Mobile library: ✓
Religious services: ✓
Transport: ✓
Activities: *Coordinator.* ✓ • *Examples:* Board games, skittles, reminiscence • *Outings:* ✓
Meetings: ✓

Registered places: 6
Guide weekly rate: Undisclosed
Specialist care: Respite
Medical services: Podiatry, dentist, optician, physiotherapy
Qualified staff: Meets standard

Home details

Location: Residential area, 2 miles from Cirencester
Communal areas: Lounge/dining room, conservatory,
    patio and garden
Accessibility: *Floors:* 2 • *Access:* Stair lift • *Wheelchair access:* Good
Smoking: ✗
Pets: ✓
Routines: Flexible

Room details

Single: 6
Shared: 0
En suite: 1
Facilities: TV, telephone

Door lock: ✓
Lockable place: ✗

Services provided

Beauty services: Hairdressing
Mobile library: ✗
Religious services: Monthly Communion service
Transport: ✓
Activities: *Coordinator:* ✗ • *Examples:* Armchair exercises,
    board games, puzzles • *Outings:* ✓
Meetings: ✗

Zapuzino

Manager: Rosemary Kilby
Owner: Rosemary Kilby
Contact: 205 Alexander Drive,
Cirencester, Gloucestershire, GL7 1UH

☏ 01285 651057

@ postmaster@
    charlienicholas.plus.com

Zapuzino is a small care home in a quiet cul-de-sac on a large housing estate outside Cirencester town. There is a large lounge/dining room and a smaller separate dining area in the conservatory. The home also has a garden with a patio area. The home offers a personalised service as there are only six residents. Communion is held monthly and a hairdresser comes weekly. The home organises daily activities such as puzzles and outings to the theatre.

Ashley House

Manager: Susan Timbrell
Owner: South West Care Homes Ltd
Contact: The Avenue, Langport,
Somerset TA10 9SA
☏ 01458 250386

Situated in a residential area, less than half a mile from Langport, Ashley House prides itself on creating a homely atmosphere with approachable staff. Currently, four cats live in the home and other pets would be permitted at the manager's discretion. There is a residents meeting every three to four months and a Communion services takes place on a monthly basis. The home also has its own library facilities.

Registered places: 25
Guide weekly rate: £382–£412
Specialist care: Day care, dementia
Medical services: Podiatry, optician
Qualified staff: Exceeds standard: 77% at NVQ level 2

Home details
Location: Residential area, 0.3 miles from Langport
Communal areas: Lounge, dining room, library facilities, conservatory, garden
Accessibility: *Floors:* 2 • *Access:* Stair lift • *Wheelchair access:* None
Smoking: In designated area
Pets: At manager's discretion
Routines: Flexible

Room details
Single: 21
Shared: 2
En suite: 21
Facilities: TV point, telephone point

Door lock: ✓
Lockable place: ✓

Services provided
Beauty services: Hairdressing
Mobile library: Library facilities
Religious services: Monthly Communion service
Transport: ✗
Activities: *Coordinator.* ✗ • *Examples:* Discussions, gentle exercise, singalongs • *Outings:* ✗
Meetings: ✓

Banbridge House

Manager: Tina Boswell
Owner: Tina Boswell
Contact: 3 The Esplanade, Minehead,
Somerset TA24 5QS
☏ 01643 702275

In a prime position on Minehead seafront, Banbridge House permits attractive sea views and is a few minutes' walk from the local train station. All areas of the home are well maintained and furnished to a high standard. The home is approximately half a mile away from the town centre. The home arranges a variety of activities for the residents which include arts and crafts and quizzes. There are also outings on offer.

Registered places: 19
Guide weekly rate: £340–£460
Specialist care: Respite
Medical services: Podiatry, dentist, optician
Qualified staff: Exceeds standard: 57% at NVQ level 2

Home details
Location: Residential area, 0.6 miles from Minehead
Communal areas: Lounge, dining room, conservatory, garden
Accessibility: *Floors:* 3 • *Access:* Lift • *Wheelchair access:* Good
Smoking: ✗
Pets: ✓
Routines: Flexible

Room details
Single: 19
Shared: 0
En suite: 19
Facilities: TV

Door lock: ✓
Lockable place: ✓

Services provided
Beauty services: Hairdressing, massage
Mobile library: ✗
Religious services: ✗
Transport: ✗
Activities: *Coordinator.* ✗ • *Examples:* Arts and crafts, bingo, quizzes • *Outings:* ✓
Meetings: ✗

Registered places: 40
Guide weekly rate: £700–£1,200
Specialist care: Nursing
Medical services: Podiatry, dentist, optician
Qualified staff: Exceeds standard: 94% at NVQ level 2

Home details

Location: Village location, 7 miles from Taunton
Communal areas: Lounge, dining room, patio and garden
Accessibility: *Floors:* 2 • *Access:* Lift • *Wheelchair access:* Good
Smoking: x
Pets: x
Routines: Flexible

Room details

Single: 40
Shared: 0
En suite: Undisclosed
Facilities: TV

Door lock: ✓
Lockable place: ✓

Services provided

Beauty services: Hairdressing
Mobile library: x
Religious services: x
Transport: x
Activities: *Coordinator.* ✓ • *Examples*: Art, exercise, musical
   entertainment • *Outings:* ✓
Meetings: x

Beauchamp Country House Care

Manager: Patricia Britten
Owner: David Kohlman
Contact: Village Road, Hatch Beauchamp, Taunton, Somerset TA3 6SG
☎ 01823 480276

The home is a large detached property, which is situated in a village seven miles from Taunton. All the communal areas, such as the lounge and dining rooms are well preserved. The home also has a garden with a patio area for residents to use in the summer months. The home has an activities coordinator who offers art and exercise sessions to the residents, as well as arranging musical entertainment. There are also outings available for residents to partake in.

Registered places: 28
Guide weekly rate: £450–£550
Specialist care: Day care, respite
Medical services: Podiatry, hygienist, optician
Qualified staff: Exceeds standard: 90% at NVQ level 2

Home details

Location: Residential area, 1.6 miles from Yeovil
Communal areas: 2 lounges, 2 dining rooms,
   2 conservatories, garden
Accessibility: *Floors:* 1 • *Wheelchair access:* Good
Smoking: x
Pets: At manager's discretion
Routines: Flexible

Room details

Single: 26
Shared: 1
En suite: 27
Facilities: TV point, telephone point

Door lock: ✓
Lockable place: ✓

Services provided

Beauty services: Hairdressing
Mobile library: ✓
Religious services: Monthly Anglican Communion service
Transport: Car
Activities: *Coordinator.* ✓ • *Examples*: Flower arranging, gardening
   Outings: ✓
Meetings: ✓

Beechwood House Retirement Home

Manager: Sandra Barclay
Owner: Beechwood House Ltd
Contact: 60 West Coker Road, Yeovil, Somerset BA20 2JA
☎ 01935 472793
@ beechwood@homecall.co.uk

Beechwood House Retirement Home is set back on a main road one and a half miles from Yeovil town centre. The home has a peaceful garden with sitting areas and a wild area with a pond. There is a quadrangle with a central fountain. There is a residents meeting twice a year and the home arranges an Anglican Communion service once a month. The home has its own car and often takes residents on outings. There are also daily activities which include gardening and quizzes and the home is visited by a mobile library.

Belmont Villa Nursing & Residential Home

Manager: Sharon Welsh
Owner: Belmont Villa Residential & Nursing Home Ltd
Contact: 58–62 Weymouth Road, Frome, Somerset BA11 1HJ
) 01373 471093
@ belmontvilla@aol.com

A family-run home situated in a residential area, Belmont Villa is opposite a park, and close to shops, pubs, and the hospital. The home has landscaped private gardens with a patio seating area. Inside the home there are four lounges and two dining rooms providing ample communal space. There is a residents meeting which takes place every two months and the home arranges a monthly Communion service. The residents are given the chance to go on outings and there are internal activities such as exercise sessions and games on offer.

Registered places: 30
Guide weekly rate: £450–£625
Specialist care: Nursing
Medical services: Podiatry, optician, physiotherapy
Qualified staff: Exceeds standard: 80% at NVQ level 2

Home details
Location: Residential area, 0.3 miles from Frome
Communal areas: 4 lounges, 2 dining rooms, conservatory, patio and 3 gardens
Accessibility: *Floors:* 3 • *Access:* Lift • *Wheelchair access:* Good
Smoking: In designated area
Pets: ✗
Routines: Flexible

Room details
Single: 29
Shared: 1
En suite: 30
Facilities: TV point, telephone point
Door lock: ✓
Lockable place: ✗

Services provided
Beauty services: Hairdressing
Mobile library: ✗
Religious services: Monthly Communion service
Transport: ✗
Activities: *Coordinator:* ✗ • *Examples:* Exercise, flower arranging
  Outings: ✓
Meetings: ✓

Brambledene Rest Home

Manager: Mrs Munday
Owner: Alutarius Ltd
Contact: 20–22 Moorland Road, Weston-super-Mare, North Somerset, BS23 4HN
) 01934 633711

Brambledene Rest Home consists of two semi-detached Victorian houses located in a residential area, one mile from Weston-super-Mare. The home has a lounge and a dining room as well as a conservatory and a garden. There is a range of activities on offer including board games, video afternoon and performances by visiting entertainers. The residents are also given the opportunity to go on outings in the local area.

Registered places: 14
Guide weekly rate: Undisclosed
Specialist care: Respite
Medical services: Podiatry, dentist, optician
Qualified staff: Meets standard

Home details
Location: Residential area, 1 mile from Weston-super-Mare
Communal areas: Lounge, dining room, conservatory, garden
Accessibility: *Floors:* 2 • *Access:* Stair lift
  Wheelchair access: Good
Smoking: ✗
Pets: At manager's discretion
Routines: Flexible

Room details
Single: 12
Shared: 1
En suite: 2
Facilities: TV, telephone point
Door lock: ✓
Lockable place: ✓

Services provided
Beauty services: Hairdressing
Mobile library: ✓
Religious services: ✓
Transport: ✓
Activities: *Coordinator:* ✓ • *Examples:* Videos, visiting entertainers
  Outings: ✓
Meetings: ✓

Registered places: 9
Guide weekly rate: £360
Specialist care: Emergency admissions, learning disability
Medical services: Podiatry, dentist, optician
Qualified staff: Meets standard

Home details

Location: Village location, 1 mile from Yeovil
Communal areas: Lounge, dining room, conservatory, garden
Accessibility: *Floors:* 2 • *Access:* Lift • *Wheelchair access:* Good
Smoking: ✗
Pets: ✓
Routines: Flexible

Room details

Single: 9
Shared: 0   Door lock: ✓
En suite: 9   Lockable place: ✓
Facilities: None

Services provided

Beauty services: Hairdressing
Mobile library: ✗
Religious services: ✗
Transport: ✗
Activities: *Coordinator.* ✗ • *Examples*: Bingo, exercises, singing
    performances • *Outings:* ✓
Meetings: ✗

Braunton

Manager: Alexandra Vickery
Owner: Braunton Residential Home Ltd
Contact: 23 Grove Avenue, Yeovil,
Somerset BA20 2BD
☎ 01935 422176

At Braunton the emphasis is on providing a homely environment where residents are encouraged to maintain good links with the community. The home is located in a village, approximately one mile from Yeovil. The home has a garden and a conservatory for residents to relax in, as well as a lounge and a separate dining room. The home arranges a variety of activities for the residents such as bingo and exercise sessions. There are also outings arranged to places of local interest.

Registered places: 10
Guide weekly rate: £361–£450
Specialist care: Respite
Medical services: Podiatry, dentist, optician
Qualified staff: Undisclosed

Home details

Location: Residential area, 1 mile from Burnham-on-Sea
Communal areas: 2 lounges, dining room, conservatory, garden
Accessibility: *Floors:* 2 • *Access:* Lift • *Wheelchair access:* Good
Smoking: ✗
Pets: ✓
Routines: Flexible

Room details

Single: 10
Shared: 0   Door lock: ✓
En suite: 4   Lockable place: ✓
Facilities: None

Services provided

Beauty services: Hairdressing
Mobile library: ✗
Religious services: ✗
Transport: ✗
Activities: *Coordinator.* ✗ • *Examples*: Bingo, knitting • *Outings:* ✓
Meetings: ✗

Broughton Lodge

Manager: Michael Matthews
Owner: Michael and Mandy Matthews
Contact: 88 Berrow Road,
Burnham-on-Sea, Somerset TA8 2HN
☎ 01278 782133

Situated close to the seafront and the town centre, Broughton Lodge is set in its own grounds. The home is approximately one mile from the centre of Burnham-on-sea. The home has a garden and a conservatory for residents to relax in and there are two lounges inside the home. There are a range of activities on offer such as bingo and knitting and the home also arranges outings in the local area.

Burnworthy House

Manager: Claire Smith
Owner: Somerset Care Ltd
Contact: South Street, South Petherton, Somerset TA13 5AD

☏ 01460 240116
@ claire.smith@somersetcare.co.uk
🖱 www.somersetcare.co.uk

Burnworthy House is situated in the large village of South Petherton offering a countryside location, but within 10 miles of Yeovil. The home is run by Somerset Care, a 'not for profit' organisation. There are residents meetings held every two months and the home arranges for a mobile library to visit on a regular basis. There are a variety of activities on offer such as arts and crafts and exercise, as well as one-to-one sessions. There is a Communion service held on a monthly basis.

Registered places: 37
Guide weekly rate: £373–£460
Specialist care: Day care, respite
Medical services: Podiatry, dentist, optician
Qualified staff: Exceeds standard: 70% at NVQ level 2

Home details
Location: Village location, 10 miles from Yeovil
Communal areas: 3 lounges, 2 dining room, garden
Accessibility: *Floors:* 2 • *Access:* Lift • *Wheelchair access:* Good
Smoking: ✗
Pets: ✓
Routines: Flexible

Room details
Single: 31
Shared: 3
En suite: 17
Facilities: TV point, telephone point

Door lock: ✓
Lockable place: ✓

Services provided
Beauty services: Hairdressing
Mobile library: ✓
Religious services: Monthly Communion service
Transport: ✗
Activities: *Coordinator:* ✗ • *Examples:* Arts and crafts, exercises, music • *Outings:* ✗
Meetings: ✓

Cary Brook

Manager: Judith Pullen
Owner: Somerset Care Ltd
Contact: Millbrook Gardens, Castle Cary, Somerset BA7 7EE

☏ 01963 350641

Situated at the top of a small hill, Cary Brook is a purpose-built home with an easily accessible, level garden. The home is found in a residential area, approximately half a mile from Castle Cary. There is an extension planned for the near future. Currently the home has a conservatory and a garden for residents to relax in, as well as a lounge. The home has an activities coordinator who arranges performances from visiting entertainers. There are also outings on offer to the residents.

Registered places: 35
Guide weekly rate: Undisclosed
Specialist care: Dementia
Medical services: Podiatry, hygienist, optician
Qualified staff: Meets standard

Home details
Location: Residential area, 0.3 miles from Castle Cary
Communal areas: Lounge, dining room, conservatory, garden
Accessibility: *Floors:* 2 • *Access:* Lift • *Wheelchair access:* Good
Smoking: In designated area
Pets: ✓
Routines: Structured

Room details
Single: 35
Shared: 0
En suite: 0
Facilities: TV point, telephone point

Door lock: ✓
Lockable place: ✓

Services provided
Beauty services: Hairdressing.
Mobile library: ✗
Religious services: ✗
Transport: ✗
Activities: *Coordinator:* ✓ • *Examples:* Visiting entertainers *Outings:* ✓
Meetings: ✗

Registered places: 22
Guide weekly rate: £600
Specialist care: Nursing, day care, emergency admissions, respite
Medical services: Podiatry, dentist, optician, physiotherapy
Qualified staff: Undisclosed

Home details

Location: Village location, 4 miles from Somerton
Communal areas: Lounge, dining room, garden
Accessibility: *Floors:* 1 • *Wheelchair access:* Good
Smoking: ✗
Pets: At manager's discretion
Routines: Flexible

Room details

Single: 20
Shared: 1
En suite: 21
Facilities: TV point, telephone point

Door lock: ✓
Lockable place: ✓

Services provided

Beauty services: Hairdressing, aromatherapy
Mobile library: ✓
Religious services: Monthly nondenominational Communion service
Transport: ✗
Activities: *Coordinator.* ✓ • *Examples:* Arts and crafts, painting
    Outings: ✓
Meetings: ✗

Castle House

Manager: Catherine Hinch
Owner: Catherine Hinch
Contact: Castle Street, Keinton
Mandeville, Somerton, Somerset
TA11 6DX
✆ 01458 223780
@ castlehnh@aol.com

A single-storey purpose-built home in the centre of Keinton Mandeville village, Castle House is a homely property set on a level site five minutes' walk from a pub, church, post office and local shops. Permitting views of the surrounding countryside, the home's gardens are spacious and attractive. With the manager living on site, Castle House is a pet-friendly environment which is home to the owner's dog. Actively encouraging 'open visiting', hairdressing is also included in the fees.

Registered places: 13
Guide weekly rate: £373
Specialist care: Day care
Medical services: Podiatry, hygienist, optician, physiotherapy
Qualified staff: Exceeds standard: 90% at NVQ level 2

Home details

Location: Residential area, 1 mile from Shepton Mallet
Communal areas: 2 lounges, dining room, library,
    conservatory, garden
Accessibility: *Floors:* 1 • *Wheelchair access:* Good
Smoking: ✗
Pets: ✓
Routines: Flexible

Room details

Single: 11
Shared: 1
En suite: 1
Facilities: TV point, telephone point

Door lock: ✓
Lockable place: ✓

Services provided

Beauty services: Hairdressing, aromatherapy, massage
Mobile library: Library facilities
Religious services: Monthly Anglican Communion service
Transport: ✗
Activities: *Coordinator.* ✓ • *Examples:* Games, exercises, quizzes
    Outings: ✓
Meetings: ✓

Centenary House

Manager: Deborah Reynolds
Owner: Deborah Reynolds
Contact: 70 Charlton Road,
Shepton Mallet, Somerset BA4 5PD
✆ 01749 342727
@ reydebor@aol.com

An older-style property that has been extended, Centenary House is located in a residential area, one mile from Shepton Mallet. The home has a small garden with a greenhouse. The home grows some of its own produce. With a garage next door that sells basic goods and a supermarket nearby, the home is also within walking distance of the centre of town. There is a residents meeting held once a month and there is also an Anglican Communion service held on a monthly basis. The home has an activities coordinator who arranges games and gentle exercises for the residents.

Clare Hall Nursing Home

Manager: Keeley Simpson
Owner: BUPA Care Homes Ltd
Contact: Ston Easton, Bath,
Somerset BA3 4DE
) 01761 241626
@ ClareHallALL@BUPA.com
⌖ www.bupacarehomes.co.uk

Clare Hall is set in the countryside, south-west of Bath, in landscaped gardens with two patio areas. Originally a private house, it has been extended and converted into a care home. There are three lounge and dining rooms and two conservatories. The bedrooms are all furnished, and some offer en suite facilities. Daily activities include art groups, games, gardening, singalongs, and outings. Clare Hall also offers care to younger people with physical disabilities, to people with Parkinson's and motor neurone disease, those who have had stroke, those requiring palliative and terminal care, and day care to local older people.

Registered places: 57
Guide weekly rate: Undisclosed
Specialist care: Nursing, day care, palliative care, respite, terminal care
Medical services: Podiatry, physiotherapy
Qualified staff: Undisclosed

Home details
Location: Village location, 8 miles from Bath
Communal areas: 3 lounge/dining rooms, 2 conservatories, garden
Accessibility: *Floors:* 2 • *Access:* Lift • *Wheelchair access:* Good
Smoking: ✗
Pets: ✗
Routines: Flexible

Room details
Single: 57
Shared: 0
En suite: 17
Facilities: TV point, telephone point

Door lock: ✓
Lockable place: ✗

Services provided
Beauty services: Hairdressing
Mobile library: ✓
Religious services: ✓
Transport: ✗
Activities: *Coordinator:* ✓ • *Examples:* Bingo, flower arranging, visiting entertainers • *Outings:* ✓
Meetings: ✓

Compton View Care Home

Manager: Lindsey Haimes
Owner: Paul and Lindsey Haimes
Contact: 267 St Michael's Avenue,
Yeovil, Somerset BA21 4NB
) 01935 476203

Compton View is located in a residential area, approximately one and a half miles from Yeovil. Residents have necessary access to appropriate healthcare professionals and it is a pleasing house which provides a comfortable environment. All areas are maintained to a high standard of repair. There is also a planned extension to the downstairs bedrooms. The home arranges for a mobile library to visit and there are religious services on offer. The home also organises activities for the residents which include singalongs and quizzes.

Registered places: 16
Guide weekly rate: Undisclosed
Specialist care: None
Medical services: Undisclosed
Qualified staff: Meets standard

Home details
Location: Residential area, 1.6 miles from Yeovil
Communal areas: 2 lounges, dining room, conservatory, garden
Accessibility: *Floors:* 2 • *Access:* Lift • *Wheelchair access:* Good
Smoking: ✗
Pets: ✗
Routines: Flexible

Room details
Single: 16
Shared: 0
En suite: 5
Facilities: None

Door lock: ✗
Lockable place: ✗

Services provided
Beauty services: Hairdressing
Mobile library: ✓
Religious services: ✗
Transport: ✗
Activities: *Coordinator:* ✗ • *Examples:* Singalongs, quizzes *Outings:* ✗
Meetings: Undisclosed

Registered places: 50
Guide weekly rate: £361–£430
Specialist care: Day care, dementia, respite
Medical services: Podiatry, optician, physiotherapy
Qualified staff: Exceeds standard: 78% at NVQ level 2

Home details

Location: Residential area, 1 mile from Frome
Communal areas: 5 lounges, 2 dining rooms, garden
Accessibility: *Floors:* 1 • *Wheelchair access:* Good
Smoking: In designated area
Pets: At manager's discretion
Routines: Flexible

Room details

Single: 36
Shared: 7
En suite: 4
Facilities: TV point, telephone point

Door lock: ✓
Lockable place: ✓

Services provided

Beauty services: Hairdressing
Mobile library: ✓
Religious services: Monthly Communion service
Transport: ✗
Activities: *Coordinator.* ✓ • *Examples:* Doll therapy • *Outings:* ✓
Meetings: ✓

Critchill Court

Manager: Sue Steeds
Owner: Somerset Care Ltd
Contact: Lynwood Close, Frome,
Somerset BA11 4DP
☎ 01373 461686
@ carol.mohide@somersetcare.co.uk
🖰 www.somersetcare.co.uk

A purpose-built home located away from the main road in a residential area of Frome, Critchill Court is split into two distinct units. Those requiring dementia support reside in a self-contained area called Cedar and Oaks. The home's pond and flowerbeds can be seen from windows overlooking the courtyard and there is a summerhouse in Cedar Oaks' garden. The home also has five lounges and two dining rooms providing ample communal space for the residents. The home arranges outings for the residents and there are also regular residents meetings.

Registered places: 25
Guide weekly rate: £415–£430
Specialist care: Day care, respite
Medical services: Podiatry, dentist, optician, physiotherapy
Qualified staff: Meets standard

Home details

Location: Rural area, 2 miles from Glastonbury
Communal areas: Lounge, dining room, garden
Accessibility: *Floors:* 2 • *Access:* Stair lift • *Wheelchair access:* Good
Smoking: ✗
Pets: ✗
Routines: Flexible

Room details

Single: 25
Shared: 0
En suite: 25
Facilities: TV point, telephone point

Door lock: ✓
Lockable place: ✗

Services provided

Beauty services: Hairdressing
Mobile library: ✓
Religious services: Monthly Anglican Communion service
Transport: ✗
Activities: *Coordinator.* ✗ • *Examples:* Bingo, exercise, quizzes
    Outings: ✓
Meetings: ✓

The Cyder Barn

Manager: Mrs Nutt
Owner: The Cyder Barn Ltd
Contact: West Pennard,
Glastonbury, Somerset BA6 8NH
☎ 01458 834945
@ cyderbarn@aol.com
🖰 www.cyderbarn.co.uk

A converted, detached blacksmith's shop, cottage and barn, The Cyder Barn offers a fresh alternative to more typical retirement developments. Situated close to West Pennard village, it is a five-minute walk to the centre where there are shops, a pub and the village hall. The home is also on a bus route which can take residents into Glastonbury. Inside the home, windows are double-glazed and relay beautiful views of the home's gardens and nearby Mendip hills. Any resident is welcome to tend to a patch of the garden and there is also an orchard.

Dunster Lodge

Manager: Margaret Hayes
Owner: Margaret and Anne Clarke
Contact: off Manor Road, Alcombe,
Minehead, Somerset TA24 6EW

☎ 01643 703007

@ info@dunsterlodge.co.uk

🖱 www.dunsterlodge.co.uk

Set in three and a half acres of expansive land at the top of a hill, Dunster Lodge offers residents panoramic views of both Minehead and the Bristol Channel. The owners living on site and the home employs a full-time activities coordinator. Activities are a very important part of life at Dunster Lodge and residents are encouraged to be sociable at events such as theme lunches and other events. Recent themes have included a 1940s lunch and a Somerset theme. There is a residents meeting held every two months.

Registered places: 19
Guide weekly rate: £375–£500
Specialist care: Day care, respite
Medical services: Podiatry, hygienist, optician, physiotherapy
Qualified staff: Exceeds standard: 80% at NVQ level 2

Home details
Location: Rural location, 1.5 miles from Minehead
Communal areas: 2 lounges, dining room, library,
conservatory, garden
Accessibility: *Floors:* 3 • *Access:* Lift • *Wheelchair access:* Good
Smoking: In designated area
Pets: ✓
Routines: Flexible

Room details
Single: 15
Shared: 2
En suite: 9
Facilities: TV point, telephone point

Door lock: ✓
Lockable place: ✓

Services provided
Beauty services: Hairdressing
Mobile library: Library facilities
Religious services: Monthly Communion service
Transport: x
Activities: *Coordinator.* ✓ • *Examples:* Resident's band, ballroom dancing, quizzes • *Outings:* ✓
Meetings: ✓

Elliscombe House Nursing Home

Manager: Melanie Smith
Owner: Park Healthcare Ltd
Contact: Higher Holton, Wincanton,
Somerset BA9 8EA

☎ 01963 33370

A country house where the property is set in large grounds which lead onto open countryside, Elliscombe House is found three miles from Wincanton. Containing many original features the home has two lounges and a large garden. The home arranges a variety of activities for the residents, both individual sessions and group activities like bingo and quizzes. There are also outings on offer to places of local interest or shopping.

Registered places: 41
Guide weekly rate: £540–£705
Specialist care: Nursing, respite
Medical services: Podiatry
Qualified staff: Exceeds standard: 72% at NVQ level 2

Home details
Location: Rural area, 3 miles from Wincanton
Communal areas: 2 lounges, dining room, garden
Accessibility: *Floors:* 2 • *Access:* Lift • *Wheelchair access:* Good
Smoking: x
Pets: x
Routines: Flexible

Room details
Single: 41
Shared: 0
En suite: 0
Facilities: TV point

Door lock: x
Lockable place: x

Services provided
Beauty services: Hairdressing
Mobile library: x
Religious services: ✓
Transport: x
Activities: *Coordinator.* ✓ • *Examples:* Bingo, one-to-one sessions, quizzes • *Outings:* ✓
Meetings: x

Registered places: 16
Guide weekly rate: £373–£405
Specialist care: Day care
Medical services: Podiatry, dentist, optician
Qualified staff: Meets standard

Home details

Location: Rural area, 2 miles from Yeovil
Communal areas: Lounge, dining room, garden
Accessibility: *Floors:* 1 • *Wheelchair access:* Good
Smoking: In designated area
Pets: At manager's discretion
Routines: Flexible

Room details

Single: 16
Shared: 0
En suite: 16
Facilities: TV point, telephone point

Door lock: ✓
Lockable place: ✓

Services provided

Beauty services: Hairdressing
Mobile library: ✓
Religious services: Monthly Anglican Communion service
Transport: ×
Activities: *Coordinator.* × • *Examples:* Bingo, *Outings:* ✓
Meetings: ×

The Elms

Manager: Lee Osborne
Owner: Lee Osborne
Contact: Yeovil Marsh, Yeovil,
Somerset BA21 3QG
) 01935 425440
@ osbornetheelms@aol.com

With the owner living on site, The Elms is run as a family home with residents given contact with Mrs Osborne's family and pets. The home is situated in the village of Yeovil Marsh around two miles from Yeovil town centre. The home has visits from a mobile library and there is an Anglican Communion service held once a month. The home organise activities like bingo to entertain the residents, as well as one-to-one sessions.

Registered places: 31
Guide weekly rate: Undisclosed
Specialist care: Nursing, day care, respite
Medical services: Podiatry, hygienist, optician, physiotherapy
Qualified staff: Meets standard

Home details

Location: Residential area, 1 mile from Yeovil
Communal areas: 2 lounges, dining room, conservatory, garden
Accessibility: *Floors:* 2 • *Access:* Lift • *Wheelchair access:* Good
Smoking: ×
Pets: ✓
Routines: Flexible

Room details

Single: 31
Shared: 0
En suite: 31
Facilities: TV point, telephone point

Door lock: ✓
Lockable place: ×

Services provided

Beauty services: Hairdressing
Mobile library: ✓
Religious services: Monthly Communion service
Transport: ×
Activities: *Coordinator.* ✓ • *Examples:* Baking, gardening
  Outings: ✓
Meetings: ✓

Ferns Nursing Home

Manager: Jackie Hufton
Owner: Almondsbury Care Ltd
Contact: 141 St Michaels Avenue,
Yeovil, Somerset BA21 4LW
) 01935 433115
@ ferns@almondsburycare.com
🖰 www.almondsburycare.com

A purpose-built home in a residential area of Yeovil, Ferns Nursing Home is located on a bus route, offering easy access to the town. The home lies approximately one mile from the town centre. The home produces a newsletter detailing upcoming events and there are residents meetings held every quarter. The home employs an activities coordinator who arranges gardening and baking for the residents, as well as outings in the local area.

Field House

Manager: Linda Tungate
Owner: Somerset Care
Contact: Cannards Grave Road,
Shepton Mallet, Somerset BA4 4LU

) 01749 342006

@ linda.tungate@somersetcare.co.uk

A listed building that is set back from the road, Field House is near the centre of Shepton Mallet and has access to shops. An activity coordinator provides games and pastimes, such as bingo and knitting. There are monthly church services. Residents can decide whether they have a television or telephone in their rooms, and there are four lounges to relax in during the day. The home also offers residents the opportunity to go on outings in the local area.

Registered places: 39
Guide weekly rate: Undisclosed
Specialist care: Day care, respite
Medical services: Undisclosed
Qualified staff: Exceeds standard: 60% at NVQ level 2

Home details
Location: Residential area, 0.5 miles from Shepton Mallet
Communal areas: 4 lounges, 2 dining rooms, patio and garden
Accessibility: *Floors:* 4 • *Access:* Lift • *Wheelchair access:* Good
Smoking: ✗
Pets: ✓
Routines: Flexible

Room details
Single: 37
Shared: 2
En suite: Undisclosed
Facilities: TV point, telephone point

Door lock: ✓
Lockable place: ✓

Services provided
Beauty services: Hairdressing, aromatherapy, manicures
Mobile library: ✗
Religious services: Monthly church service
Transport: ✗
Activities: *Coordinator.* ✓ • *Examples:* Bingo, knitting • *Outings:* ✓
Meetings: ✗

Fir Villa

Manager: Jane Booth
Owner: Ann Williams
Contact: Camel Street, Marston Magna,
Yeovil, Somerset BA22 8DB
) 01935 850670

A family-run business, Fir Villa is situated on a bus route five and a half miles from Yeovil and Sherborne. Home cooking emphasises the homely environment at Fir Villa. The home has its own car for transport and also arranges for a mobile library to visit. There is an Anglican Communion service held at the home on a monthly basis. The home employs an activities coordinator who arranges arts and crafts and gentle exercises for the residents.

Registered places: 20
Guide weekly rate: £373–£395
Specialist care: Day care, respite
Medical services: Podiatry, dentist, optician
Qualified staff: Meets standard

Home details
Location: Village location, 5.5 miles from Yeovil
Communal areas: 2 lounges, 2 dining rooms, garden
Accessibility: *Floors:* 2 • *Access:* Stair lift
  Wheelchair access: Limited
Smoking: In designated area
Pets: At manager's discretion
Routines: Flexible

Room details
Single: 19
Shared: 1
En suite: 13
Facilities: TV point, telephone point

Door lock: ✓
Lockable place: ✓

Services provided
Beauty services: Hairdressing
Mobile library: ✓
Religious services: Monthly Anglican Communion service
Transport: Car
Activities: *Coordinator.* ✓ • *Examples:* Arts and crafts, bingo, gentle exercise • *Outings:* ✗
Meetings: ✗

Registered places: 28
Guide weekly rate: £560
Specialist care: Nursing
Medical services: Podiatry, dentist, optician, physiotherapy
Qualified staff: Exceeds standard: 99% at NVQ level 2

Home details

Location: Residential area, 1.5 miles from Taunton
Communal areas: 2 lounges, dining room, conservatory,
 patio and garden
Accessibility: *Floors:* 2 • *Access:* Lift • *Wheelchair access:* Good
Smoking: ✗
Pets: ✗
Routines: Structured

Room details

Single: 28
Shared: 0
En suite: 28
Facilities: TV point

Door lock: ✓
Lockable place: ✗

Services provided

Beauty services: Hairdressing, aromatherapy, manicures
Mobile library: ✓
Religious services: Visits from clergy
Transport: ✗
Activities: *Coordinator.* ✓ • *Examples*: Exercises, games
 Outings: ✓
Meetings: ✓

The First Nursing Home

Manager: Kathleen Vound
Owner: Care West Country Ltd
Contact: 251 Staplegrove Road, Taunton, Somerset TA2 6AQ
☎ 01823 275927
@ nursingho@aol.com

The Firs is located on the busy Staplegrove Road, one and a half miles from Taunton. It is in a residential area with access to shops via a bus. The home has indoor activities for the residents and also has visits from the local donkey sanctuary. Though pets are not allowed to stay, they are welcome to visit. The home is undergoing a refurbishment that will provide 10 additional bedrooms looking over the garden. A registered nurse is on duty 24 hours a day.

Registered places: 58
Guide weekly rate: £420–£515
Specialist care: Day care, respite
Medical services: Podiatry, dentist, optician
Qualified staff: Exceeds standard: 60% at NVQ level 2

Home details

Location: Rural area, 0.7 miles from Wells
Communal areas: 4 lounges, 2 dining rooms, bar, hairdressing salon,
 conservatory, garden
Accessibility: *Floors:* 2 • *Access:* Lift • *Wheelchair access:* Good
Smoking: ✗
Pets: At manager's discretion
Routines: Flexible

Room details

Single: 58
Shared: 0
En suite: 35
Facilities: TV point, telephone point

Door lock: ✓
Lockable place: ✓

Services provided

Beauty services: Hairdressing
Mobile library: ✓
Religious services: Weekly Anglican service,
 monthly Communion service
Transport: ✗
Activities: *Coordinator.* ✓ • *Examples*: Bingo, singalongs, talks
 Outings: ✓
Meetings: ✗

Fletcher House

Manager: Mrs Mohide
Owner: Somerset Care Ltd
Contact: Glastonbury Road, Wells, Somerset BA5 1TN
☎ 01749 678068
@ enquiries@somersetcare.co.uk
🖥 www.somersetcare.co.uk

Located on the main Glastonbury road, Fletcher House is situated in a rural area, almost one mile from Wells town centre. The home's gardens include a summerhouse. Inside the home there is a hairdressing salon in addition to four lounges and two dining rooms. The home arranges an Anglican service once a week and a Communion service takes place on a monthly basis. There is an activities coordinator at the home who arranges a variety of activities as well as outings for the residents.

Frethey House Nursing Home

Manager: Susan Hull
Owner: Affirmative Care Ltd
Contact: Frethey Lane, Bishops Hull, Taunton, Somerset TA4 1AB

) 01823 253071
@ info@affirmativecare.co.uk

Situated in the outskirts of the village of Bishops Hull a few miles from Taunton town centre, Frethey House offers a quiet country setting close to a variety of local amenities. Although the country lane leading to the home is not ideal for wheelchairs, there is generally good access inside the home and a bus stop 400 yards away. Pets are welcome to visit and the Donkey sanctuary pays a visit two or three times a year. A regular monthly newsletter is provided for all residents and relatives.

Registered places: 41
Guide weekly rate: £485–£775
Specialist care: Nursing, emergency admissions, respite
Medical services: Podiatry, dentist, physiotherapy
Qualified staff: Exceeds standard: 80% at NVQ level 2

Home details
Location: Village location, 3 miles from Taunton
Communal areas: Lounge, dining room, courtyard, garden
Accessibility: *Floors:* 2 • *Access:* 2 lifts • *Wheelchair access:* Limited
Smoking: x
Pets: x
Routines: Flexible

Room details
Single: 41
Shared: 0
En suite: 41
Facilities: TV point, telephone point

Door lock: ✓
Lockable place: ✓

Services provided
Beauty services: Hairdressing, aromatherapy
Mobile library: Library facilities
Religious services: Monthly Communion service, Anglican service every 6 weeks
Transport: x
Activities: *Coordinator:* ✓ • *Examples:* Arts and crafts, gardening club, musical events • *Outings:* ✓
Meetings: ✓

Friarn House Residential Care Home

Manager: Alan Farkas
Owner: Westcare Ltd
Contact: 35 Friarn Street, Bridgwater, Somerset, TA6 3LJ

) 01278 445115
@ admin@friarsgatecarehome. freeserve.co.uk

A terraced house situated in Bridgwater a few minutes' walk from to local amenities, Friarn House has enclosed gardens which residents can enjoy in the summer months. The home shares its minibus with its sister home Beech Tree House and often takes the residents on outings in the local area. The home employs an activities coordinator who arranges board games and performances by visiting entertainers as part of the activities programme.

Registered places: 16
Guide weekly rate: £380–£500
Specialist care: Day care, dementia, respite
Medical services: Podiatry, dentist, optician
Qualified staff: Meets standard

Home details
Location: Residential area, 0.2 miles from Bridgwater
Communal areas: Lounge, dining room, conservatory, garden
Accessibility: *Floors:* 2 • *Access:* Stair lift *Wheelchair access:* Limited
Smoking: In designated area
Pets: At manager's discretion
Routines: Flexible

Room details
Single: 14
Shared: 1
En suite: 11
Facilities: TV point

Door lock: ✓
Lockable place: x

Services provided
Beauty services: Hairdressing
Mobile library: x
Religious services: x
Transport: Minibus
Activities: *Coordinator:* ✓ • *Examples:* Board games, visiting entertainers • *Outings:* ✓
Meetings: ✓

Registered places: 11
Guide weekly rate: £360–£400
Specialist care: Day care, respite
Medical services: Podiatry, dentist, occupational therapy, optician, physiotherapy
Qualified staff: Exceeds standard: 76% at NVQ level 2

Home details
Location: Residential area, 0.4 miles from Minehead
Communal areas: Lounge, dining room, garden
Accessibility: *Floors:* 3 • *Access:* Lift • *Wheelchair access:* Good
Smoking: x
Pets: In designated area
Routines: Flexible

Room details
Single: 11
Shared: 0
En suite: 11
Facilities: TV point, telephone point

Door lock: ✓
Lockable place: ✓

Services provided
Beauty services: Hairdressing, aromatherapy
Mobile library: x
Religious services: Monthly Communion service
Transport: Car
Activities: *Coordinator.* x • *Examples:* Arts and crafts, baking, films
Outings: ✓
Meetings: ✓

Glen Lyn Residential Care Home For The Elderly

Manager: Melanie Reaney
Owner: Mr and Mrs Reaney
Contact: 2 Tregonwell Road, Minehead, Somerset, TA24 5DT
) 01643 702415
@ reaney.glenlyn@virgin.net

Set back from the road in a quiet residential area in the heart of Minehead, this attractive semi-detached property is situated a few minutes' walk from local amenities such as shops and a post office. The seafront is also a short walk away. Although the garden is small, it is level and mainly paved with flowers, shrubs and a pond. There is a varied activities programme in place at the home which includes gardening, gentle exercise and reminiscence sessions.

Registered places: 58
Guide weekly rate: Undisclosed
Specialist care: Nursing, respite
Medical services: Podiatry, physiotherapy
Qualified staff: Undisclosed

Home details
Location: Rural location, 4 miles from Shepton Mallet
Communal areas: 4 lounges, 3 dining rooms, hairdressing salon, patio and garden
Accessibility: *Floors:* 3 • *Access:* Lift • *Wheelchair access:* Good
Smoking: x
Pets: ✓
Routines: Flexible

Room details
Single: 45
Shared: 6
En suite: 47
Facilities: TV point, telephone point

Door lock: ✓
Lockable place: x

Services provided
Beauty services: Hairdressing
Mobile library: ✓
Religious services: Monthly Communion service
Transport: ✓
Activities: *Coordinator.* ✓ • Exercise: Art, visiting entertainers, yoga
Outings: ✓
Meetings: ✓

The Glen Nursing and Residential Home

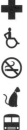

Manager: Gale Smith
Owner: BUPA Care Homes Ltd
Contact: Shapway Lane, Evercreech, Shepton Mallet, Somerset, BA4 6JS
) 01749 830369
@ TheGlenALL@BUPA.com
⌂ www.bupacarehomes.co.uk

Originally a large private house, The Glen is situated in countryside, yet with shops and amenities within walking distance and Shepton Mallet only four miles away. There is a choice of three lounges, landscaped grounds and a patio in which to meet and chat or entertain guests. Daily activities offered include art, yoga and flexercise classes and trips to local places of interest. For those who enjoy gardening, the home's greenhouse is available. The Glen also offers care to younger people with physical disabilities and to those requiring palliative or terminal care.

Glenavon Nursing Home

Manager: Susan McCallum
Owner: David and Lesley Sutcliffe
Contact: The Old Vicarage, Hambridge, Langport, Somerset, TA10 0BG
☎ 01460 281670

Glenavon is a care home providing nursing care for up to 23 residents. The home is a three-storey domestic-style building in the rural village of Hampbridge, three miles from Langport town centre. It is quite an isolated location with no public transport through the village and no village shop. The home has a bungalow in its grounds in which self-caring residents can live. The home employs an activities coordinator who puts together a programme for the residents which includes quizzes and exercise sessions.

Registered places: 23
Guide weekly rate: £487–£608
Specialist care: Nursing
Medical services: Podiatry, dentist, optician
Qualified staff: Exceeds standard: 63% at NVQ level 2

Home details
Location: Village location, 3 miles from Langport
Communal areas: 2 lounges, conservatory
Accessibility: *Floors:* 3 • *Access:* Lift • *Wheelchair access:* Good
Smoking: ✗
Pets: ✓
Routines: Flexible

Room details
Single: 23
Shared: 0
En suite: 23
Facilities: TV

Door lock: ✓
Lockable place: ✓

Services provided
Beauty services: Hairdressing
Mobile library: ✗
Religious services: ✗
Transport: ✗
Activities: *Coordinator.* ✓ • *Examples:* Exercises, quizzes, skittles
   Outings: ✗
Meetings: ✗

Gotton Manor and The Coach House Care Home

Manager: Sue Stephens
Owner: Four Seasons Healthcare Ltd
Contact: West Monkton, Taunton, Somerset, TA2 8LL
☎ 01823 413118
@ gotton.manor@fshc.co.uk
🖰 www.fshc.co.uk

A country house set in manicured lawns close to the centre of West Monkton, Gotton Manor and The Coach House is one care home that is split into two adjoining sites, allowing those individuals who require nursing care to be treated separately. Many of the bedrooms have balconies and permit lovely views of the surrounding countryside. There are quiet lounges alongside those communal areas with a TV for residents wishing to pass the time peacefully. Gotton Manor also has a mobile shop.

Registered places: 60
Guide weekly rate: Undisclosed
Specialist care: Nursing, day care, emergency admissions, respite
Medical services: Podiatry, dentist, optician
Qualified staff: Undisclosed

Home details
Location: Rural area, 4 miles from Taunton
Communal areas: 3 lounges, 2 dining rooms, conservatory, garden
Accessibility: *Floors:* 2 • *Access:* Lift • *Wheelchair access:* Good
Smoking: ✗
Pets: At manager's discretion
Routines: Flexible

Room details
Single: 60
Shared: 0
En suite: 52
Facilities: TV point

Door lock: ✓
Lockable place: ✓

Services provided
Beauty services: Hairdressing
Mobile library: Library facilities
Religious services: Monthly Anglican Communion service
Transport: ✗
Activities: *Coordinator.* ✗ • *Examples:* Exercise, films, gardening club
   Outings: ✓
Meetings: ✓

Registered places: 25
Guide weekly rate: From £450
Specialist care: Day care, respite
Medical services: Podiatry, dentist, occupational therapy, optician, physiotherapy
Qualified staff: Undisclosed

Home details

Location: Residential area, 1.5 miles from Frome
Communal areas: 2 lounges, dining room, patio and garden
Accessibility: *Floors:* 1 • *Wheelchair access:* Good
Smoking: ✗
Pets: ✗
Routines: Flexible

Room details

Single: 23
Shared: 1
En suite: 21
Facilities: TV point, telephone point

Door lock: ✓
Lockable place: ✓

Services provided

Beauty services: Hairdressing
Mobile library: Library facilities
Religious services: Weekly Communion service
Transport: ✗
Activities: *Coordinator.* ✓ • *Examples*: Arts and crafts, exercise, gardening • *Outings:* ✗
Meetings: ✓

Greenhill Grange Residential Home

Manager: Gillian Twohig
Owner: Greenhill Grange Residential Home Ltd
Contact: Catherston Close, Frome, Somerset, BA11 4HR
☎ 01373 471688

Situated in its own grounds and overlooking some beautiful countryside, Greenhill Grange is a single storey building that is only a bus ride away from Frome town centre and close to a nearby corner shop. A family-run business, Mr Twohig and his son assist with gardening and driving while Mrs Twohig is responsible for the day-to-day management. Residents with an interest in gardening may enjoy the many potted displays and greenhouse while the home allows resident's pets to visit. With a lounge dedicated to quiet, the gardens with enclosed patio area also provide a peaceful place for residents to sit.

Registered places: 26
Guide weekly rate: £373–£420
Specialist care: Respite
Medical services: Podiatry, dentist, optician
Qualified staff: Exceeds standard: 70% at NVQ level 2

Home details

Location: Residential area, 0.5 miles from Cheddar
Communal areas: 2 lounges, dining room, conservatory, patio and garden
Accessibility: *Floors:* 1 • *Wheelchair access:* Good
Smoking: ✗
Pets: ✗
Routines: Flexible

Room details

Single: 22
Shared: 2
En suite: Undisclosed
Facilities: None

Door lock: ✓
Lockable place: ✓

Services provided

Beauty services: Hairdressing
Mobile library: ✗
Religious services: ✗
Transport: ✗
Activities: *Coordinator.* ✓ • *Examples*: Games, gentle exercise
Outings: ✗
Meetings: ✗.

Greenhill House

Manager: Alison Difford
Owner: Somerset Care Ltd
Contact: Tweentown, Cheddar, Somerset, BS27 3HY
☎ 01934 742280

A purpose-built home located on the outskirts of Cheddar, Greenhill House is approximately half a mile from the town centre. The home has a garden with a patio area and a conservatory for residents to enjoy in the summer months. The home also has two lounges for residents to relax in. The activities coordinator puts together a varied programme of activities for the residents, which includes games and gentle exercises. The home is laid out across one level, providing excellent access for the residents.

Highfield House Residential Care Home

Manager: Mr Biddlecombe
Owner: Mr and Mrs Biddlecombe
Contact: High Street, Castle Cary, Somerset, BA7 7AN

) 01963 350697
@ highfieldhouse@yahoo.co.uk
⌐ www.high-field.co.uk

Highfield House is an attractive country town house set in the centre of Castle Cary and two minutes' walk from a variety of local amenities that include shops and a post office. Run by Mr and Mrs Biddlecombe since 1988, the owners now reside in the house next door to the property. With a bright and sunny interior and sprawling lawns, Highfield House provides an attractive prospect.

Registered places: 22
Guide weekly rate: £380–£450
Specialist care: Day care, respite
Medical services: Podiatry, dentist, optician
Qualified staff: Exceeds standard: 75% at NVQ level 2

Home details
Location: Village location, in Castle Carey
Communal areas: Lounge, dining room, conservatory, patio and garden
Accessibility: *Floors:* 2 • *Access:* Lift • *Wheelchair access:* Limited
Smoking: ✗
Pets: ✓
Routines: Flexible

Room details
Single: 22
Shared: 0
En suite: 15
Facilities: TV point

Door lock: ✓
Lockable place: ✓

Services provided
Beauty services: Hairdressing
Mobile library: ✗
Religious services: Monthly Anglican Communion service
Transport: 7-seater vehicle
Activities: *Coordinator.* ✗ • *Examples*: Bingo, musical mornings, yoga *Outings:* ✓
Meetings: ✓

The Hollies

Manager: Judith Adams
Owner: M & J Care Homes Ltd
Contact: Florida Street, Castle Cary, Somerset, BA7 7AE

) 01963 350709

Situated in a quiet residential area, The Hollies is around 250 metres from the town centre and lies 13 miles from Yeovil. The home has a conservatory and a garden for residents to enjoy as well as two lounges. There is an Anglican Communion service held at the home every month for residents to attend if they wish. The home arranges a variety of activities for the residents including chair exercises and singalongs.

Registered places: 13
Guide weekly rate: £365–£430
Specialist care: Day care, respite
Medical services: Podiatry, dentist, optician
Qualified staff: Meets standard

Home details
Location: Residential area, 0.2 miles from Castle Cary
Communal areas: 2 lounges, dining room, conservatory, garden
Accessibility: *Floors:* 2 • *Access:* Stair lift *Wheelchair access:* Limited
Smoking: ✗
Pets: At manager's discretion
Routines: Flexible

Room details
Single: 16
Shared: 1
En suite: 6
Facilities: TV point, telephone point

Door lock: ✓
Lockable place: ✓

Services provided
Beauty services: Hairdressing
Mobile library: ✗
Religious services: Monthly Anglican Communion service
Transport: ✗
Activities: *Coordinator.* ✗ • *Examples*: Chair exercises, games, singalongs • *Outings:* ✗
Meetings: ✗

Registered places: 7
Guide weekly rate: Undisclosed
Specialist care: Respite
Medical services: Podiatry, dentist, optician
Qualified staff: Fails standard

Home details

Location: Residential area, 0.7 miles from Ilminster
Communal areas: Lounge, dining room
Accessibility: *Floors:* 2 • *Access:* Lift • *Wheelchair access:* Good
Smoking: ×
Pets: ✓
Routines: Flexible

Room details

Single: 6
Shared: 1
En suite: 2
Facilities: None

Door lock: ✓
Lockable place: ✓

Services provided

Beauty services: Hairdressing
Mobile library: ×
Religious services: ×
Transport: ×
Activities: *Coordinator.* ✓ • *Examples:* Exercises, games • *Outings:* ×
Meetings: ×

Holway House

Manager: Jane Noina
Owner: Jane Noina
Contact: 130 Station Road, Ilminster, Somerset, TA19 9PW
☎ 01460 53781

Situated close to local amenities, Holway House is situated in a residential area, under a mile from Ilminster. The house has been registered as a care home since 1990. Having recently come under new management, several changes are anticipated, which includes a refurbishment of the home. The home employs an activities coordinator who arranges a variety of activities for the residents.

Registered places: 25
Guide weekly rate: £525–£550
Specialist care: Nursing
Medical services: Podiatry, optician
Qualified staff: Meets standard

Home details

Location: Village location, 3 miles from Highbridge
Communal areas: 2 lounges, dining room, garden
Accessibility: *Floors:* 2 • *Access:* Lift • *Wheelchair access:* Good
Smoking: ×
Pets: ✓
Routines: Flexible

Room details

Single: 17
Shared: 4
En suite: 11
Facilities: None

Door lock: ✓
Lockable place: ✓

Services provided

Beauty services: Hairdressing
Mobile library: ×
Religious services: ×
Transport: ×
Activities: *Coordinator.* ✓ • *Examples:* Cards • *Outings:* ✓
Meetings: ✓

Holywell Nursing Home

Manager: Sarah Joyce
Owner: Sarah Joyce
Contact: Brent Street, Brent Knoll, Somerset, TA9 4BB
☎ 01278 760601

With ample parking and pleasant gardens, Holywell Nursing Home is a large property situated in the village of Brent Knoll. It has views of the surrounding countryside and lies three miles from Highbridge. Monthly meetings take place for family and friends. The home is well used by the local community and has good community links. The home employs an activities coordinator who arranges a programme for the residents which includes cards and outings in the local area.

Hurds Hill Residential Home Ltd

Manager: Diana Pride
Owner: Diana Pride
Contact: Westover, Langport, Somerset, TA10 0ND

) 01458 252 609
@ www.hurdshill.co.uk

Set within its own landscaped gardens, Hurd's Hill Residential Home is a large Regency period house with places for 31 residents. Some of the staff have been at the home for over 10 years. The home is situated on the outskirts of Langport, one mile from the town centre. The home has a mobile library which visits and has its own transport. There are also religious services available. External activities coordinators come to the home to arrange reminiscence sessions and singalongs for the residents.

Registered places: 31
Guide weekly rate: From £350
Specialist care: Respite
Medical services: Podiatry, dentist, optician
Qualified staff: Meets standard

Home details
Location: Residential area, 1 mile from Langport
Communal areas: Lounge, dining room, conservatory, garden
Accessibility: *Floors:* 2 • *Access:* Stair lift • *Wheelchair access:* Good
Smoking: ×
Pets: At manager's discretion
Routines: Flexible

Room details
Single: 31
Shared: 0
En suite: 31
Facilities: TV, telephone

Door lock: ✓
Lockable place: ✓

Services provided
Beauty services: Hairdressing, manicures
Mobile library: ✓
Religious services: ✓
Transport: ✓
Activities: *Coordinator.* ✓ • *Examples:* Arts and crafts, reminiscence, singalongs • *Outings:* ✓
Meetings: ✓

Hurst Manor

Manager: Ada Aldworth
Owner: Hurst Manor Ltd
Contact: Hurst, Martock, Somerset, TA12 6JU

) 01935 823467
@ info@hurstmanor.co.uk
⌂ www.hurstmanor.co.uk

A Grade III listed Georgian house, Hurst Manor is situated in the centre of Hurst village in landscaped grounds. Positioned a five-minute walk away from the local pub and 10 minutes from shops, the home is also serviced by regular buses. On 13 September 2006, the home received a visit from The Princess Royal commemorating the opening of the new Garden Wing – an area providing extra bedrooms with patio doors leading to the gardens. As well as a comprehensive activities programme and monthly outings, the home also receives visits from Pets As Therapy.

Registered places: 36
Guide weekly rate: From £600
Specialist care: Nursing, day care, respite
Medical services: Podiatry, dentist, optician
Qualified staff: Undisclosed

Home details
Location: Village location, 0.5 miles from Martock
Communal areas: 2 lounges, dining room, garden
Accessibility: Floors 3 • *Access:* Lift • *Wheelchair access:* Good
Smoking: In designated area
Pets: At manager's discretion
Routines: Flexible

Room details
Single: 30
Shared: 3
En suite: 20
Facilities: TV point, telephone point

Door lock: ✓
Lockable place: ✓

Services provided
Beauty services: Hairdressing, aromatherapy
Mobile library: ✓
Religious services: Fortnightly Anglican Communion service
Transport: ×
Activities: *Coordinator.* ✓ • *Examples:* Armchair exercises, bingo *Outings:* ✓
Meetings: ×

Registered places: 23
Guide weekly rate: £375–£440
Specialist care: Day care
Medical services: Podiatry, dentist, optician
Qualified staff: Fails standard: 40% at NVQ level 2

Home details

Location: Residential area, 0.7 miles from Burnham-on-Sea
Communal areas: 2 lounges, dining room, garden
Accessibility: *Floors:* 2 • *Access:* Stair lift • *Wheelchair access:* Good
Smoking: ✗
Pets: ✓
Routines: Flexible

Room details

Single: 23
Shared: 0
En suite: 7
Facilities: None

Door lock: ✓
Lockable place: ✓

Services provided

Beauty services: Hairdressing, reflexology
Mobile library: ✗
Religious services: ✗
Transport: ✗
Activities: *Coordinator:* ✗ • *Examples:* Exercise sessions • *Outings:* ✗
Meetings: ✗

Kingsleigh

Manager: Marissa Spearing
Owner: EZ4 Life Ltd
Contact: 78 Berrow Road,
Burnham-on-Sea, Somerset, TA8 2HJ
) 01278 792768
@ Kingsleigh78@btinternet.com

Kingsleigh is a large detached house in Burnham-on-Sea, under a mile from the town centre. The building is traditional in style, with some modern extensions. The home has pleasant gardens situated to the front of the property. It is close to local amenities and the seafront. There is no activities coordinator in the home, but a dedicated member of staff organises various activities, including reflexology and keep fit sessions. There are two lounges which can be joined into one lounge. One of the lounges has access onto the garden.

Registered places: 20
Guide weekly rate: £393–£450
Specialist care: Respite
Medical services: Podiatry, dentist, optician
Qualified staff: Meets standard

Home details

Location: Village location, 6 miles from Wincanton
Communal areas: Lounge, hairdressing salon, garden
Accessibility: *Floors:* 2 • *Access:* Stair lift
    Wheelchair access: Good
Smoking: ✗
Pets: At manager's discretion
Routines: Flexible

Room details

Single: 20
Shared: 0
En suite: 16
Facilities: TV, telephone point

Door lock: ✓
Lockable place: ✓

Services provided

Beauty services: Hairdressing
Mobile library: Library facilities
Religious services: ✓
Transport: ✗
Activities: *Coordinator:* ✓ • *Examples:* Seasonal events, visiting
    entertainers • *Outings:* No
Meetings: ✓

Knights Templar Court

Manager: Lorraine Hill
Owner: Greenview Care Ltd
Contact: Throop Road, Templecombe,
Somerset, BA8 0HR
) 01963 370317

The Knights Templar Court is situated in the village of Templecombe, approximately six miles from Wincanton. The home has large gardens for residents to relax in, in addition to a lounge. There is one room in the home that can be used at double capacity for a married couple. The home has its own hairdressing room and there are religious visits from local clergy. There is a varied activities programme on offer including performances by visiting entertainers and seasonal events such as a Halloween party.

Linden House Nursing Home

Manager: Linda Bennett
Owner: S Joyce
Contact: Lower Westford, Wellington, Somerset, TA21 0DW
☎ 01823 667711
@ enquiries@linden-house.net
🖰 www.linden-house.net

Residing in landscaped grounds and accessed by way of two private roads, Linden House is a converted property with a newly built nursing wing. The home is set seven acres of ground, from which you are able to see the Wellington Monument. There is also a conservatory so the garden and views can be appreciated all year round. Outdoor facilities include a sensory garden and an area where the home grows its own vegetables. The home's kitchen has been awarded a five-star rating. The home produces a newsletter called 'Linden Latest'.

Registered places: 34
Guide weekly rate: £700
Specialist care: Nursing, respite
Medical services: Podiatry, dentist, optician, physiotherapy
Qualified staff: Exceeds standard: 65% at NVQ level 2

Home details

Location: Residential area, 8 miles from Taunton
Communal areas: 2 lounges, dining room, conservatory, patio and garden
Accessibility: *Floors:* 2 • *Access:* Lift • *Wheelchair access:* Good
Smoking: ✗
Pets: At manager's discretion
Routines: Flexible

Room details

Single: 30
Shared: 2
En suite: 22
Facilities: TV point, telephone point

Door lock: ✓
Lockable place: ✓

Services provided

Beauty services: Hairdressing, aromatherapy
Mobile library: ✗
Religious services: Monthly Communion service
Transport: ✗
Activities: *Coordinator:* ✗ • *Examples:* Exercise, singalongs, visiting entertainers • *Outings:* ✓
Meetings: ✓

Mamsey House Nursing Home

Manager: Barbara Kinzett
Owner: Clinida Care Ltd
Contact: Priest Street, Williton, Somerset, TA4 4NJ
☎ 01984 633712
@ mamseyhouse@hotmail.com

A converted vicarage with extension, Mamsey House is situated a few hundred yards from local facilities including a post office, bank, pub and supermarket. The home is located in a village, 15 and a half miles from Taunton town centre. The home boasts a raised garden, a gazebo, pergola and a small fishpond. The home also has its own library facilities and organises an Anglican service every two weeks. The home has its own minibus and often takes the residents on outings in the local area. The activities coordinator puts together a varied programme for the residents, which includes exercise and reminiscence sessions.

Registered places: 33
Guide weekly rate: Undisclosed
Specialist care: Nursing, physical disability
Medical services: Podiatry, dentist
Qualified staff: Meets standard

Home details

Location: Village location, 15.5 miles from Taunton
Communal areas: 2 lounges, 2 dining rooms, library, patio and garden
Accessibility: *Floors:* 2 • *Access:* Lift • *Wheelchair access:* Good
Smoking: ✗
Pets: ✓
Routines: Flexible

Room details

Single: 33
Shared: 0
En suite: 32
Facilities: TV point, telephone point

Door lock: ✗
Lockable place: ✗

Services provided

Beauty services: Hairdressing
Mobile library: Library facilities
Religious services: Fortnightly Anglican service
Transport: Minibus
Activities: *Coordinator:* ✓ • *Examples:* Arts and crafts, quizzes, music *Outings:* ✓
Meetings: ✗

Registered places: 54
Guide weekly rate: £373
Specialist care: Day care, respite
Medical services: Dentist, optician
Qualified staff: Exceeds standard: 66% at NVQ level 2

Home details

Location: Residential area, 2 miles from Taunton
Communal areas: 2 lounges
Accessibility: *Floors:* 2 • *Access:* Lift • *Wheelchair access:* Good
Smoking: ✗
Pets: ✓
Routines: Flexible

Room details

Single: 54
Shared: 0
En suite: 23
Facilities: None

Door lock: ✓
Lockable place: ✗

Services provided

Beauty services: Hairdressing
Mobile library: ✗
Religious services: ✗
Transport: Minibus
Activities: *Coordinator:* ✗ • *Examples:* Bingo, gardening club
　　Outings: ✓
Meetings: ✓

Moorhaven

Manager: Jo Fenn
Owner: Somerset Care Ltd
Contact: Normandy Drive, Taunton, Somerset, TA1 2JT
☎ 01823 331524
@ diane.allen@somersetcare.co.uk

Situated in a residential area two miles from Taunton, Moorhaven provides care for 54 residents. Moorhaven has a special treatment room, where residents are able to privately meet healthcare professionals outside of their bedrooms. Moorhaven is adapted for its purpose, allowing easy access to all areas for wheelchair users. There is also a good range of activities and social events. These include bingo, a gardening club and quizzes. There are also outings on offer to the residents.

Registered places: 11
Guide weekly rate: From £360
Specialist care: None
Medical services: Podiatry, dentist, optician, physiotherapy
Qualified staff: Fails standard

Home details

Location: Residential area, 1 mile from Burnham-on-Sea
Communal areas: Lounge, dining room, conservatory, garden
Accessibility: *Floors:* 2 • *Access:* Stair lift
　　Wheelchair access: Good
Smoking: ✗
Pets: At manager's discretion
Routines: Flexible

Room details

Single: 12
Shared: 0
En suite: 2
Facilities: TV point, telephone point

Door lock: ✓
Lockable place: ✓

Services provided

Beauty services: Hairdressing
Mobile library: ✗
Religious services: ✗
Transport: ✗
Activities: *Coordinator:* ✗ • *Examples:* Puzzles, visiting entertainers
　　Outings: ✓
Meetings: ✓

Newton Lodge

Manager: Mrs Taylor House
Owner: C&K Homes Ltd
Contact: 139 Berrow Road, Burnham-on-Sea, Somerset, TA8 2PN
☎ 01278 787321
@ newtonlodge@btconnect.com

Newton Lodge is located one mile from Burnham-on-Sea in a residential area. The home has a lounge with a dining area and there is a conservatory and a garden for residents to enjoy in the warmer weather. The home arranges outings for the residents, for example to local garden centres and pubs. There are also internal activities such as puzzles. There are regular residents meetings to discuss any issues the residents may have.

Nynehead Court

Manager: Diana Hathaway
Owner: Nynehead Care Ltd
Contact: Nynehead, Wellington, Somerset, TA21 0BW

) 01823 662481
@ nyneheadcare@aol.com
⌂ www.tssg.co.uk

A Grade II listed manor house from the 17th century, Nynehead Court is situated in the heart of the village of Nynehead, seven miles from Taunton. Residents are granted exceptional views as the home lies in 13 acres of parkland and the formal gardens feature such magnificent sites as a walled arboretum, ice house and croquet lawn. Open to the public, these gardens are maintained by three full-time gardeners. Nynehead Court prides itself on offering a hotel style of living, sourcing fresh produce including fish from local suppliers.

Registered places: 35
Guide weekly rate: £555–£1,000
Specialist care: None
Medical services: Podiatry, optician
Qualified staff: Fails standard

Home details
Location: Rural area, 7 miles from Taunton
Communal areas: Lounge, dining room, sitting room, library, garden
Accessibility: *Floors:* 3 • *Access:* Lift • *Wheelchair access:* Good
Smoking: In designated area
Pets: ×
Routines: Flexible

Room details
Single: 27
Shared: 4
En suite: 31
Facilities: TV point, telephone point

Door lock: ✓
Lockable place: ✓

Services provided
Beauty services: Hairdressing, reflexology
Mobile library: ✓
Religious services: Monthly Anglican Communion service
Transport: Minibus and car
Activities: *Coordinator.* ✓ • *Examples:* Arts and crafts, bridge, gentle exercise • *Outings:* ✓
Meetings: ×

The Old Vicarage

Manager: Susan Thomas
Owner: Sean and Samantha O'Brien
Contact: Stockland, Bridgwater, Somerset, TA5 2PZ

) 01278 652352
@ enquiries@restcare.co.uk

A large property set in extensive grounds, The Old Vicarage is located on high ground and is near the sea. Residents can plant flowers in the garden and local school children regularly visit the home. The Old Vicarage has a good reputation in the community, with the local doctors and nurses. The home employs an activities coordinator who provides residents with a varied programme including bingo and gardening. There are also outings on offer and the home has its own minibus. A mobile library comes to the home and there are also visits from Anglican ministers.

Registered places: 26
Guide weekly rate: £420–£498
Specialist care: Day care, respite
Medical services: Podiatry, hygienist, optician, physiotherapy
Qualified staff: Exceeds standard: 80% at NVQ level 2

Home details
Location: Rural area, 7.5 miles from Bridgwater
Communal areas: Lounge, dining room, conservatory, garden
Accessibility: *Floors:* 2 • *Access:* Stair lift *Wheelchair access:* Good
Smoking: ×
Pets: ✓
Routines: Flexible

Room details
Single: 26
Shared: 0
En suite: 10
Facilities: TV, telephone

Door lock: ✓
Lockable place: ✓

Services provided
Beauty services: Hairdressing, aromatherapy, manicures
Mobile Library: ✓
Religious services: Anglican visits, Communion service
Transport: Minibus
Activities: *Coordinator.* ✓ • *Examples:* Bingo, gardening, poetry *Outings:* ✓
Meetings: ✓

Registered places: 21
Guide weekly rate: £365–£450
Specialist care: Day care, respite
Medical services: Podiatry, dentist, optician
Qualified staff: Fails standard

Home details

Location: Residential area, 1.5 miles from Weston-super-Mare
Communal areas: 2 lounges, dining room, garden
Accessibility: *Floors:* 2 • *Access:* Stair lift • *Wheelchair access:* Good
Smoking: x
Pets: At manager's discretion
Routines: Flexible

Room details

Single: 20
Shared: 0
En suite: 11
Facilities: TV, telephone

Door lock: ✓
Lockable place: ✓

Services provided

Beauty services: Hairdressing
Mobile library: ✓
Religious services: x
Transport: ✓
Activities: *Coordinator:* ✓ • *Examples:* Jigsaws, visiting entertainers
   Outings: ✓
Meetings: ✓

Pine Lodge

Manager: Rebecca Kingston
Owner: Orchard Care Ltd
Contact: 13 Hazeldene Road, Weston-super-Mare, North Somerset, BS23 2XL
) 01934 622539
@ pinelodge@orchardcare.co.uk
🖱 www.orchardcare.co.uk

Pine Lodge is located in a residential area, one and a half miles from Weston-super-Mare. All of the rooms in the home are used for single occupancy but shared rooms are available on request. There is also a lounge and a quiet lounge for residents to relax in. The home arranges daily activities for the residents including jigsaws and performances by visiting entertainers.

Registered places: 74
Guide weekly rate: Undisclosed
Specialist care: None
Medical services: Podiatry, dentist, optician, physiotherapy
Qualified staff: Meets standard

Home details

Location: Residential area, 7 miles from Taunton
Communal areas: Lounge, dining room, large garden
Accessibility: *Floors:* 2 • *Access:* Lift • *Wheelchair access:* Good
Smoking: x
Pets: x
Routines: Flexible

Room details

Single: 74
Shared: 0
En suite: 7
Facilities: TV point

Door lock: ✓
Lockable place: ✓

Services provided

Beauty services: Hairdressing
Mobile library: x
Religious services: ✓
Transport: Minibus
Activities: *Coordinator:* ✓ • *Examples:* Arts and crafts, bingo
   Outings: ✓
Meetings: x

Popham House

Manager: Hazel Jones
Owner: Somerset Care Ltd
Contact: Courtland Road, Wellington, Somerset, TA21 8NF
) 01823 662513
@ hazel.jones@somersetcare.co.uk
🖱 www.somersetcare.co.uk

Situated opposite a community park, Popham Home is a listed building which was formerly a purpose-built home for the blind. The home has large gardens and is located near to the town centre. A TV point can be arranged for the residents and there is a public telephone. The home has an activities coordinator who arranges activities such as bingo and arts and crafts. There are also outings arranged to the local garden centre. The home has its own cat but pets are generally not allowed.

Pulsford Lodge

Manager: Sonya Matthias
Owner: Somerset Care Ltd
Contact: North Street, Wiveliscombe, Somerset, TA4 2LA
☎ 01984 623569
@ sonya.matthias@somersetcare.co.uk
🖱 www.somersetcare.co.uk

A modern, purpose-built home situated in the market town of Wiveliscombe, Pulsford Lodge is approximately 150 yards from all the modern amenities that the town has to offer. Residents benefit from the views the home offers of the surrounding countryside. With a comprehensive activities programme that includes outings, Pulsford Lodge also has an in-house shop where residents may purchase sweets and toiletries. The home is set in landscaped grounds and residents with an interest in gardening can tend to their own patch in the grounds.

Registered places: 50
Guide weekly rate: £470–£560
Specialist care: Day care, emergency admissions, respite
Medical services: Podiatry, dentist, optician
Qualified staff: Meets standard

Home details
Location: Residential area, 0.3 miles from **Wiveliscombe**
Communal areas: 7 lounges, 2 dining rooms, hairdressing salon, library, patio and garden
Accessibility: *Floors:* 2 • *Access:* Lift • *Wheelchair access:* Good
Smoking: In designated area
Pets: At manager's discretion
Routines: Flexible

Room details
Single: 50
Shared: 0
En suite: 42
Facilities: TV point, telephone point

Door lock: ✓
Lockable place: ✓

Services provided
Beauty services: Hairdressing
Mobile library: Library facilities
Religious services: Weekly Catholic visits, weekly church service
Transport: x
Activities: *Coordinator.* ✓ • *Examples:* Arts and crafts, exercise *Outings:* ✓
Meetings: ✓

Riverview General Nursing Home

Manager: Mary Burford
Owner: Riverview Care Ltd
Contact: Styles Hill, Frome, Somerset, BA11 5JR
☎ 01373 473113
@ riverviewcare@yahoo.co.uk

A purpose-built home set in a sloped wooded area, Riverview General Nursing Home is a family-owned home one and a half miles from the town of Frome. There is a bus service near the home. The home has its own activities coordinator who organises one-to-one activities for the residents. The home arranges a hairdressing and manicure service and there is an interdenominational religious service once a month.

Registered places: 24
Guide weekly rate: £500
Specialist care: Nursing, physical disability
Medical services: Podiatry, dentist, optician, physiotherapy
Qualified staff: Meets standard

Home details
Location: Residential area, 1.5 miles from Frome
Communal areas: Lounge, dining room, garden
Accessibility: *Floors:* 2 • *Access:* Lift • *Wheelchair access:* Good
Smoking: ✓
Pets: ✓
Routines: Flexible

Room details
Single: 24
Shared: 0
En suite: 24
Facilities: TV, telephone point

Door lock: ✓
Lockable place: ✓

Services provided
Beauty services: Hairdressing, manicures
Mobile library: x
Religious services: ✓
Transport: x
Activities: *Coordinator.* ✓ • *Examples:* Games, one-to-one activities *Outings:* x
Meetings: x

Registered places: 61
Guide weekly rate: Undisclosed
Specialist care: Nursing, respite
Medical services: Podiatry, dentist, optician, physiotherapy
Qualified staff: Undisclosed

Home details

Location: Rural area, 7 miles from Taunton
Communal areas: 2 lounges, 2 dining rooms, patio and garden
Accessibility: *Floors:* 3 • *Access:* Lift • *Wheelchair access:* Good
Smoking: In designated area
Pets: ✗
Routines: Flexible

Room details

Single: 61
Shared: 0
En suite: 61   Door lock: ✓
Facilities: TV, telephone   Lockable place: ✓

Services provided

Beauty services: Hairdressing, aromatherapy, manicures
Mobile library: ✓
Religious services: ✓
Transport: Minibus
Activities: *Coordinator.* ✓ • *Examples:* Bowling, reminiscence, singing • *Outings:* ✓
Meetings: ✓

Robins Close Nursing Home

Manager: Mathilda Ngomane
Owner: Majestic Number One Ltd
Contact: Middle Green Road, Wellington, Somerset, TA21 9NS
☎ 01823 662032
@ robinscare@majesticcare.co.uk

Surrounded by large gardens, which include a sensory garden, Robins Close Nursing Home is located on the outskirts of Wellington. Each resident receives a warm welcome and is given an individual care plan to suit their needs. The home has two activities coordinators who arrange a new activities programme every month including reminiscence sessions and bowling. There are also organised outings in the home's minibus. Pets are allowed to visit and smoking is permitted outside in a designated area. There are regular residents meetings and the visiting hours are flexible.

Registered places: 63
Guide weekly rate: £567–£610
Specialist care: Nursing, day care, respite
Medical services: Podiatry, hygienist, optician, physiotherapy
Qualified staff: Meets standard

Home details

Location: Residential area, 1.5 miles from Bridgwater
Communal areas: 2 lounges, 2 dining rooms, TV lounge, garden
Accessibility: *Floors:* 2 • *Access:* Lift • *Wheelchair access:* Good
Smoking: In designated area
Pets: At manager's discretion
Routines: Flexible

Room details

Single: 61
Shared: 1
En suite: 59   Door lock: ✓
Facilities: TV point, telephone point   Lockable place: ✓

Services provided

Beauty services: Hairdressing
Mobile library: ✓
Religious services: Monthly Anglican Communion service
Transport: ✗
Activities: *Coordinator.* ✓ • *Examples:* Flower arranging, reminiscence, quizzes • *Outings:* ✓
Meetings: ✓

The Rosary Nursing Home

Manager: Lyn Taylor
Owner: Sanctuary Care Ltd
Contact: Mayfield Drive, Durleigh, Bridgwater, Somerset, TA6 7JQ
☎ 01278 431164
🖱 www.sanctuary-housing.co.uk

A refurbished and extended convent, The Rosary Nursing Home boasts large gardens with a greenhouse, gazebo and raised gardens. The home publishes a newsletter, '*The Rosary Newsletter*' every month. Work has begun to extend the home further, adding another 40 beds. The home employs an activities coordinator who arranges a varied programme for the residents and there are also outings on offer. There are also regular residents meetings.

Ruishton Court Nursing & Residential Home

Manager: Carol Palmer
Owner: Jane Harris, Graham and Susan Ford, Valerie Pauling-Canvin
Contact: Henlade, Taunton, Somerset, TA3 5LT
) 01823 443443
@ ruishtoncourt@aol.com

Formed from a converted house which has stood for more than 100 years, Ruishton Court sits in large grounds. The home is located in a residential area, four miles from Taunton. The gardens boast a greenhouse, a pond and a gazebo is erected for the summer. The home employs an activities coordinator who arranges activities such as bingo as well as outings for the residents. There is a mobile library which visits the home and a Communion service is held once a month.

Registered places: 33
Guide weekly rate: £308–£780
Specialist care: Nursing, day care, respite
Medical services: Podiatry, hygienist, optician
Qualified staff: Fails standard

Home details
Location: Residential area, 4 miles from Taunton
Communal areas: 2 lounges, dining rooms, garden
Accessibility: *Floors:* 3 • *Access:* Lift • *Wheelchair access:* Good
Smoking: In designated area
Pets: ✓
Routines: Flexible

Room details
Single: 22
Shared: 4
En suite: 26
Facilities: TV point, telephone point

Door lock: ✓
Lockable place: ✓

Services provided
Beauty services: Hairdressing
Mobile library: ✓
Religious services: Monthly Communion service
Transport: ✗
Activities: *Coordinator.* ✓ • *Examples:* Bingo • *Outings:* ✓
Meetings: ✗

South Cary House

Manager: Christine Garden
Owner: Christine and Roderick Garden
Contact: South Street, Castle Cary, Somerset, BA7 7ES
) 01963 350272
@ rory.garden@btinternet.com

A Grade II listed Georgian house set in approximately one acre of ground, South Cary House is in a prime location for more active and independent residents. Within a 10-minute walk of local amenities, it is also on a regular bus route, with buses departing hourly from near the home. South Cary House has a large garden which overlooks the attractive countryside and is a good spot for fêtes and outdoor gatherings. Residents with an interest in horticulture are also free here to garden.

Registered places: 18
Guide weekly rate: From £410
Specialist care: Day care, respite
Medical services: Podiatry, dentist, optician, physiotherapy
Qualified staff: Exceeds standard: 80% at NVQ level 2

Home details
Location: Rural area, 0.5 miles from Castle Cary
Communal areas: Lounge, dining room, library, garden
Accessibility: *Floors:* 2 • *Access:* Lift • *Wheelchair access:* Good
Smoking: ✗
Pets: At manager's discretion
Routines: Flexible

Room details
Single: 18
Shared: 0
En suite: 18
Facilities: TV point, telephone point

Door lock: ✓
Lockable place: ✓

Services provided
Beauty services: Hairdressing, manicures
Mobile library: Library facilities
Religious services: Weekly Catholic Communion service, monthly Anglican Communion service
Transport: ✗
Activities: *Coordinator.* ✗ • *Examples:* Arts and crafts, sherry evenings, walks • *Outings:* ✓
Meetings: ✗

Registered places: 40
Guide weekly rate: £420–£450
Specialist care: Day care, respite
Medical services: Podiatry, dentist, optician
Qualified staff: Exceeds standard: 59% at NVQ level 2

Home details

Location: Residential area, 1 mile from Street
Communal areas: Lounge, dining room, conservatory, garden
Accessibility: *Floors:* 2 • *Access:* Lift • *Wheelchair access:* Good
Smoking: In designated area
Pets: ✗
Routines: Structured

Room details

Single: 40
Shared: 0
En suite: 20
Facilities: None

Door lock: ✓
Lockable place: ✓

Services provided

Beauty services: Hairdressing
Mobile library: ✗
Religious services: Monthly Communion service
Transport: ✗
Activities: *Coordinator.* ✓ • *Examples:* Bingo, music and movement, quizzes • *Outings:* ✗
Meetings: ✓

Southlawns

Manager: Vera Fellows
Owner: Somerset Care Ltd
Contact: Highfield Road, Street, Somerset, BA16 0JJ
☎ 01458 443635

Close to the high street with all its amenities, Southlawns is located in a residential area of Street, one mile from the town centre. The home has a shop where residents can buy small items and there is a garden and a conservatory for residents to relax in the summer months. There is a residents meeting every six months and a Communion service takes place on a monthly basis. The home employs an activities coordinator who arranges a variety of activities for the residents, such as quizzes and music and movement.

Registered places: 20
Guide weekly rate: £399–£424
Specialist care: Respite
Medical services: Podiatry, dentist, optician
Qualified staff: Undisclosed

Home details

Location: Village location, 7.5 miles from Taunton
Communal areas: Lounge, dining room, garden
Accessibility: *Floors:* 2 • *Access:* Lift • *Wheelchair access:* Good
Smoking: ✗
Pets: ✗
Routines: Flexible

Room details

Single: 18
Shared: 1
En suite: 19
Facilities: None

Door lock: ✓
Lockable place: ✓

Services provided

Beauty services: Hairdressing
Mobile library: ✗
Religious services: Monthly Communion service
Transport: ✗
Activities: *Coordinator.* ✓ • *Examples:* Exercise, games • *Outings:* ✗
Meetings: ✓

St George's Residential Home

Manager: Anne Moyle
Owner: Mr and Mrs Moyle
Contact: 17 Wilton Street, Taunton, Somerset, TA1 3JR
☎ 01823 275268

St George's comprises a main building and a new block that faces onto an attractive courtyard. The home is situated in a village, seven and a half miles from Taunton. The home arranges a monthly Communion service for residents to attend and the activities coordinator put together a programme which includes games and exercise sessions. There are also regular residents meetings.

Stratton House

Manager: Claire Nicholls
Owner: Christine Watson
Contact: 15 Rectory Road,
Burnham-on-Sea, Somerset, TA8 2BZ
) 01278 787735

Situated in a residential area close to the seafront and the facilities of the town centre Stratton House lies almost a mile from Burnham-on-Sea. The home has a lounge and a quiet lounge as well as a dining room and a garden with a patio area. The home arranges activities for the residents such as playing musical instruments and drawing. There is a communal safe in the home for valuables. The home also offers day care.

Registered places: 24
Guide weekly rate: £375–£395
Specialist care: Day care, dementia
Medical services: Podiatry, dentist, optician
Qualified staff: Exceeds standard: 75% at NVQ level 2

Home details
Location: Residential area, 0.7 miles from Burnham-on-Sea
Communal areas: Lounge, quiet lounge, dining room,
   patio and garden
Accessibility: *Floors:* 2 • *Access:* Lift and stair lift
   Wheelchair access: Good
Smoking: In designated area
Pets: ✗
Routines: Flexible

Room details
Single: 24
Shared: 0
En suite: 24
Facilities: TV

Door lock: ✗
Lockable place: ✗

Services provided
Beauty services: Hairdressing, manicures
Mobile library: ✗
Religious services: ✗
Transport: ✗
Activities: *Coordinator:* ✗ • *Examples:* Drawing, singing • *Outings:* ✗
Meetings: ✗

Sunningdale Lodge

Manager: Patricia Ellesmere
Owner: Somerset Care Ltd
Contact: Sunningdale Road, Yeovil,
Somerset, BA21 5LD
) 01935 422980
@ patricia.ellesmere@
   somersetcare.co.uk
⌂ www.somersetcare.co.uk

Located in a residential area of Yeovil, Sunningdale Lodge is close to the town's facilities which include shops, a post office and church. The home has quiet areas for residents and their families to enjoy some privacy and a conservatory has recently been built. The home has several lounges and a dining room as well as a patio area and a conservatory. The home has its own library facilities and the books are changed every three months. Pets would be allowed at the manager's discretion and smoking is permitted outside the building only.

Registered places: 38
Guide weekly rate: Up to £450
Specialist care: Podiatry, dentist, optician
Medical services: None
Qualified staff: Exceeds standard: 66% at NVQ level 2

Home details
Location: Residential area, 1.5 miles from Yeovil
Communal areas: Lounges, dining room, conservatory, quiet areas,
   patio and garden
Accessibility: *Floors:* 3 • *Access:* Lift • *Wheelchair access:* Good
Smoking: ✗
Pets: At manager's discretion
Routines: Flexible

Room details
Single: 38
Shared: 0
En suite: Undisclosed
Facilities: TV

Door lock: ✗
Lockable place: ✓

Services provided
Beauty services: Hairdressing
Mobile library: Library facilities
Religious services: ✓
Transport: ✓
Activities: *Coordinator:* ✓ • *Examples:* Cooking, painting,
   reminiscence • *Outings:* ✓
Meetings: Meetings

Registered places: 50
Guide weekly rate: Undisclosed
Specialist care: Respite, dementia
Medical services: Podiatry, dentist, optician
Qualified staff: Exceeds standard: 80% at NVQ level 2

Home details

Location: Residential area, 0.3 miles from Chard
Communal areas: Dining room, garden
Accessibility: *Floors:* 2 • *Access:* None • *Wheelchair access:* Limited
Smoking: ✗
Pets: ✓
Routines: Flexible

Room details

Single: 50
Shared: 0
En suite: 6
Facilities: TV

Door lock: ✓
Lockable place: ✓

Services provided

Beauty services: Hairdressing, manicures
Mobile library: ✗
Religious services: ✗
Transport: ✗
Activities: *Coordinator.* ✗ • *Examples:* Ball games, card games, quizzes
    Outings: ✗
Meetings: ✓

Sunnymeade

Manager: Nicola Passant
Owner: Somerset Care Ltd
Contact: Helliers Close, Chard, Somerset, TA20 1LJ
☏ 01460 63563

Sunnymeade is a purpose-built residential care home operated by Somerset Care Ltd. The home is situated in a residential area, approximately half a mile from Chard. It has five ground floor units of eight places and some upper floor accommodation for those who are sufficiently mobile to climb stairs. The home arranges activities for the residents, such as ball games and quizzes and there are regular residents meetings held.

Registered places: 14
Guide weekly rate: £382–£450
Specialist care: Day care, respite
Medical services: Podiatry, dentist, optician
Qualified staff: Exceeds standard: 100% at NVQ level 2

Home details

Location: Residential area, 0.5 miles from Chard
Communal areas: Lounge, dining room, garden
Accessibility: *Floors:* 2 • *Access:* Lift • *Wheelchair access:* Good
Smoking: ✗
Pets: ✗
Routines: Flexible

Room details

Single: 14
Shared: 0
En suite: 14
Facilities: TV, telephone

Door lock: ✓
Lockable place: ✓

Services provided

Beauty services: Hairdressing
Mobile library: ✓
Religious services: ✓
Transport: ✓
Activities: *Coordinator.* ✗ • *Examples:* Board games, word games
    Outings: ✓
Meetings: ✓

Sunnyside Residential Home

Manager: Shirley Pontefract
Owner: Shirley Pontefract
Contact: Crewkerne Road, Chard, Somerset, TA20 1EZ
☏ 01460 61623
@ annponty3@yahoo.co.uk

Sunnyside Residential Home is located half a mile from the centre of Chard and provides care for 14 residents. The home also offers respite and day care. There is a bus service to the town centre but the home also has its own transport. The home prides itself on the flexibility of the residents' daily routines. Although there are set meal times these too are very flexible. The home arranges daily activities such as scrabble and board games and there are also outings to the theatre. There are residents meetings every two months.

Sydenham House

Manager: Michael Vickery
Owner: Somerset Care Ltd
Contact: Bridgwater, Somerset, TA6 4NG
) 01278 422763
@ Mike.vickery@somersetcare.co.uk

Sydenham House is a modern, purpose-built home in a residential development in Bridgwater. The town of Bridgwater boasts shops and a rugby club and can easily be reached on foot. The town centre is approximately one and a half miles away. The home prides itself on its airy and spacious rooms and its regular programme of social events which includes regular informal meetings. Split into two parts, the home also has an intermediate care facility, called The Willows, which provides care for up to six people.

Registered places: 51
Guide weekly rate: £373–£485
Specialist care: Day care, respite
Medical services: Undisclosed
Qualified staff: Exceeds standard: 82% at NVQ level 2

Home details
Location: Residential area, 1.5 miles from Bridgwater
Communal areas: Lounge, dining room, conservatory, garden
Accessibility: *Floors:* 2 • *Access:* Lift • *Wheelchair access:* Good
Smoking: ✗
Pets: At manager's discretion
Routines: Flexible

Room details
Single: 49
Shared: 1
En suite: 24
Facilities: TV point, telephone point

Door lock: ✓
Lockable place: ✓

Services provided
Beauty services: Hairdressing, manicures
Mobile library: ✓
Religious services: Monthly Anglican Communion service
Transport: Minibus
Activities: *Coordinator.* ✓ • *Examples*: Movement and music, quizzes *Outings:* ✓
Meetings: ✓

Tudor Lodge

Manager: Judith Arnold
Owner: JDA Care Ltd
Contact: 8 Brightstowe Road,
Burnham-on-Sea, Somerset, TA8 2HW
) 01278 784277
@ mail@tudorlodge.net
⌐⊟ www.tudorlodge.net

An older-style property set back from the road in a residential area, Tudor Lodge is attractively located in close proximity to both the sea and the town centre, approximately one mile away. The home has an attractive sun terrace as well as a garden and conservatory. There are a range of activities on offer such as arts and crafts and exercises. There are performances by visiting entertainers and the residents benefit from the location of the home with trips to the nearby seaside and shopping trips to Street.

Registered places: 27
Guide weekly rate: £373–£490
Specialist care: Respite
Medical services: Podiatry, dentist, optician
Qualified staff: Exceeds standard: 60% at NVQ level 2

Home details
Location: Residential area, 1 mile from Burnham-on-sea
Communal areas: Lounge, dining room, conservatory, patio and garden
Accessibility: *Floors:* 2 • *Access:* Lift • *Wheelchair access:* Good
Smoking: In designated area
Pets: ✗
Routines: Flexible

Room details
Single: 23
Shared: 2
En suite: 0
Facilities: TV, telephone

Door lock: ✓
Lockable place: ✓

Services provided
Beauty services: Hairdressing, aromatherapy
Mobile library: ✗
Religious services: Fortnightly Methodist or Anglican Communion service
Transport: ✗
Activities: *Coordinator.* ✓ • *Examples*: Arts and crafts, keep fit, visiting entertainers • *Outings:* ✓
Meetings: ✗

Registered places: 27
Guide weekly rate: £665–£958
Specialist care: Nursing, day care, respite
Medical services: Podiatry, hygienist, optician
Qualified staff: Meets standard

Home details

Location: Residential area, 0.7 miles from Yeovil
Communal areas: 2 lounges, dining room, patio and garden
Accessibility: *Floors:* 2 • *Access:* Lift • *Wheelchair access:* Good
Smoking: ✗
Pets: At manager's discretion
Routines: Structured

Room details

Single: 17
Shared: 5
En suite: 3
Facilities: Telephone point

Door lock: ✓
Lockable place: ✓

Services provided

Beauty services: Hairdressing
Mobile library: ✗
Religious services: Monthly visit from vicar
Transport: Minibus
Activities: *Coordinator:* ✓ • *Examples:* Arts and crafts, bingo, film club
　　　　Outings: ✗
Meetings: ✗

Tyndale Nursing Home

Manager: Pauline Purnell
Owner: Christopher Wharton
Contact: 36 Preston Road, Yeovil, Somerset, BA21 3AQ
) 01935 472102
@ janipaul@aol.com

Situated in Yeovil on a site that includes a residential care home and sheltered housing complex, Tyndale is a converted house with purpose-built extension. It is located close to local shops and a bus ride away from the town centre. The home has two gardens including a quiet, courtyard garden that can be accessed from the lounge. The home produces a newsletter and there are visits from a vicar once a month. The home also has its own minibus.

Registered places: 96
Guide weekly rate: From £780
Specialist care: Nursing, dementia, physically disabled, respite
Medical services: Podiatry, dentist, optician, physiotherapy
Qualified staff: Meets standard

Home details

Location: Residential area, 2.5 miles from Yeovil
Communal areas: Lounge, dining room, hairdressing salon, garden
Accessibility: *Floors:* 2 • *Access:* Lift • *Wheelchair access:* Good
Smoking: ✗
Pets: ✓
Routines: Flexible

Room details

Single: 90
Shared: 3
En suite: 93
Facilities: No

Door lock: ✗
Lockable place: ✓

Services provided

Beauty services: Hairdressing
Mobile library: ✓
Religious services: ✓
Transport: ✓
Activities: *Coordinator:* ✓ • *Examples:* Arts and crafts, music, visiting entertainers • *Outings:* ✓
Meetings: ✓

West Abbey House

Manager: Beverley Davies
Owner: Barchester Healthcare Ltd
Contact: Stourton Way, Yeovil, Somerset, BA21 3UA
) 01935 411136
🖱 www.barchester.com

West Abbey House is situated in a residential area, two and a half miles from Yeovil. The home has recently undergone a refurbishment and now contains a lounge, a dining room and a garden with raised flowerbeds. There is also a separate lounge for younger residents. The home employs three activities coordinators who arrange outings to the theatre and local garden centre as well as internal activities such as arts and crafts and performances by visiting entertainers.

Winash Rest Home

Manager: Heather House
Owner: Heather House
Contact: 9 Albert Road, Clevedon, North Somerset, BS21 7RP

☎ 01275 873129

🖰 heatherhouse87@hotmail.com

Winash Rest Home is a converted Victorian property, located in a residential area, half a mile from Clevedon. The home has a lounge and a dining room as well as a garden and a conservatory. There are regular activities held including games, cards and musical entertainment. The home also offers outings to the residents, including to the local shops. There are residents meetings held every three months.

Registered places: 32
Guide weekly rate: From £360
Specialist care: Undisclosed
Medical services: Podiatry, optician, physiotherapy
Qualified staff: Meets standard

Home details
Location: Residential area, 0.5 miles from Clevedon
Communal areas: Lounge, dining room, conservatory, garden
Accessibility: *Floors:* 3 • *Access:* Lift • Wheelchair access: Good
Smoking: ✗
Pets: At manager's discretion
Routines: Flexible

Room details
Single: 32
Shared: 0
En suite: 23
Facilities: TV, telephone

Door lock: ✓
Lockable place: ✓

Services provided
Beauty services: Hairdressing
Mobile library: ✓
Religious services: Communion service
Transport: ✗
Activities: *Coordinator:* ✓ • *Examples:* Games, singing • *Outings:* ✓
Meetings: Yes

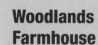

Woodlands Farmhouse

Manager: Emma Purvis
Owner: Emma Purvis
Contact: Wrantage, Taunton, Somerset, TA3 6DF

☎ 01823 481036

@ woodlandsfarmhouse@hotmail.com

Woodlands Farmhouse is situated in the countryside, a bus ride away from shops and six and a half miles from Taunton. This is a small house that does not feel like an institution. The countryside forms a calm atmosphere and presents beautiful views. It is perfect for those who enjoy the countryside, as there are acres of grounds to walk around in. The home arranges outings for the residents as well as internal activities such as visiting entertainers and music. The residents have regular meetings to discuss any issues they may have.

Registered places: 13
Guide weekly rate: £450–£595
Specialist care: Day care, respite
Medical services: Podiatry, hygienist, optician, physiotherapy
Qualified staff: Exceeds standard: 90% at NVQ level 2

Home details
Location: Rural area, 6.5 miles from Taunton
Communal areas: 2 lounges, dining room, patio and garden
Accessibility: *Floors:* 2 • *Access:* Stair lift • *Wheelchair access:* Good
Smoking: ✗
Pets: ✓
Routines: Flexible

Room details
Single: 10
Shared: 2
En suite: 12
Facilities: TV, telephone

Door lock: ✓
Lockable place: ✓

Services provided
Beauty services: Hairdressing
Mobile library: ✗
Religious services: ✗
Transport: ✗
Activities: *Coordinator:* ✗ • Examples: Knitting, music, visiting entertainers • *Outings:* ✓
Meetings: ✓

Registered places: 5
Guide weekly rate: £550–£600
Specialist care: Day care, dementia, respite
Medical services: Podiatry, optician
Qualified staff: Fails standard

Home details

Location: Rural area, 1.4 miles from Chard
Communal areas: Lounge, dining room, garden
Accessibility: *Floors:* 2 • *Access:* Stair lift
    Wheelchair access: Limited
Smoking: ×
Pets: At manager's discretion
Routines: Flexible

Room details

Single: 5
Shared: 0 | Door lock: ✓
En suite: 5 | Lockable place: ✓
Facilities: TV point, telephone point

Services provided

Beauty services: Hairdressing
Mobile library: ×
Religious services: Monthly Anglican Communion service
Transport: Car
Activities: *Coordinator.* × • *Examples:* Word searches • *Outings:* ✓
Meetings: ×

Yew Tree Cottage Residential Home

Manager: Brenda Seaby
Owner: Brenda Seaby
Contact: Hornsbury Hill, Chard, Somerset, TA20 3DB
☏ 01460 64735

Yew Tree Cottage is a very small care home where the manager lives on site. An annex is attached to the main house and holds a lounge, kitchenette and en suite twin bedroom. The home prides itself on its substantial gardens to the front and rear of the property. The gardens are landscaped and contain a greenhouse and vegetable plot which residents are free to use. The home has its own transport and often arranges outings for residents in the local area.

Registered places: 21
Guide weekly rate: £380–£450
Specialist care: Day care, dementia, respite
Medical services: Podiatry, hygienist, optician
Qualified staff: Exceeds standard: 75% at NVQ level 2

Home details

Location: Village location, 8 miles from Shaftesbury
Communal areas: Lounge, dining room, conservatory,
    patio and garden
Accessibility: *Floors:* 2 • *Access:* Lift • *Wheelchair access:* Good
Smoking: In designated area
Pets: ✓
Routines: Flexible

Room details

Single: 21
Shared: 0 | Door lock: ✓
En suite: 21 | Lockable place: ✓
Facilities: TV point, telephone point

Services provided

Beauty services: Hairdressing
Mobile library: ✓
Religious services: Fortnightly Communion service
Transport: ×
Activities: *Coordinator.* ✓ • *Examples:* Art classes • *Outings:* ✓
Meetings: ✓

Albany House

Manager: Janet Matthews
Owner: BM Care Ltd
Contact: The Square, Tisbury, Salisbury, Wiltshire SP3 6HA
☏ 01747 870313
@ albanyhouse@bmcare.plus.com
🖱 www.bmcare.plus.com

Situated in the centre of Tisbury village, Albany House is an older Victorian building that benefits from its close proximity to the village facilities, including shops and a mainline railway station with services to London Waterloo. This residential home offers care for the elderly, those with dementia and respite care. There are also day care facilities that people in the village make use of. An activities coordinator organises in-house activities and outings for residents and a number of services are provided at the home, including a mobile library and hairdressing.

Aldbourne Nursing Home

Manager: Guy Montezuma
Owner: Aldbourne Nursing Home Ltd
Contact: South Street, Aldbourne, Marlborough, Wiltshire SN8 2DW
☎ 01672 540919

A purpose-built home set in its own grounds, Aldbourne Nursing Home is located in Aldbourne village, which is easily accessed by the M4 and around eight miles from Swindon town. The home provides care for 40 residents and cares for a few residents who are terminally ill or have dementia. All rooms are on the ground floor and there are helpful mobility devices around the floor, such as handrails. Therefore, the home has good wheelchair access throughout.

Registered places: 40
Guide weekly rate: From £600
Specialist care: Nursing, physical disability, respite, terminal care
Medical services: Podiatry, dentist, optician, physiotherapy
Qualified staff: Exceeds standard: 80% at NVQ level 2

Home details
Location: Village location, 8 miles from Swindon
Communal areas: Dining room, conservatory, patio and garden
Accessibility: *Floors:* 1 • *Wheelchair access:* Good
Smoking: ✗
Pets: ✓
Routines: Flexible

Room details
Single: 40
Shared: 0
En suite: 40
Facilities: None

Door lock: ✓
Lockable place: ✓

Services provided
Beauty services: Hairdressing
Mobile library: Library facilities
Religious services: ✓
Transport: ✗
Activities: *Coordinator:* ✓ • *Examples:* Bingo, crosswords
　　　　　Outings: ✗
Meetings: ✓

Registered places: 55
Guide weekly rate: £625–£850
Specialist care: Podiatry
Medical services: Nursing, dementia, physical disability
Qualified staff: Meets standard

Home details

Location: Village location, 7 miles from Salisbury
Communal areas: 2 lounges, 2 dining rooms, patio and garden
Accessibility: *Floors:* 2 • *Access:* Lift • *Wheelchair access:* Good
Smoking: ✗
Pets: ✓
Routines: Flexible

Room details

Single: 43
Shared: 6
En suite: 34
Facilities: None

Door lock: ✓
Lockable place: ✓

Services provided

Beauty services: Hairdressing
Mobile library: ✗
Religious services: Monthly Communion service
Transport: ✗
Activities: *Coordinator.* ✗ • *Examples:* Visiting entertainers
   Outings: ✗
Meetings: ✗

Ashley Grange Nursing Home

Manager: Mrs Dempster
Owner: Mr and Mrs Ashley
Contact: Lode Hill, Downton, Salisbury, Wiltshire SP5 3PP
☏ 01725 512811
@ trevorashley@ashleycarehomes.co.uk
🖱 www.ashleycarehomes.co.uk

Ashley Grange is a purpose-built nursing home situated in the village of Downton, seven miles from Salisbury. There are numerous communal areas, including two lounges, two dining rooms and a pleasant garden. Residents can bring their own furniture to make their room feel more homely. Furthermore, residents are allowed to bring their own pets. Facilities are available for family or friends to stay overnight .

Registered places: 60
Guide weekly rate: Undisclosed
Specialist care: Nursing, emergency admissions, palliative care, physical disability, respite, terminal care
Medical services: Podiatry, physiotherapy, occupational therapy, optician, speech therapy
Qualified staff: Exceeds standard: 70% at NVQ level 2

Home details

Location: Residential area, one mile from Chippenham centre
Communal areas: 4 lounges, 2 dining rooms, conservatory, hairdressing salon, kitchenette, garden
Access *Floors:* 2 • *Access:* Lift • *Wheelchair access:* Good
Smoking: ✗
Pets: ✗
Routines: Flexible

Room details

Single: 60
Shared: 0
En suite: 60
Facilities: TV point, telephone point

Door lock: ✓
Lockable place: ✗

Services provided

Beauty services: Hairdressing, aromatherapy
Mobile library: ✓
Religious services: Monthly Communion service
Transport: ✗
Activities: *Coordinator.* ✓ • *Examples:* Arts and crafts, bingo, music
   Outings: ✓
Meetings: ✓

Avon Court

Manager: Elissa Beaven
Owner: BUPA Care Homes Ltd
Contact: St Francis Avenue, Rowden Hill, Chippenham, Wiltshire SN15 2SE
☏ 01249 660055
@ AvonCourtEveryone@BUPA.com
🖱 www.bupacarehomes.co.uk

Avon Court is centrally located in Rowden Hill, a short distance from Chippenham town centre, and offers views over the Wiltshire countryside. It is adjacent to Chippenham Community Hospital and has easy access from the M4 motorway. The two-storey home was built in 1990 and was specifically designed to meet the needs of elderly residents who require either nursing or residential care. Both floors are wheelchair accessible, with a lift to the first floor. Each bedroom has en suite facilities, and some have garden views. Regular activities are arranged, including arts and crafts, exercise, music and entertainers.

Bethesda House

Manager: Rebecca Wheeler
Owner: The Gospel Bethesda Fund
Contact: Derry Hill, Calne,
Wiltshire, SN11 9NN
☎ 01249 816666

A purpose-built property, Bethesda House is a small home that is one of a number managed by the Gospel Bethesda Fund. The home is situated in the village of Derry Hill, four miles from Chippenham. It is a condition of residency at the home that residents continually attend a Gospel chapel, with special arrangements made for those too ill. The home does not permit televisions although radios and similar equipment are permitted in residents bedrooms at allocated times. There is a summerhouse in the garden.

Registered places: 13
Guide weekly rate: £385–£443
Specialist care: Physical disability
Medical services: Podiatry, optician
Qualified staff: Meets standard

Home details
Location: Village location, 4 miles from Chippenham
Communal areas: Lounge, dining room, library, garden
Accessibility: *Floors:* 1 • *Wheelchair access:* Good
Smoking: ✗
Pets: ✗
Routines: Flexible

Room details
Single: 11
Shared: 1
En suite: 11
Facilities: Telephone point

Door lock: ✓
Lockable place: ✓

Services provided
Beauty services: Hairdressing
Mobile library: Library facilities
Religious services: Daily gospel services
Transport: Minibus
Activities: *Coordinator:* ✗ • *Examples:* Arts and crafts, exercise group
Outings: ✓
Meetings: ✓

Bluebells

Manager: Alison Turner
Owner: Abitalib Ebrahimjee
Contact: 152 Moredon Road, Swindon,
Wiltshire, SN25 3EP
☎ 01793 611014

Bluebells is a large bungalow in the Moredon area of Swindon. The home is a quarter of a mile from the local shops and is on a bus route. The home is open-plan, with two lounges and a dining room. There are three double rooms and 10 single rooms. The home has recently been refurbished and the garden now has a patio area and has been landscaped. The home has visits from a reminiscence therapist and has its own activities coordinator. The home also organises outings for the residents to the coast.

Registered places: 16
Guide weekly rate: Undisclosed
Specialist care: Respite
Medical services: Podiatry, dentist, optician, physiotherapy
Qualified staff: Meets standard

Home details
Location: Residential area, 2.5 miles from Swindon centre
Communal areas: 2 lounges, dining room, conservatory,
patio and garden
Accessibility: *Floors:* 1 • *Wheelchair access:* Good
Smoking: ✗
Pets: At manager's discretion
Routines: Flexible

Room details
Single: 10
Shared: 3
En suite: 0
Facilities: TV point, telephone

Door lock: ✓
Lockable place: ✓

Services provided
Beauty services: Hairdressing
Mobile library: ✗
Religious services: Monthly church service
Transport: Car
Activities: *Coordinator:* ✓ • *Examples:* Arts and crafts, cooking, films
Outings: ✓
Meetings: ✓

Registered places: 55
Guide weekly rate: £695–£990
Specialist care: Nursing
Medical services: Podiatry
Qualified staff: Meets standard

Home details

Location: Residential area, 1.5 miles from Salisbury
Communal areas: 3 lounges, hairdressing salon, computer room, garden and patio
Accessibility: *Floors:* 3 • *Access:* Lift • *Wheelchair access:* Good
Smoking: ×
Pets: ×
Routines: Flexible

Room details

Single: Undisclosed
Shared: Undisclosed
En suite: 55
Facilities: TV, telephone

Door lock: Undisclosed
Lockable place: ×

Services provided

Beauty services: Hairdressing
Mobile library: ✓
Religious services: Twice monthly Communion
Transport: Minibus
Activities: *Coordinator:* ✓ • *Examples:* One-to-one sessions
   Outings: ✓
Meetings: ✓

Braemar Lodge

Manager: Irene Gray
Owner: Colten Care Ltd
Contact: Stratford Road, Salisbury, Wiltshire SP1 3JH
☎ 01722 439700
@ braemarlodge@coltencare.co.uk
🖰 www.coltencare.co.uk

Braemar Lodge is situated in a residential area, approximately one and a half miles from Salisbury. The home has a lounge on each floor as well as a large entrance hall and a patio garden. There is also a computer room. The home arranges Communion twice month and there are also outings in the home's minibus. The home employs an activities coordinator who arranges both group and one-to-one sessions.

Registered places: 37
Guide weekly rate: Undisclosed
Specialist care: Dementia, physical disability, respite
Medical services: Podiatry, optician, physiotherapy
Qualified staff: Exceeds standard: 75% at NVQ level 2

Home details

Location: Village location, 4 miles from Gillingham
Communal areas: 2 lounges, dining room, garden
Accessibility: *Floors:* 2 • *Access:* Lift • *Wheelchair access:* Good
Smoking: ×
Pets: ×
Routines: Flexible

Room details

Single: 37
Shared: 0
En suite: Undisclosed
Facilities: TV point, telephone point

Door lock: ✓
Lockable place: ✓

Services provided

Beauty services: Hairdressing
Mobile library: ✓
Religious services: Monthly Communion service
Transport: Car
Activities: *Coordinator.* × • *Examples:* Bingo, theme days
   Outings: ✓
Meetings: ✓

Bramley House

Manager: Elizabeth Miller
Owner: Gerald and Barbara Saunt
Contact: Castle Street, Mere, Warminster, Wiltshire, BA12 6JN
☎ 01747 860192

Bramley House is in the village of Mere, very close to the A303 and four miles from Gillingham town. Situated five minutes' walk from village amenities, it is well located so that able residents can remain independent. There is a pleasant garden and a vegetable garden where the gardener grows many of the vegetables used in the home's cooking.

Bybrook House Nursing Home

Manager: Janet Rowland
Owner: Avon Care Homes Ltd
Contact: Middlehill, Box, Wiltshire, SN13 8QP
☎ 01225 743672
🖰 www.bybrookhouse.co.uk

Situated in a rural area surrounded by countryside, Bybrook House Nursing Home is an old country house set in seven acres of land. The home has a trout stream in the grounds and there is the opportunity for bird watching. The home has its own activities coordinator who arranges bingo, flower arranging and visiting entertainers. There are also visits in the summer months to local garden centres. The home has visits from a mobile library once a month and there is Communion every two weeks.

Registered places: 30
Guide weekly rate: £795–£1,188
Specialist care: Nursing, day care, physical disability, respite,
Medical services: Podiatry, dentist, optician, physiotherapy
Qualified staff: Exceeds standard: 80% at NVQ Level 2

Home details
Location: Rural area, 5 miles from Bath
Communal areas: 2 lounges, dining room, conservatory, garden
Accessibility: *Floors:* 3 • *Access:* Lift • *Wheelchair access:* Good
Smoking: ✗
Pets: At manager's discretion
Routines: Flexible

Room details
Single: 24
Shared: 3
En suite: 7
Facilities: TV, telephone

Door lock: ✓
Lockable place: ✓

Services provided
Beauty services: Hairdressing, manicures
Mobile library: ✓
Religious services: ✓
Transport: ✗
Activities: *Coordinator.* ✓ • *Examples*: Bingo, flower arranging, visiting entertainers • *Outings:* ✓
Meetings: ✓

Castle View Nursing Home

Manager: Jennifer Walker
Owner: Frederick and Gill Brewer
Contact: 8 Old Castle Road, Salisbury, Wiltshire, SP1 3SF
☎ 01722 328243
@ castleviewnh@btinternet.com

On an elevated position on the outskirts of Salisbury city centre, Castle View stays true to its name and permits views of Old Sarum and the surrounding countryside. The home is located about a mile and a half from Salisbury city centre, with its shops and the cathedral. Although pets are not allowed to live in the home, they are welcome to visit. An impressively maintained garden is to the rear of the home and spacious parking is at the front.

Registered places: 25
Guide weekly rate: £550
Specialist care: Nursing
Medical services: Podiatry, optician, physiotherapy
Qualified staff: Exceeds standard: 60% at NVQ level 2

Home details
Location: Residential area, 1.5 miles from Salisbury centre
Communal areas: Lounge, conservatory, garden
Accessibility: *Floors:* 3 • *Access:* Lift • *Wheelchair access:* Good
Smoking: In designated area
Pets: ✗
Routines: Flexible

Room details
Single: 25
Shared: 0
En suite: 2
Facilities: TV point, telephone point

Door lock: ✓
Lockable place: ✓

Services provided
Beauty services: Hairdressing, massage
Mobile library: Library facilities
Religious services: Weekly nondenominational service
Transport: ✗
Activities: *Coordinator.* ✓ • *Examples*: Arts and crafts, bingo, musical entertainment • *Outings:* ✗
Meetings: ✗

Registered places: 71
Guide weekly rate: £550–£850
Specialist care: Nursing, dementia, physical disability, respite
Medical services: Podiatry, hygienist, optician, physiotherapy
Qualified staff: Meets standard

Home details

Location: Rural area, 10 miles from Salisbury
Communal areas: Lounge, dining room, conservatory, garden
Accessibility: *Floors:* 2 • *Access:* Lift • *Wheelchair access:* Good
Smoking: In designated area
Pets: ✓
Routines: Flexible

Room details

Single: 69
Shared: 1
En suite: 66
Facilities: TV point, telephone point

Door lock: ✓
Lockable place: ✓

Services provided

Beauty services: Hairdressing
Mobile library: ✓
Religious services: Monthly Communion service
Transport: Car
Activities: *Coordinator.* ✓ • *Examples:* Art classes, poetry reading, singalongs • *Outings:* ✓
Meetings: ✓

The Cedars Nursing Home

Manager: Marilyn Bulmer
Owner: Alphacare Holdings Ltd
Contact: Northlands, Landford, Salisbury, Wiltshire, SP5 2EJ
📞 01794 390284

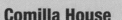

An older building in a rural location, The Cedars Nursing Home is situated on the edge of the New Forest in 40 acres of well maintained grounds. The home is relatively isolated, and is 10 miles to the city of Salisbury. The home does, however, have its own car to facilitate transport. The home has recently been renovated to offer 40 more beds.

Registered places: 38
Guide weekly rate: £515–£599
Specialist care: Nursing, respite
Medical services: Podiatry, dentist, optician
Qualified staff: Meets standard

Home details

Location: Residential area, in Amesbury
Communal areas: 3 lounges, dining room, garden
Accessibility: *Floors:* 2 • *Access:* Lift • *Wheelchair access:* Good
Smoking: ✗
Pets: ✗
Routines: Flexible

Room details

Single: 38
Shared: 2
En suite: 40
Facilities: TV point

Door lock: ✓
Lockable place: ✓

Services provided

Beauty services: Hairdressing
Mobile library: ✗
Religious services: ✗
Transport: ✗
Activities: *Coordinator.* ✓ • *Examples:* Bingo, discussion groups, pottery *Outings:* ✗
Meetings: ✗

Comilla House

Manager: Louisa Smigielska
Owner: Cornelia Care Homes
Contact: 1 Countess Road, Amesbury, Wiltshire, SP4 7DW
📞 01980 625498

A partially listed building with a newer wing, Comilla House is on the same site as Countess House. Approximately 20 minutes' drive from Salisbury train station, and near the centre of Amesbury, the home also has good bus links. The home's garden has raised flowerbeds so that residents can garden if they wish. Facilities are available for family or friends to stay overnight. Residents may bring their own furniture to personalise their rooms.

Countess House

Manager: Yvette Jones
Owner: Cornelia Care Homes
Contact: 1 Countess Road, Amesbury, Wiltshire, SP4 7DW
☎ 01980 625549

A purpose-built care home that is situated on the same campus as its sister home, Comilla House, Countess House is centrally located, approximately 20 minutes' drive from Salisbury train station. Coffee mornings offer residents the opportunity to socialise with other residents, and a church service is offered as well. The home shares its garden with Comilla House and has raised flowerbeds so that residents can easily join in gardening activities.

Registered places: 19
Guide weekly rate: £549–£640
Specialist care: Nursing, physical disability
Medical services: Podiatry
Qualified staff: Fails standard

Home details
Location: Residential area, in Amesbury
Communal areas: Lounge, dining room, patio and garden
Accessibility: *Floors:* 2 • *Access:* Lift • *Wheelchair access:* Good
Smoking: ×
Pets: ✓
Routines: Flexible

Room details
Single: 19
Shared: 0
En suite: 19
Facilities: None

Door lock: ✓
Lockable place: ✓

Services provided
Beauty services: Hairdressing
Mobile library: ×
Religious services: ✓
Transport: ×
Activities: *Coordinator.* ✓ • *Examples:* Coffee mornings • *Outings:* ×
Meetings: ×

Dauntsey House

Manager: Mair Rowles
Owner: Avenue Care Ltd
Contact: 9 Church Street, West Lavington, Devizes, Wiltshire, SN10 4LB
☎ 01380 812340

Dauntsey House is located within the village of West Lavington, close to village facilities and around five and a half miles from Devizes. The home cares for 20 residents and offers a good number of communal areas, including a lounge, conservatory and separate dining room. There is also a pleasant garden accessible for residents and wheelchair access throughout the home. There is no activities coordinator at the home, but staff ensure residents are stimulated.

Registered places: 20
Guide weekly rate: Undisclosed
Specialist care: Dementia, mental disorder, respite
Medical services: Podiatry, dentist, optician
Qualified staff: Exceeds standard: 90% at NVQ level 2

Home details
Location: Village location, 5.5 miles from Devizes
Communal areas: Lounge, dining room, conservatory, garden
Accessibility: *Floors:* 2 • *Access:* Lift • *Wheelchair access:* Good
Smoking: ×
Pets: ✓
Routines: Flexible

Room details
Single: 18
Shared: 1
En suite: 1
Facilities: TV point, telephone point

Door lock: ✓
Lockable place: ✓

Services provided
Beauty services: Hairdressing
Mobile library: ✓
Religious services: Monthly Communion service
Transport: ×
Activities: *Coordinator.* × • *Examples:* Videos, visiting entertainers
Outings: ✓
Meetings: ✓

Registered places: 20
Guide weekly rate: £400–£480
Specialist care: Dementia, respite
Medical services: Podiatry, dentist, optician
Qualified staff: Undisclosed

Home details

Location: Residential area, 1 mile from Salisbury centre
Communal areas: 2 lounges, dining room, hairdressing salon, garden
Accessibility: *Floors:* 2 • *Access:* Lift • *Wheelchair access:* x
Smoking: In designated area
Pets: At manager's discretion
Routines: Flexible

Room details

Single: 20
Shared: 0   Door lock: ✓
En suite: 12   Lockable place: x
Facilities: TV point, telephone point

Services provided

Beauty services: Hairdressing.
Mobile library: x
Religious services: Monthly Communion service, weekly bible study
Transport: Car
Activities: *Coordinator.* x • *Examples:* Keep fit • *Outings:* ✓
Meetings: ✓

Fairfax House

Manager: Mrs Butchers
Owner: Mr and Mrs Butchers
Contact: 85 Castle Road, Salisbury, Wiltshire, SP1 3RW
📞 01722 332846
@ dianabutchers@btconnect.com

A large detached house overlooking Victoria Park, Fairfax House is situated approximately one mile from the centre of Salisbury, easily accessed by buses which run regularly from near the front door. The home is also a 10-minute walk from the nearby supermarket. Fairfax House is a Christian residential home, and prides itself on offering 'flexible, attentive and non-discriminatory' care. With attractive gardens which feature a seating area and pond, the home also offers facilities for able residents to make their own snacks and tries to accompany residents out of the home on regular occasions.

Registered places: 38
Guide weekly rate: £735–£890
Specialist care: Nursing, physical disability, respite
Medical services: None
Qualified staff: Exceeds standard: 96% at NVQ level 2

Home details

Location: Village location, 2.5 miles from Bradford-on-Avon
Communal areas: 2 lounges, 2 dining rooms, garden
Accessibility: *Floors:* 2 • *Access:* Lift • *Wheelchair access:* Good
Smoking: In designated area
Pets: x
Routines: Flexible

Room details

Single: 38
Shared: 0   Door lock: ✓
En suite: 28   Lockable place: ✓
Facilities: TV, telephone point

Services provided

Beauty services: Hairdressing, aromatherapy
Mobile library: ✓
Religious services: Monthly Anglican Communion service
Transport: Minibus
Activities: *Coordinator.* ✓ • *Examples:* Art classes, games, music therapy • *Outings:* x
Meetings: x

Firlawn House Nursing Home

Manager: Penelope Jarvis
Owner: Firlawn Nursing Home Ltd
Contact: The Street, Holt, Trowbridge, Wiltshire, BA14 6QH
📞 01225 783333
@ enquiries@firlawn.com
🖰 www.firlawn.com

Comprised of two homes on one site, Firlawn is set in large gardens and is found in the village of Holt, two and a half miles from Bradford-on-Avon. The home has good views of the surrounding countryside, including 'The Courts', a site maintained by the National Trust. The Courts offers free entry to residents of Firlawn. The 38 residents have the choice of two lounges and two dining rooms in which to sit with other residents.

Greenacre Residential Home

Manager: Rosalind Vine
Owner: Rosalind Vine
Contact: Cleveland Gardens, Trowbridge, Wiltshire, BA14 7LX

) 01225 764935

Built in the 1960s, Greenacre Residential Home has been extended and adapted to house 14 residents. The home is situated in a residential area of the town of Trowbridge. A programme of activities is displayed in the hallway. Activities include art therapy, aromatherapy, music for health, church services and singers. Residents use a hairdressing salon in town when they need their hair done.

Registered places: 14
Guide weekly rate: £400–£460
Specialist care: Dementia
Medical services: Podiatry, dentist, optician
Qualified staff: Undisclosed

Home details
Location: Residential area, in Trowbridge
Communal areas: Lounge, dining room, conservatory, garden
Accessibility: *Floors:* 1 • *Wheelchair access:* Good
Smoking: ×
Pets: ✓
Routines: Flexible

Room details
Single: 8
Shared: 3
En suite: 5
Facilities: TV

Door lock: ✓
Lockable place: ×

Services provided
Beauty services: Aromatherapy
Mobile library: ×
Religious services: Church service
Transport: ×
Activities: *Coordinator.* × • *Examples:* Art therapy, visiting entertainers • *Outings:* ×
Meetings: ×

Greengates

Manager: Chong Siam Yeoh
Owner: Greengates Care Home Ltd
Contact: Redland Lane, Westbury, Wiltshire, BA13 3QA

) 01373 822727

Greengates is located in a residential area of Westbury, 15 minutes' walk from the town's train station and shops. Ideally placed for active residents wishing to maintain a life outside the home, there is also a bus stop at the end of the road. The home cares for 54 residents and offers residential care for the elderly as well as some dementia care. The home employs a handyman who will respond to issues of maintenance quickly.

Registered places: 54
Guide weekly rate: £236–£395
Specialist care: Dementia, mental disorder
Medical services: Podiatry, hygienist, optician
Qualified staff: Undisclosed

Home details
Location: Residential area, in Westbury
Communal areas: 3 lounges, dining room, library, garden
Accessibility: *Floors:* 2 • *Access:* Stair lift • *Wheelchair access:* Good
Smoking: In designated area
Pets: At manager's discretion
Routines: Flexible

Room details
Single: 26
Shared: 14
En suite: 2
Facilities: TV point, telephone point

Door lock: ×
Lockable place: ×

Services provided
Beauty services: Hairdressing
Mobile library: ×
Religious services: Monthly Communion service
Transport: Car
Activities: *Coordinator.* ✓ • *Examples:* Exercises, games *Outings:* ✓
Meetings: ✓

Registered places: 13
Guide weekly rate: From £400
Specialist care: Day care, dementia, respite
Medical services: Podiatry, dentist, optician
Qualified staff: Fails standard

Home details
Location: Residential area, 0.5 miles from Trowbridge centre
Communal areas: Lounge, dining room, garden
Accessibility: *Floors:* 2 • *Access:* Lift • *Wheelchair access:* Good
Smoking: ×
Pets: At manager's discretion
Routines: Structured

Room details
Single: 9
Shared: 2
En suite: 4
Facilities: TV point, telephone point

Door lock: ×
Lockable place: ×

Services provided
Beauty services: Hairdressing
Mobile library: ✓
Religious services: ×
Transport: ×
Activities: *Coordinator.* ✓ • *Examples*: Bingo, quizzes • *Outings:* ×
Meetings: ×

Greenwood House

Manager: Fredericka Davis
Owner: Fredericka Davis
Contact: 7 Green Lane, Trowbridge, Wiltshire, BA14 7DA
☏ 01225 754622

A semi-detached Victorian house, Greenwood House is located around half a mile from the centre of Trowbridge. The home is reasonably small, caring for 13 residents. There is an activities coordinator in the home who regularly organises games and quizzes for residents. There is a day care facility at the home and a mobile library visits.

Registered places: 27
Guide weekly rate: Up to £440
Specialist care: Dementia, respite
Medical services: Podiatry, hygienist, optician, physiotherapy
Qualified staff: Meets standard

Home details
Location: Residential location, in Highworth
Communal areas: Lounge, dining room, conservatory, garden
Accessibility: *Floors:* 3 • *Access:* Lift • *Wheelchair access:* Good
Smoking: In designated area
Pets: At manager's discretion
Routines: Flexible

Room details
Single: 13
Shared: 7
En suite: 0
Facilities: TV point, telephone point

Door lock: ✓
Lockable place: ✓

Services provided
Beauty services: Hairdressing
Mobile library: ✓
Religious services: Weekly Anglican service
Transport: Car
Activities: *Coordinator.* ✓ • *Examples*: Games, gardening
    Outings: ✓
Meetings: ×

Grove Hill Residential Home

Manager: James Dunn
Owner: James Dunn
Contact: Grove Hill, Highworth, Swindon, Wiltshire, SN6 7JN
☏ 01793 765317

Grove Hill Residential Home offers easy access to the local facilities of Highworth which is located approximately six miles from the centre of Swindon. There is a lounge, a dining room and two small sitting areas on each floor. The sitting area on the second floor is a designated smoking area for residents. There are choices at breakfast with set meals at lunch and teatimes although alternatives are provided. A range of activities is provided which residents can participate in if they wish.

Harnham Croft Nursing Home

Manager: Nicky Maguire
Owner: BUPA Care Homes Ltd
Contact: 76 Harnham Road,Salisbury, Wiltshire, SP2 8JN
) 01722 327623
⑤ HarnhamCroftNursingHomeEveryone@BUPA.com
⌂ www.bupacarehomes.co.uk

Harnham Croft is situated in the residential area of Harnham, on the banks of the River Nadder with views over Salisbury Cathedral and the water meadows. It is one mile from Salisbury city centre and on a main bus route into the city, with local shops, post office and church all within walking distance. Originally built in 1898, Harnham Croft has been extended and converted to meet the needs of elderly residents who require nursing care. There is a hairdressing salon, and regular activities are arranged, including arts and crafts, entertainers and trips to local places of interest.

Registered places: 44
Guide weekly rate: Undisclosed
Specialist care: Nursing, palliative care, physical disability, respite, terminal care
Medical services: Podiatry, physiotherapy
Qualified staff: Undisclosed

Home details
Location: Residential area, 1 mile from Salisbury centre
Communal areas: Lounge, dining room, hairdressing salon, garden
Accessibility: *Floors:* 3 • *Access:* Lift • *Wheelchair access:* Good
Smoking: ✕
Pets: ✕
Routines: Flexible

Room details
Single: 36
Shared: 4
En suite: 40
Facilities: TV point, telephone point

Door lock: ✓
Lockable place: ✕

Services provided
Beauty services: Hairdressing, aromatherapy
Mobile library: ✓
Religious services: ✓
Transport: ✓
Activities: *Coordinator.* ✓ • *Examples:* Arts and crafts, visiting entertainers • *Outings:* ✓
Meetings: ✕

Henford House Nursing Home

Manager: Vacant
Owner: Barchester Healthcare Ltd
Contact: Lower Marsh Road,Warminster, Wiltshire, BA12 9PB
) 01985 212430
@ henford@barchester.com
⌂ www.barchester.com/henford

Situated in a residential area of Warminster, Henford House is an extended period property which offers views of the Wiltshire countryside. As part of the activities programme, Henford House sometimes has visits from Pets As Therapy as well as local entertainers and pottery classes. There is also a library at the home with a selection of books that is changed regularly.

Registered places: 56
Guide weekly rate: £426–£1,200
Specialist care: Nursing, physical disability, respite
Medical services: Podiatry, hygienist, optician
Qualified staff: Meets standard

Home details
Location: Residential area, in Warminster
Communal areas: 2 lounges, dining room, library, garden
Accessibility: *Floors:* 2 • *Access:* Lift • *Wheelchair access:* Good
Smoking: ✕
Pets: At manager's discretion
Routines: Flexible

Room details
Single: 50
Shared: 3
En suite: 53
Facilities: TV, telephone point

Door lock: ✓
Lockable place: ✓

Services provided
Beauty services: Hairdressing
Mobile library: Library facilities
Religious services: Monthly Communion service
Transport: ✕
Activities: *Coordinator.* ✓ • *Examples:* Cooking, pottery classes, visiting entertainers • *Outings:* ✕
Meetings: ✓

Registered places: 26
Guide weekly rate: £560–£645
Specialist care: Respite
Medical services: Podiatry
Qualified staff: Meets standard

Home details

Location: Residential area, in Marlborough
Communal areas: Lounge, dining room, garden
Accessibility: *Floors:* 3 • *Access:* Lift • *Wheelchair access:* Good
Smoking: ✗
Pets: ✗
Routines: Flexible

Room details

Single: 23
Shared: 2
En suite: 22
Facilities: TV point, telephone point

Door lock: ✓
Lockable place: ✓

Services provided

Beauty services: Hairdressing
Mobile library: ✓
Religious services: Monthly Communion service
Transport: ✗
Activities: *Coordinator.* ✓ • *Examples*: Reading, reminiscence, yoga
   Outings: ✓
Meetings: ✗

Highfield

Manager: Vanessa Hillier
Owner: Anthony and Andrea Leeson
Contact: The Common, Marlborough, Wiltshire, SN8 1DL
☏ 01672 512671
@ enquiries@highfieldresidentialhome.co.uk
🖱 www.highfieldresidentialhome.co.uk

Highfield is a Victorian property that has been extended over the years and is situated in a residential area of Marlborough. The home is situated around five minutes' walk from the centre of town with its shops and local amenities. The home offers panoramic views of the countryside over Marlborough Common. There is a designated activities coordinator who organises outings and in-house activities such as reminiscence sessions and yoga.

Registered places: 20
Guide weekly rate: £396–£465
Specialist care: Nursing, mental disorder, respite
Medical services: Podiatry, dentist, optician, physiotherapy
Qualified staff: Meets standard

Home details

Location: Residential area, in Salisbury
Communal areas: 2 lounges, dining room, conservatory, garden
Accessibility: *Floors:* 3 • *Access:* Lift • *Wheelchair access:* Good
Smoking: ✗
Pets: At manager's discretion
Routines: Flexible

Room details

Single: 20
Shared: 0
En suite: 19
Facilities: None

Door lock: ✗
Lockable place: ✓

Services provided

Beauty services: Hairdressing, manicures
Mobile library: ✓
Religious services: Communion service
Transport: ✗
Activities:Coordinator: ✗ • Examples: Games, keep fit, one-to-one
   sessions • Outings: ✓
Meetings: ✗

Inwood House

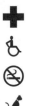

Manager: Alan Butchers
Owner: Alan and Diana Butchers
Contact: 10 Bellamy Lane, Salisbury, Wiltshire, SP1 2SP
☏ 01722 331980
@ admin.inwood@btiternet.com

Inwood House is location in a residential area in Salisbury, around half a mile from the city centre. At Inwood House, residents follow their own routines. There is an activities programme each week, which is offered and many of the residents regularly take a trip into town. There are ample communal areas, including two lounges, a dining room and a conservatory as well as a pleasant garden.

Kimberly House

Manager: Margaret Coyle
Owner: Wessex Care Ltd
Contact: 1 Fowlers Hill, Salisbury, Wiltshire, SP1 2JF
☎ 01722 322494

Kimberly House is a red-bricked home set back from the road and close to a bus route with services running into Salisbury. Owned by Wessex Care Ltd it is also less than a mile from one of its twin homes, Little Manor and 100 yards from a local store. Kimberly House also has its own cat and though pets are not usually allowed to stay they are welcome to visit. The home employs a welfare assistant who helps those more frail residents with tasks such as shopping. There are also resident/relatives meetings three times a year.

Registered places: 21
Guide weekly rate: £460–£560
Specialist care: Nursing, dementia
Medical services: Podiatry, dentist, optician
Qualified staff: Undisclosed

Home details
Location: Residential area, 1 mile from Salisbury
Communal areas: Lounge and dining room, garden
Accessibility: *Floors:* 3 • *Access:* Lift • *Wheelchair access:* Good
Smoking: ✗
Pets: At manager's discretion
Routines: Flexible

Room details
Single: 19
Shared: 1
En suite: 0
Facilities: TV, telephone point

Door lock: ✗
Lockable place: ✓

Services provided
Beauty services: Hairdressing.
Mobile library: ✓
Religious services: Monthly nondenominational Communion service
Transport: ✗
Activities: *Coordinator:* ✗ • *Examples:* Arts and crafts, games, one-to-one sessions • *Outings:* ✓
Meetings: ✓

Kings Court Care Centre

Manager: Helen Marshall
Owner: Life Style Care Plc
Contact: Kent Road, Swindon, Wiltshire, SN1 3NP
☎ 01793 715480

The Kings Court Care Centre is situated in the Old Town in Swindon, and is well serviced by bus routes. With each of the two floors housing separate general nursing units and dementia units, the home has many spacious rooms, including a sensory stimulation room. There is a portable telephone that residents can use. A newsletter is produced monthly. The home has two rabbits that live in the garden. The Kings Court also has four kitchenettes set up with fridge and microwave, providing an opportunity for residents to exercise their independence.

Registered places: 60
Guide weekly rate: From £700
Specialist care: Nursing, dementia, respite
Medical services: Podiatry, dentist, optician, physiotherapy
Qualified staff: Exceeds standard: 70% at NVQ level 2

Home details
Location: Residential area, in Swindon
Communal areas: 8 lounges, 2 dining rooms, 4 kitchenettes, sensory room, patio and garden
Accessibility: *Floors:* 2 • *Access:* Lift • *Wheelchair access:* Good
Smoking: In designated area
Pets: At manager's discretion
Routines: Flexible

Room details
Single: 60
Shared: 0
En suite: 60
Facilities: None

Door lock: ✓
Lockable place: ✓

Services provided
Beauty services: Hairdressing
Mobile library: ✓
Religious services: Monthly Anglican visits
Transport: ✗
Activities: *Coordinator:* ✓ • *Examples:* Arts and crafts, games, musical entertainment • *Outings:* ✓
Meetings: ✗

Registered places: 43
Guide weekly rate: Undisclosed
Specialist care: Nursing, dementia, mental disorder, respite
Medical services: Podiatry, hygienist, optician
Qualified staff: Meets standard

Home details

Location: Residential area, in Swindon
Communal areas: 3 lounges, 2 dining rooms, patio and garden
Accessibility: *Floors:* 2 • *Access:* Lift • *Wheelchair access:* Good
Smoking: In designated area
Pets: ✓
Routines: Structured

Room details

Single: 41
Shared: 2
En suite: Undisclosed
Facilities: TV, telephone point

Door lock: ✗
Lockable place: ✗

Services provided

Beauty services: Hairdressing
Mobile library: ✓
Religious services: Anglican visits
Transport: ✗
Activities: *Coordinator.* ✓ • *Examples:* One-to-one sessions
   Outings: ✗
Meetings: ✓

Kingsmead Care Home

Manager: Gillian Whiter
Owner: Four Seasons Healthcare Ltd
Contact: 63 Prospect Place, Old Town, Swindon, Wiltshire, SN1 3LJ
) 01793 422333
@ kingsmead@fshc.co.uk
🖰 www.fshc.co.uk

Kingsmead Care Home is situated in the Old Town of Swindon, a short distance from the centre. A modern building, the home is split into three sections which denote a residential unit as well as a nursing and dementia/mental health unit. Each unit has its own lounge in which activities happen. With a comprehensive weekly activities programme, this home offers a safe and interesting environment.

Registered places: 34
Guide weekly rate: From £410
Specialist care: Respite
Medical services: Podiatry, optician, physiotherapy
Qualified staff: Meets standard

Home details

Location: Village location, 3.5 miles from Chippenham
Communal areas: 2 lounges, dining room, art room, library, garden
Accessibility: *Floors:* 2 • *Access:* Lift and stair lift
   Wheelchair access: Good
Smoking: ✗
Pets: At manager's discretion
Routines: Flexible

Room details

Single: 34
Shared: 0
En suite: 34
Facilities: TV point, telephone point

Door lock: ✓
Lockable place: ✓

Services provided

Beauty services: Hairdressing, manicures
Mobile library: ✓
Religious services: Weekly Anglican service
Transport: ✗
Activities: *Coordinator.* ✓ • *Examples:* Art classes, bingo, puzzles
   Outings: ✓
Meetings: ✓

Kingston House

Manager: Carol Mather
Owner: Greensleeves Homes Trust
Contact: Lansdowne Crescent, Derry Hill, Calne, Wiltshire, SN11 9NT
) 01249 815555
@ kingston@greensleeves.org.uk
🖰 www.greensleeves.org.uk

Kingston House is a purpose-built home situated in its own grounds in the peaceful village of Derry Hill, which is mid-way between Calne and Chippenham. The home was built by the British Red Cross as a convalescent home and was acquired by WRVS in 1978 when it became a residential care home for older people. Since 1997, the home has been owned and managed by Greensleeves Homes Trust. The home has a 'link system' where volunteers take residents shopping or to nearby towns. There are two large lounges as well as an art room, used for activities, and library area.

Kington St Michael Residential Home

Manager: Mrs Teelucksingh-Tirbhowan
Owner: Mr and Mrs Teelucksingh-Tirbhowan
Contact: 81 Kington St Michael, Chippenham, Wiltshire, SN14 6JB

📞 01249 750737

Kington St Michael Residential Home is located in the heart of Kington St Michael village next to the local pub. With parts of the building dating back to the middle of the 17th century, the home is steeped in history. Residents have the opportunity to exercise choice and control over their lives. The laid back approach allows them to choose where to spend their time and whether to take part in the home's activities.

Registered places: 9
Guide weekly rate: £350–£450
Specialist care: Dementia, respite
Medical services: Podiatry, dentist
Qualified staff: Meets standard

Home details
Location: Village location, 3 miles from Chippenham
Communal areas: Lounge, dining room, garden
Accessibility: *Floors:* 2 • *Access:* Stair lift
    Wheelchair access: Limited
Smoking: ✗
Pets: ✗
Routines: Flexible

Room details
Single: 9
Shared: 0
En suite: 8
Facilities: None

Door lock: ✓
Lockable place: ✓

Services provided
Beauty services: Hairdressing, manicures
Mobile library: ✗
Religious services: ✗
Transport: ✗
Activities: *Coordinator:* ✗ • *Examples:* Games, skittles • *Outings:* ✓
Meetings: ✗

Ladymead Nursing Home

Manager: Anne Rouse
Owner: Four Seasons Healthcare Ltd
Contact: Moormead Road, Wroughton, Swindon, Wiltshire, SN4 9BY

📞 01793 845063
@ ladymead@fshc.co.uk
🖱 www.fshc.co.uk

Ladymead is a purpose-built home situated in Wroughton village, within easy reach of shops and other amenities, public transport and the M4. Specifically, Swindon town centre is only a mile away. The home has two lounges with televisions, a quiet room and a summerhouse which overlooks the home's grounds. An activities coordinator is employed 29 hours a week and organises games, gentle exercise and some outings.

Registered places: 40
Guide weekly rate: £650–£700
Specialist care: Nursing, day care, respite, terminal care
Medical services: Podiatry
Qualified staff: Undisclosed

Home details
Location: Village location, 1 mile from Swindon centre
Communal areas: 2 lounges, 2 dining rooms, quiet room, garden
Accessibility: *Floors:* 2 • *Access:* Lift • *Wheelchair access:* Good
Smoking: ✗
Pets: ✓
Routines: Flexible

Room details
Single: 30
Shared: 4
En suite: Undisclosed
Facilities: TV

Door lock: ✗
Lockable place: ✗

Services provided
Beauty services: Hairdressing
Mobile library: ✗
Religious services: Monthly church service
Transport: ✗
Activities: *Coordinator:* ✓ • *Examples:* Exercises, quizzes
    Outings: ✓
Meetings: ✓

Registered places: 21
Guide weekly rate: £455–£554
Specialist care: Dementia, respite
Medical services: Podiatry, dentist, optician, dietician
Qualified staff: Meets standard

Home details
Location: Residential area, 0.5 miles from Lymington centre
Communal areas: 2 lounges, dining room, patio and garden
Accessibility: *Floors:* 2 • *Access:* Lift • *Wheelchair access:* Limited
Smoking: ×
Pets: ×
Routines: Flexible

Room details
Single: 18
Shared: 1
En suite: 0
Facilities: None

Door lock: ×
Lockable place: ×

Services provided
Beauty services: Weekly Protestant service
Mobile library: ×
Religious services: ×
Transport: ×
Activities: *Coordinator:* × • *Examples:* Armchair exercises,
arts and crafts, games • *Outings:* ✓
Meetings: ✓

Leonora

Manager: Gaie Marshall
Owner: Pilgrim Homes
Contact: Wood Lane, Chippenham,
Wiltshire, SN15 3DY
) 01249 651613
@ chippenham@pilgrimhomes.org.uk
🖰 www.pilgrimhomes.org.uk

Located in a residential area half a mile from Chippenham, Leonora is a home in the Pilgrim Homes group. Pilgrim Homes are run according to a Protestant Christian doctrine, and have a strong set of beliefs. Devotions are held every day except Sunday and Monday, when worship services take place. The home offers residential care. The building is a detached old stone house with a patio area and garden. Radios and televisions are not permitted in communal areas of the home, but are allowed in rooms.

Registered places: 9
Guide weekly rate: £380–£450
Specialist care: Respite
Medical services: Podiatry, optician, physiotherapy
Qualified staff: Meets standard

Home details
Location: Residential area, in Calne
Communal areas: Lounge/dining room, patio and garden
Accessibility: *Floors:* 1 • *Wheelchair access:* Good
Smoking: In designated area
Pets: ✓
Routines: Flexible

Room details
Single: 5
Shared: 2
En suite: 7
Facilities: TV point, telephone point

Door lock: ✓
Lockable place: ✓

Services provided
Beauty services: Hairdressing
Mobile library: ✓
Religious services: Monthly Communion service
Transport: Car
Activities: *Coordinator:* × • *Examples:* Bingo, games, singalongs
Outings: ×
Meetings: ×

The Lilacs

Manager: Trudy Taylor
Owner: Ronald Taylor
Contact: 2a Lickhill Road,
Calne, Wiltshire, SN11 9DD
) 01249 821422
@ Trudy1taylor@aol.com

A purpose-built family-run care home, The Lilacs is 10 minutes' walk from Calne town centre where there are a variety of local facilities. The home is small, caring for only nine residents, and is set on one floor, aiding access for the more frail. The home has a garden with a patio area and a pleasant lounge and dining space. Staff run activities to suit residents' abilities, and these include games and singalongs.

Little Manor

Manager: Asha Tonse
Owner: Wessex Care Ltd
Contact: Manor Farm Road, Salisbury, Wiltshire, SP1 2RS
☎ 01722 333114

Little Manor is a modern building set on the main road, with beautiful, secure gardens. Owned by Wessex Care Ltd, it is also less than a mile from one of its twin home, Kimberly House, and a 15-minute walk from the centre of Salisbury where there are numerous shops and facilities. With hourly buses offering active residents further opportunities to explore the city centre, the home's gardens are an attraction themselves and some of the resident's bedrooms have direct access through patio doors. A full-time maintenance person is employed to ensure the home is always in full running order.

Registered places: 26
Guide weekly rate: £460–£600
Specialist care: Nursing
Medical services: Podiatry, dentist, optician
Qualified staff: Undisclosed

Home details
Location: Residential area, 0.5 mile from Salisbury centre
Communal areas: 2 lounges, 2 dining rooms, garden
Accessibility: *Floors:* 4 • *Access:* Lift • *Wheelchair access:* Good
Smoking: In designated area
Pets: ✗
Routines: Flexible

Room details
Single: 22
Shared: 2
En suite: 21
Facilities: TV point, telephone point

Door lock: ✓
Lockable place: ✗

Services provided
Beauty services: Hairdressing
Mobile library: ✗
Religious services: Fortnightly nondenominational Communion service
Transport: ✗
Activities: *Coordinator:* ✓ • *Examples:* Bingo, keep fit, one-to-one sessions • *Outings:* ✗
Meetings: ✓

Longbridge Deverill House

Manager: Jean Proctor
Owner: Equality Care Ltd
Contact: Church Street, Longbridge Deverill, Warminster, Wiltshire, BA12 7DJ
☎ 01985 214040

A 300-year-old listed building, Longbridge Deverill House is situated on the A350 close to limited local amenities with a bus stop right outside. The town of Warminster is just over two miles away. Caring for up to 25 residents, there is ample communal space and a separate hairdressing salon. Residents are encouraged to keep active and outings and activities are organised at the home.

Registered places: 25
Guide weekly rate: £460–£650
Specialist care: Day care, dementia, respite
Medical services: Podiatry, massage
Qualified staff: Exceeds standard: 67% at NVQ level 2

Home details
Location: Village location, 2.5 miles from Warminster
Communal areas: 2 lounges, dining room, hairdressing salon, garden
Accessibility: *Floors:* 2 • *Access:* Lift and stair lift *Wheelchair access:* Good
Smoking: In designated area
Pets: ✓
Routines: Flexible

Room details
Single: 23
Shared: 2
En suite: 24
Facilities: TV point

Door lock: ✓
Lockable place: ✓

Services provided
Beauty services: Hairdressing
Mobile library: ✗
Religious services: Monthly Anglican service
Transport: ✗
Activities: *Coordinator:* ✗ • *Examples:* Visiting entertainers *Outings:* ✓
Meetings: ✗

Registered places: 17
Guide weekly rate: From £650
Specialist care: Nursing, day care, physical disability, respite, terminal care
Medical services: Podiatry, dentist, optician, physiotherapy
Qualified staff: Exceeds standard: 100% at NVQ Level 2

Home details

Location: Residential area, 0.5 miles from Salisbury centre
Communal areas: Lounge, dining room, patio and garden
Accessibility: *Floors:* 2 • *Access:* Lift • *Wheelchair access:* Good
Smoking: ×
Pets: At manager's discretion
Routines: Flexible

Room details

Single: 15
Shared: 1
En suite: 5
Facilities: TV, telephone

Door lock: ×
Lockable place: ✓

Services provided

Beauty services: Hairdressing, manicures
Mobile library: Library facilities
Religious services: ✓
Transport: ×
Activities: *Coordinator.* ✓ • *Examples*: Music, videos, visiting entertainers • *Outings:* ✓
Meetings: ×

Maristow House Nursing Home

Manager: Lindsey Wallace
Owner: Lindsey Wallace
Contact: 16 Bourne Avenue, Salisbury, Wiltshire, SP1 1LT
☏ 01722 322970
@ Maristow16@hotmail.co.uk

Maristow House is an older building that has been converted into a nursing home. The home is located in a quiet area of Salisbury, a five-minute walk to the town centre. The activities coordinator tends to the needs of each resident including individual outings. There are also group activities such as visiting entertainers. The home allows pets at the manager's discretion and has its own library facilities. The home has a lounge, a dining room and a garden with a patio area. An outdoor lift has recently been installed allowing all residents access to the garden.

Registered places: 87
Guide weekly rate: Undisclosed
Specialist care: Nursing, dementia, palliative care, physical disability, respite, terminal care
Medical services: Podiatry, physiotherapy, occupational therapy, speech therapy
Qualified staff: Undisclosed

Home details

Location: Village location, 6 miles from Devizes
Communal areas: 3 lounges, 3 dining rooms, hairdressing salon, kitchenette, garden
Accessibility: *Floors:* 2 • *Access:* Lift • *Wheelchair access:* Good
Smoking: ×
Pets: ×
Routines: Flexible

Room details

Single: 79
Shared: 4
En suite: 76
Facilities: TV point, telephone point

Door lock: ×
Lockable place: ×

Services provided

Beauty services: Hairdressing
Mobile library: ✓
Religious services: ✓
Transport: Minibus
Activities: *Coordinator.* ✓ • *Examples:* Bingo, Arts and crafts, visiting entertainers • *Outings:* ✓
Meetings: ×

Market Lavington Nursing and Residential Centre

Manager: Debs Tilney
Owner: BUPA Care Homes Ltd
Contact: 39 High Street, Market Lavington, Devizes, Wiltshire, SN10 4AG
☏ 01380 812282
@ MarketLavington@BUPA.com
⌂ www.bupacarehomes.co.uk

Situated in the heart of the Wiltshire countryside, within easy reach of Devizes, Marlborough, Salisbury and Bath, Market Lavington is a nursing home providing care for elderly residents and those with dementia. Originally a private house Market Lavington has been carefully converted over two floors. The home has large, landscaped grounds that during the summer provide the perfect place for residents to relax and enjoy the weather. The home's activities organiser ensures a stimulating programme including reminiscence therapy, outings to local places of interest and visits from local entertainers.

Marlborough Lodge

Manager: Susan Harper
Owner: Susan and David Harper
Contact: 83–84 London Road,
Marlborough, Wiltshire, SN8 2AN
☎ 01672 512288

Comprising of two Victorian houses which have been made into one building, Marlborough Lodge is situated just off the A4, 15 minutes' walk from the town centre. A bus stop can also be found close to the home and this passes through the town centre. An extension has been built at the home, adding three en suite bedrooms and a conservatory.

Registered places: 18
Guide weekly rate: £390–£600
Specialist care: Day care, respite
Medical services: Podiatry, optician
Qualified staff: Meets standard

Home details
Location: Residential area, 0.5 miles from Marlborough centre
Communal areas: Lounge, lounge/dining room, conservatory, garden
Accessibility: *Floors:* 2 • *Access:* Stair lift • *Wheelchair access:* Good
Smoking: In designated area
Pets: ✗
Routines: Flexible

Room details
Single: 10
Shared: 4
En suite: 5
Facilities: TV point, telephone point

Door lock: ✓
Lockable place: ✓

Services provided
Beauty services: Hairdressing
Mobile library: ✓
Religious services: Monthly Communion service
Transport: ✗
Activities: *Coordinator:* ✓ • *Examples:* Exercise sessions, games
Outings: ✓
Meetings: ✓

Mavern House Nursing Home

Manager: Sara Young
Owner: Mavern Care Ltd
Contact: Corsham Road, Shaw,
Melksham, Wiltshire, SN12 8EH
☎ 01225 708168
@ sara@marvencare.co.uk
🖱 www.marvencare.co.uk

In a village location, approximately two miles from Melksham, Mavern Care Ltd, a family-owned business, owns Mavern House Nursing Home. There is an activities coordinator, who facilitates games and socialising. Residents also have the opportunity of watching films. The home is set in the countryside, and provides entertainment and activities for the residents. There is a garden at the front of it with a patio to enjoy the area. Pets such as birds are allowed, and other pets are allowed to visit, this is at the manager's discretion.

Registered places: 48
Guide weekly rate: Undisclosed
Specialist care: Nursing
Medical services: Podiatry, hygienist, optician, physiotherapy
Qualified staff: Exceeds standard: 80% at NVQ level 2

Home details
Location: Village location, 2 miles from Melksham
Communal areas: 2 lounges, dining room, conservatory,
patio and garden
Accessibility: *Floors:* 2 • *Access:* Lift • *Wheelchair access:* Good
Smoking: ✗
Pets: At manager's discretion
Routines: Structured

Room details
Single: 44
Shared: 4
En suite: 48
Facilities: TV, telephone point

Door lock: ✓
Lockable place: ✓

Services provided
Beauty services: Hairdressing
Mobile library: ✓
Religious services: Monthly visits
Transport: ✗
Activities: *Coordinator:* ✓ • *Examples:* Films, musical entertainment,
visiting entertainers • *Outings:* ✗
Meetings: ✓

Registered places: 66
Guide weekly rate: £665–£775
Specialist care: Nursing, dementia, respite
Medical services: Podiatry, dentist, optician, physiotherapy
Qualified staff: Meets standard

Home details

Location: Residential area, 0.75 miles from Marlborough centre
Communal areas: 4 lounges, 3 dining rooms, patio and garden
Accessibility: *Floors:* 2 • *Access:* 2 lifts • *Wheelchair access:* Good
Smoking: ✗
Pets: ✓
Routines: Flexible

Room details

Single: 62
Shared: 2
En suite: 64
Facilities: TV

Door lock: ✓
Lockable place: ✗

Services provided

Beauty services: Hairdressing
Mobile library: Library facilities
Religious services: Weekly Communion service
Transport: ✗
Activities: *Coordinator.* ✗ • *Examples:* Exercise sessions, walks
    Outings: ✓
Meetings: ✓

Merlin Court

Manager: Amanda Short
Owner: Southern Cross Healthcare Ltd
Contact: Hyde Lane, Marlborough,
Wiltshire, SN8 1JT
☎ 01672 512454
🖱 www.schealthcare.co.uk

A purpose-built home that is divided into three distinct units, with one committed to residents with dementia, Merlin Court is situated approximately three quarters of a mile from Marlborough town centre, where there are a range of amenities. There is a bus service to the town centre. The home has its own activities coordinator who arranges exercise sessions and games. The residents are taken out for walks in addition to these activities. The home offers a range of communal facilities including one room dedicated to quiet. There are two lifts in the home providing access for the residents.

Registered places: 80
Guide weekly rate: £668–£965
Specialist care: Physical disability, respite, terminal care
Medical services: Podiatry
Qualified staff: Undisclosed

Home details

Location: Residential area, 1 mile from Salisbury
Communal areas: Lounge, dining room, garden
Accessibility: *Floors:* 2 • *Access:* Lift • *Wheelchair access:* Good
Smoking: ✗
Pets: ✓
Routines: Flexible

Room details

Single: 76
Shared: 4
En suite: Undisclosed
Facilities: TV

Door lock: ✓
Lockable place: ✗

Services provided

Beauty services: Hairdressing
Mobile library: ✗
Religious services: ✓
Transport: ✗
Activities: *Coordinator.* ✓ • *Examples:* Exercises, games
    Outings: ✓
Meetings: ✓

Milford House

Manager: Catherine Fountain
Owner: Barchester Healthcare Ltd
Contact: Milford Mill Road, Milford,
Salisbury, Wiltshire, SP1 1NJ
☎ 01722 322737

Milford House, run by Barchester Healthcare, is a nursing home located on the outskirts of the city of Salisbury. It is split into two parts with the Cathedral Wing joining them. The home provides large garden areas which are all accessible to wheelchairs. As well as organising appropriate activities for residents, the activities coordinator facilitates outings for those who wish to leave the home. There is also a group involving residents which meets regularly called 'Friends of Milford House'.

Milford Manor

Manager: Tracey Morris
Owner: Wessex Care Ltd
Contact: Milford Manor Gardens,
Salisbury, Wiltshire, SP1 2RN
☎ 01722 338652

Situated in a quiet residential area five minutes from the centre of Salisbury and near a bus stop, Milford manor is set an old building. The garden has recently had a wooden decking area added which provides access to the garden for all the residents. The home has its own activities coordinator who organises a daily activities schedule for the residents. There are also organised outings. Pets are allowed at the manager's discretion and smoking is permitted outside in a designated area.

Registered places: 29
Guide weekly rate: £360–£600
Specialist care: Dementia, respite
Medical services: Podiatry, dentist, optician.
Qualified staff: Meets standard

Home details

Location: Residential area, 1 mile from Salisbury centre
Communal areas: Lounge, dining room, conservatory, garden
Accessibility: *Floors:* 2 • *Access:* Lift • *Wheelchair access:* Good
Smoking: In designated area
Pets: At manager's discretion
Routines: Flexible

Room details

Single: 27
Shared: 1
En suite: 1
Facilities: TV point

Door lock: ✓
Lockable place: ✓

Services provided

Beauty services: Hairdressing
Mobile library: ✓
Religious services: ✓
Transport: ✗
Activities: *Coordinator.* ✓ • *Examples*: Bingo, musical entertainment • *Outings:* ✓
Meetings: ✓

Moormead House Nursing Home

Manager: Steven Sharp
Owner: Steven and Zandra Sharp
Contact: 67 Moormead Road,
Wroughton Swindon,
Wiltshire, SN4 9BU
☎ 01793 814259

Situated close to the centre of Wroughton, with easy access to amenities including shops and a pub, Moormead House is also located close to a bus stop for less mobile but still active residents. The home offers nursing care to 21 residents, with a few of the bedrooms having en suite facilities. Hairdressing and manicures regularly takes place at the home, and an activities coordinator assures that every resident is spent time with individually.

Registered places: 21
Guide weekly rate: Undisclosed
Specialist care: Nursing
Medical services: Dentist, optician
Qualified staff: Exceeds standard: 80% at NVQ level 2

Home details

Location: Residential area, 2.5 miles from Swindon
Communal areas: Lounge, dining room, conservatory, garden
Accessibility: *Floors:* 2 • *Access:* Lift • *Wheelchair access:* Good
Smoking: ✗
Pets: ✓
Routines: Flexible

Room details

Single: 19
Shared: 1
En suite: 5
Facilities: TV point

Door lock: ✗
Lockable place: ✗

Services provided

Beauty services: Hairdressing, manicures
Mobile library: ✗
Religious services: ✗
Transport: ✗
Activities: *Coordinator.* ✓ • *Examples*: Bingo, one-to-one sessions, themed events • *Outings:* ✗
Meetings: ✗

Registered places: 15
Guide weekly rate: Undisclosed
Specialist care: Nursing, physical disability, terminal care
Medical services: Occupational therapy
Qualified staff: Undisclosed

Home details

Location: Village location, 5 miles from Salisbury
Communal areas: Lounge, dining room, garden
Accessibility: *Floors:* 2 • *Access:* Lift • *Wheelchair access:* Good
Smoking: ×
Pets: ×
Routines: Structured

Room details

Single: 15
Shared: 0 | Door lock: ×
En suite: 15 | Lockable place: ×
Facilities: None

Services provided

Beauty services: Hairdressing
Mobile library: ×
Religious services: ✓
Transport: ×
Activities: *Coordinator.* ✓ • *Examples:* Social groups • *Outings:* ×
Meetings: Undisclosed

Newton House

Manager: Krystyna Romain
Owner: Glenside Manor Healthcare Services Ltd
Contact: South Newton, Salisbury, Wiltshire, SP2 0QD
☎ 01722 742066
@ newtonhouse@glensidemanor.co.uk
🖳 www.glensidemanor.co.uk

Located on a shared site in South Newton, Newton House is an older building with a newer extension. The home is one of six on the same campus. The six registered homes are owned by Glenside Manor Health Care Services Ltd. Newton House is able to share social events and activities with the other homes. The home benefits from a large well-maintained garden, and several bedrooms have patio doors leading onto it. As well as older people, the home also accommodates a number of younger high-dependency users.

Registered places: 20
Guide weekly rate: £380–£465
Specialist care: None
Medical services: Podiatry, optician, physiotherapy
Qualified staff: Meets standard

Home details

Location: Residential area, in Chippenham
Communal areas: 2 lounges, dining room, patio and garden
Accessibility: *Floors:* 2 • *Access:* Lift • *Wheelchair access:* Limited
Smoking: In designated area
Pets: ✓
Routines: Flexible

Room details

Single: 20
Shared: 0 | Door lock: ✓
En suite: 20 | Lockable place: ✓
Facilities: TV point, telephone point

Services provided

Beauty services: Hairdressing
Mobile library: Library facilities
Religious services: Monthly Communion service
Transport: ×
Activities: *Coordinator.* ✓ • *Examples:* Courses, piano recitals, singing • *Outings:* ×
Meetings: ✓

The Old Vicarage

Manager: Cheryl Williams
Owner: The Old Vicarage Ltd
Contact: St Mary's Street, Chippenham, Wiltshire, SN15 3JW
☎ 01249 653838
@ oldvicwilliams@hotmail.com

A period property located opposite the church, The Old Vicarage has a large garden that leads down towards the River Avon. The Grade II listed building is set in an acre of its own grounds in central Chippenham, 200 yards from a local library. The home participates in the University of the Third Age programme which creates learning cooperatives which draw upon the talents and expertise of members and volunteers to provide creative, educational and leisure opportunities. Courses run at the home include history, poetry, literature and play reading. There is a TV room with DVD facilities and a Freeview box.

The Old Vicarage

Manager: Lucy Wilcox
Owner: Equality Care Ltd
Contact: Staverton, Trowbridge,
Wiltshire, BA14 6NX
) 01225 782019

Situated in Staverton village, The Old Vicarage is approximately two miles from the town of Trowbridge. The home has a flexible daily routine with set meal times and an activities programme. There is an activities coordinator who arranges activities such as bingo, reminiscence sessions and exercise sessions. There are also outings to the shops and a Christmas lunch every year. The home has a very flexible policy regarding pets and has an individual care plan for each resident. The home arranges religious services as well as offering hairdressing and aromatherapy.

Registered places: 21
Guide weekly rate: £440
Specialist care: Dementia, mental disorder, respite
Medical services: Podiatry, dentist, optician, physiotherapy
Qualified staff: Meets standard

Home details
Location: Village location, 2 miles from Trowbridge
Communal areas: Lounge, dining room, patio and garden
Accessibility: *Floors:* 2 • *Access:* Stair lift • *Wheelchair access:* Good
Smoking: In designated area
Pets: ✓
Routines: Flexible

Room details
Single: 21
Shared: 0
En suite: 19
Facilities: TV, telephone

Door lock: ✓
Lockable place: ✓

Services provided
Beauty services: Hairdressing, aromatherapy
Mobile library: ✓
Religious services: ✓
Transport: ✗
Activities: *Coordinator:* ✓ • Examples: Bingo, reminiscence, visiting entertainers • *Outings:* ✓
Meetings: ✗

The Orchards

Manager: Pauline Buckingham
Owner: Buckland Care Ltd
Contact: 1 Perrys Lane, Wroughton,
Swindon, Wiltshire, SN4 9AX
) 01793 812242
⌂ www.buckland.co.uk

The Orchards is located in a quiet village, close to the local library and provides a comfortable atmosphere for 35 residents. The home has two lounges, a dining room, a conservatory and a garden with a patio area. The home has its own activities coordinator who arranges group activities such as reminiscence sessions and armchair exercises. There are also one-to-one sessions arranged and special events like a summer fête. The residents have a flexible daily routine and there are set meal times for the hot meals, although these can also be flexible.

Registered places: 35
Guide weekly rate: £550–£560
Specialist care: Dementia
Medical services: Undisclosed
Qualified staff: Exceeds standard: 65% at NVQ Level 2

Home details
Location: Village location, 3 miles from Swindon
Communal areas: 2 lounges, dining room, conservatory, patio and garden
Accessibility: *Floors:* 2 • *Access:* Lift • *Wheelchair access:* Good
Smoking: ✗
Pets: ✗
Routines: Flexible

Room details
Single: 35
Shared: 0
En suite: 17
Facilities: TV, telephone

Door lock: ✓
Lockable place: ✗

Services provided
Beauty services: Hairdressing
Mobile library: Library facilities
Religious services: Monthly Communion service
Transport: ✗
Activities: *Coordinator:* ✓ • *Examples:* Armchair exercises, cards, visiting entertainers • *Outings:* ✗
Meetings: ✓

Registered places: 41
Guide weekly rate: £590
Specialist care: Nursing, respite, terminal care
Medical services: Podiatry, optician
Qualified staff: Undisclosed

Home details
Location: Rural area, 5 miles from Swindon
Communal areas: Lounge, dining room, garden
Accessibility: *Floors:* 2 • *Access:* Lift • *Wheelchair access:* Good
Smoking: ✗
Pets: ✓
Routines: Flexible

Room details
Single: 39
Shared: 2
En suite: 41
Facilities: TV

Door lock: ✗
Lockable place: ✓

Services provided
Beauty services: Aromatherapy, massage, reflexology, Reiki
Mobile library: ✓
Religious services: ✓
Transport: ✗
Activities: *Coordinator.* ✓ • Examples: Games, videos • *Outings:* ✓
Meetings: ✓

Park View Nursing Home

Manager: Angela Rogers
Owner: Bothwells Ltd
Contact: Broad Bush, Blunsdon, Swindon, Wiltshire, SN26 7DH
☎ 01793 721352
@ parkviewcarehome@aol.com

Park View Nursing Home is situated in its own grounds in the village of Blundson, near Swindon town. A wide range of in-house activity is provided, which are either held in groups or with individual residents. Residents also have access to complementary therapies such as Reiki, reflexology and head massage. Forthcoming social events are displayed on a notice board and these included opportunities to get out of the home, such as a trip to a local garden centre.

Registered places: 18
Guide weekly rate: £495–£545
Specialist care: Dementia, emergency admissions, respite
Medical services: Podiatry, dentist, optician, physiotherapy
Qualified staff: Meets standard

Home details
Location: Residential area, 0.5 miles from Chippenham
Communal areas: Lounge, dining room, patio and garden
Accessibility: *Floors:* 2 • *Access:* Stair lift • *Wheelchair access:* Good
Smoking: ✗
Pets: ✗
Routines: Flexible

Room details
Single: 14
Shared: 2
En suite: 15
Facilities: TV point, telephone point

Door lock: ✓
Lockable place: ✓

Services provided
Beauty services: Hairdressing, aromatherapy, yoga
Mobile library: ✓
Religious services: Monthly Anglican Communion service
Transport: ✗
Activities: *Coordinator.* ✗ • *Examples*: Arts and crafts, exercise, *Outings:* ✓
Residents meetings: ✗

The Priory Residential Care Home

Manager: Julie Grimshaw
Owner: Lower Green Ltd
Contact: Greenway Lane, Chippenham, Wiltshire, SN15 1AA
☎ 01249 652153
@ mballworth@tinyworld.co.uk
🖥 www.thepriorycarehome.co.uk

The Priory is a large Edwardian family house that is set in its own gardens in a residential area of Chippenham. The home has attractive south-facing gardens where residents with an interest in gardening can often be found. With a regular activities programme featuring monthly outings that include pub lunches and garden visits, The Priory also organises seasonal events such as summer fêtes and Christmas parties. The owner is responsible for writing a quarterly newsletter which updates residents and their relatives on current care issues.

Quarry Mount Residential Care Home

Manager: Karen Meadowcroft
Owner: Quarry Mount Care Ltd
Contact: 83 Bath Road, Swindon, Wiltshire, SN1 4AX
) 01793 527715
@ enquiries@quarrymount.co.uk
www.quarrymount.co.uk

Quarry Mount is situated in a residential area of Swindon, close to the town centre. The home cares for 32 residents, with dementia or physical disabilities as well as elderly residents. There are two lounges, two dining rooms and a conservatory in the home, there are also two bungalows in the home's back garden which accommodate residents who are more mobile.

Registered places: 32
Guide weekly rate: £410–£580
Specialist care: Dementia, physical disability, respite
Medical services: Podiatry, occupational therapy
Qualified staff: Exceeds standard: 85% at NVQ level 2

Home details
Location: Residential area, in Swindon
Communal areas: 2 lounges, 2 dining rooms, conservatory, garden
Accessibility: *Floors:* 3 • *Access:* Lift • *Wheelchair access:* Good
Smoking: x
Pets: At manager's discretion
Routines: Structured

Room details
Single: 16
Shared: 8
En suite: 3
Facilities: TV point, telephone point

Door lock: ✓
Lockable place: ✓

Services provided
Beauty services: Hairdressing
Mobile library: x
Religious services: x
Transport: Car
Activities: *Coordinator.* ✓ • *Examples:* Bingo, gentle exercise, singalongs • *Outings:* x
Meetings: ✓

Ravenscroft Care Centre

Manager: Vacant
Owner: Southern Cross Healthcare Ltd
Contact: Hilperton Road, Trowbridge, Wiltshire, BA14 7JQ
) 01225 752087
@ ravenscroft@schealthcare.co.uk
www.schealthcare.co.uk

An older building that previously belonged to a mill owner and that has been extended over the years, Ravenscroft Care Centre is situated on the outskirts of Trowbridge, on a main bus route. The rooms to the rear of the home permit views of the surrounding countryside. The home is close to the town's amenities which include shops and a pub. Trowbridge also has its own railway station. With a comprehensive activities programme, the home also offers outings and holds a garden fête on its lawns every year.

Registered places: 46
Guide weekly rate: £442–£650
Specialist care: Nursing, emergency admissions, physical disability, respite
Medical services: Podiatry, dentist, optician, physiotherapy
Qualified staff: Undisclosed

Home details
Location: 1 mile from Trowbridge centre
Communal areas: 3 lounges, 2 dining rooms, garden
Accessibility: *Floors:* 3 • *Access:* Lift • *Wheelchair access:* Good
Smoking: x
Pets: At manager's discretion
Routines: Flexible

Room details
Single: 36
Shared: 5
En suite: 20
Facilities: TV point, telephone point

Door lock: ✓
Lockable place: ✓

Services provided
Beauty services: Hairdressing.
Mobile library:
Library facilities
Religious services: Monthly Anglican and Catholic Communion services
Transport: x
Activities: *Coordinator.* ✓ • *Examples:* Bingo, one-to-one sessions, singalongs • *Outings:* ✓
Meetings: x

Rose Cottage Nursing Home

Manager: Janet Asparassa
Owner: Hemingway Management Services Ltd
Contact: 47 High Street, Haydon Wick, Swindon, Wiltshire, SN25 1HU
☎ 01793 706876
@ Rose.cottage@btconnect.com

Rose Cottage Nursing Home is a small care home located approximately 20 minutes' walk from local facilities and four miles from the centre of Swindon. The home has two lounges, a dining room and a garden with a patio area. The home has an activities coordinator who organises games, nail painting and visiting entertainers, as well as arranging outings. Pets would be allowed at the manager's discretion but smoking is not permitted. The home offers a monthly church service and the services of a hairdresser. The home also offers nursing and respite care.

Registered places: 18
Guide weekly rate: Undisclosed
Specialist care: Nursing, respite
Medical services: Podiatry, dentist, optician, physiotherapy
Qualified staff: Exceeds standard: 60% at NVQ Level 2

Home details
Location: Residential area, 4 miles from Swindon centre
Communal areas: 2 lounges, dining room, patio and garden
Accessibility: *Floors:* 2 • *Access:* Lift • *Wheelchair access:* Good
Smoking: ✗
Pets: At manager's discretion
Routines: Flexible

Room details
Single: 16
Shared: 1
En suite: 0
Door lock: ✗
Lockable place: ✓
Facilities: TV point, telephone point

Services provided
Beauty services: Hairdressing, aromatherapy, manicures
Mobile library: ✗
Religious services: Monthly church service
Transport: ✗
Activities: *Coordinator.* ✓ • *Examples:* Games, painting, visiting entertainers • *Outings:* ✓
Meetings: ✓

Sheldon Lodge

Manager: Sateeam Arithoppah
Owner: Sateeam and Jayne Arithoppah
Contact: 150 Sheldon Road, Chippenham, Wiltshire, SN14 0BZ
☎ 01249 660001
@ Jayne150@btopenworld.com

Located within a residential area of Chippenham, Sheldon Lodge also lies on the same street as a pub and convenience store. The home is small, caring for nine residents and therefore the owners pride themselves on the homely feel of the home. The owners themselves live on the premises and provide night care. Regular activities are organised, as are outings into town.

Registered places: 9
Guide weekly rate: £367–£420
Specialist care: Day care, dementia, mental disorder
Medical services: Podiatry, optician
Qualified staff: Exceeds standard: 80% at NVQ level 2

Home details
Location: Residential area, 0.5 miles from Chippenham centre
Communal areas: Lounge, dining room, garden
Accessibility: *Floors:* 2 • *Access:* Stair lift
Wheelchair access: Good
Smoking: In designated area
Pets: At manager's discretion
Routines: Flexible

Room details
Single: 5
Shared: 2
En suite: 0
Door lock: ✓
Lockable place: ✓
Facilities: TV point, telephone point

Services provided
Beauty services: Hairdressing
Mobile library: ✗
Religious services: Monthly Methodist service
Transport: Car
Activities: *Coordinator.* ✓ • *Examples:* Art therapy, bingo, cooking, music
Outings: ✓
Meetings: ✗

Southdown Nursing & Residential Home

Manager: Deborah McHugh
Owner: Carevale Ltd
Contact: The Old Vicarage, 17 Church Road, Wanborough, Swindon, Wiltshire, SN4 0BZ
☎ 01793 790727

Southdown Nursing and Residential Home is a Grade II listed building with a purpose-built annexe. The home is located in the village of Wanborough, approximately four miles from the centre of Swindon. The home has three lounges, one of which has a dining area. There is also a garden with a patio area. The home has a dedicated activities coordinator and there are frequent outings available to the residents. The home also holds regular residents meetings to discuss any issues that may have arisen.

Registered places: 30
Guide weekly rate: £400–£575
Specialist care: Nursing, respite
Medical services: Podiatry, dentist, optician
Qualified staff: Meets standard

Home details
Location: Village location, 4 miles from Swindon
Communal areas: 3 lounges, dining area, patio and garden
Accessibility: *Floors:* 3 • *Access:* 2 lifts • *Wheelchair access: Good*
Smoking: x
Pets: At manager's discretion
Routines: Flexible

Room details
Single: 24
Shared: 3
En suite: 8
Facilities: TV, telephone point

Door lock: ✓
Lockable place: ✓

Services provided
Beauty services: Hairdressing
Mobile library: ✓
Religious services: ✓
Transport: x
Activities: *Coordinator:* ✓ • *Examples:* Barbecues, bingo
• *Outings:* ✓
Meetings: ✓

Sutton Veny Nursing Home

Manager: Patricia Gronow
Owner: Sutton Veny House Ltd
Contact: Nr Warminster, Wiltshire, BA12 7BJ
☎ 01985 840224

Sutton Veny is a period house in its own large grounds. The home is situated on the outskirts of the village of Sutton Veny, close to the Wiltshire town of Warminster, which also has a range of shops, and a railway station. Sutton Veny is about 10 minutes' drive from the A303, which links with the M3. The home does not have a dining room and residents eat their meals in their rooms or at tables in the sitting room.

Registered places: 28
Guide weekly rate: Undisclosed
Specialist care: Nursing, terminal care
Medical services: Podiatry, dentist, optician, physiotherapy
Qualified staff: Undisclosed

Home details
Location: Village location, 2.5 miles from Warminster
Communal areas: Lounge, garden
Accessibility: *Floors:* 3 • *Access:* Lift • *Wheelchair access: Good*
Smoking: x
Pets: ✓
Routines: Flexible

Room details
Single: 26
Shared: 2
En suite: 0
Facilities: TV point, telephone point

Door lock: x
Lockable place: ✓

Services provided
Beauty services: Hairdressing, aromatherapy, manicures
Mobile library: ✓
Religious services: x
Transport: x
Activities: *Coordinator.* ✓ • *Examples:* One-to-one sessions
Outings: x
Meetings: x

Registered places: 24
Guide weekly rate: From £550
Specialist care: Dementia, mental disorder, respite
Medical services: Podiatry, optician
Qualified staff: Exceeds standard: 75% at NVQ level 2

Home details

Location: Residential area, 1 mile from Salisbury
Communal areas: 3 lounges, 2 dining rooms, patio and garden
Accessibility: *Floors:* 2 • *Access:* Lift • *Wheelchair access:* Good
Smoking: In designated area
Pets: At manager's discretion
Routines: Flexible

Room details

Single: 22
Shared: 1   Door lock: ✓
En suite: 23   Lockable place: ✓
Facilities: TV point, telephone point

Services provided

Beauty services: Hairdressing
Mobile library: ✓
Religious services: Monthly Anglican service
Transport: ✗
Activities: *Coordinator.* ✓ • *Examples*: One-to-one sessions
     Outings: ✗
Meetings: ✗

Tower House

Manager: Lisa Mulholland
Owner: Eileen O'Connor-Marsh
Contact: 43 Manor Road, Salisbury, Wiltshire, SP1 1JT
❯ 0722 338395

A detached Victorian property that lies close to its two sister homes, Dunraven and Dunraven Lodge, Tower House is 10 minutes' walk from Salisbury city centre where amenities are ample. Tower House comprises of two buildings: the original Victorian building and a new purpose-built dementia unit. The two are connected by a walkway. Residents have access to a cordless phone where they can make outgoing calls free of charge. The home arranges one-to-one activity sessions for the residents and there is also a mobile library which comes to the home. An Anglican service is held on a monthly basis.

Registered places: 8
Guide weekly rate: Undisclosed
Specialist care: Dementia
Medical services: Podiatry, hygienist, optician, physiotherapy
Qualified staff: Meets standard

Home details

Location: Village location, 8 miles from Chippenham
Communal areas: Lounge, dining room, garden
Accessibility: *Floors:* 2 • *Access:* Stair lift
     Wheelchair access: Good
Smoking: ✗
Pets: At manager's discretion
Routines: Flexible

Room details

Single: 7
Shared: 2   Door lock: ✗
En suite: 2   Lockable place: ✗
Facilities: TV

Services provided

Beauty services: Hairdressing
Mobile Library: ✓
Religious services: Twice-monthly Anglican service
Transport: ✗
Activities: *Coordinator.* ✓ • *Examples*: Community-based activities
     Outings: ✗
Meetings: ✗

Trimnell House

Manager: Susan Parkinson
Owner: Susan Parkinson
Contact: Market Place, Colerne, Wiltshire, SN14 8AY
❯ 01225 742239
@ Trimnellhouse@btinternet.com

Trimnell House is a large, detached Victorian house with three floors located in a village, eight miles from Chippenham. Currently a dog and cat reside in the home. The landscaped grounds are extensive and a lot of the produce used in the kitchens in grown in the gardens around the house. Mrs Parkinson, the owner and manager also runs a domiciliary agency that provides care and meals for several elderly people in the village. Through strong connections with the village, residents are integrated socially into village life through lunch clubs.

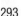

Trowbridge Oaks Nursing Home

Manager: Keeley Simpson
Owner: BUPA Care Homes Ltd
Contact: West Ashton Road, Trowbridge, Wiltshire, BA14 6DW
📞 01225 774492
@ TrowbridgeOaksALL@BUPA.com
🖰 www.bupacarehomes.co.uk

Trowbridge Oaks is set in a leafy, residential area of Trowbridge. This purpose-built home has been designed to meet the needs of elderly residents, and is surrounded by a garden and patio area. It has a choice of two lounges, one of which includes a large conservatory. There is also a large, bright traditional style dining room. Some of the bedrooms have views over the gardens, and all have en suite facilities. Among the daily activities are arts and crafts, gardening, reminiscence sessions and entertainers.

Registered places: 60
Guide weekly rate: Undisclosed
Specialist care: Nursing, palliative care, physical disability, respite, terminal care
Medical services: Podiatry, physiotherapy
Qualified staff: Undisclosed

Home details
Location: Residential area, 1 mile from Trowbridge centre
Communal areas: Lounge, 2 dining rooms, conservatory, kitchenette, patio and garden
Accessibility: *Floors:* 2 • *Access:* Lift • *Wheelchair access:* Good
Smoking: ✗
Pets: ✗
Routines: Flexible

Room details
Single: 44
Shared: 8
En suite: 52
Facilities: TV point, telephone point
Door lock: ✓
Lockable place: ✗

Services provided
Beauty services: Hairdressing
Mobile library: ✓
Religious services: ✓
Transport: ✓
Activities: *Coordinator.* ✓ • *Examples:* Arts and crafts, gardening, visiting entertainers • *Outings:* ✓
Meetings: ✗

Watersmead

Manager: Julia Matthews
Owner: The Orders Of St John Care Trust
Contact: White Horse Way, Westbury, Wiltshire, BA13 3AU
📞 01373 826503
@ manager.watersmead@ osjctwilts.co.uk
🖰 www.osj.co.uk

Watersmead is a purpose-built home located close to the centre of Westbury a five-minute walk from the shops and centre of the town. The home prides itself on the computer and internet facilities. They have adventurous outings such as going ice-skating and going to the pantomime. Inside the home the activities coordinator arranges parties for special occasions such as birthdays and anniversaries.

Registered places: 50
Guide weekly rate: £395–£460
Specialist care: Day care, dementia, respite
Medical services: Podiatry, hygienist, optician, physiotherapy
Qualified staff: Exceeds standard: 82% at NVQ level 2

Home details
Location: Residential area, 0.5 miles from Westbury
Communal areas: 2 lounges, lounge-dining room, garden
Accessibility: *Floors:* 1 • *Wheelchair access:* Good
Smoking: In designated area
Pets: At manager's discretion
Routines: Flexible

Room details
Single: 50
Shared: 0
En suite: 1
Facilities: TV, telephone point
Door lock: ✓
Lockable place: ✓

Services provided
Beauty services: Hairdressing, manicures
Mobile Library: ✓
Religious services: Anglican and Catholic visits, weekly church service
Transport: ✗
Activities: *Coordinator.* ✓ • *Examples:* Bingo, parties *Outings:* ✓
Meetings: ✓

Registered places: 53
Guide weekly rate: £595–£770
Specialist care: Nursing, dementia, physical disability
Medical services: Podiatry, hygienist, optician, physiotherapy
Qualified staff: Exceeds standard: 90% at NVQ level 2

Home details
Location: Residential area, 3 miles from Swindon
Communal areas: 2 lounges, 2 dining rooms, conservatory, garden
Accessibility: *Floors:* 2 • *Access:* Lift • *Wheelchair access:* Good
Smoking: In designated area
Pets: x
Routines: Flexible

Room details
Single: 43
Shared: 5
En suite: 48
Facilities: TV point, telephone point

Door lock: ✓
Lockable place: ✓

Services provided
Beauty services: Hairdressing
Mobile library: ✓
Religious services: Weekly Catholic Mass, monthly service
Transport: Bus
Activities: *Coordinator:* ✓ • *Examples:* Quizzes, visiting entertainers
    Outings: ✓
Meetings: ✓

Wemyss Lodge

Manager: Kay Thompson
Owner: Wemyss Lodge Ltd
Contact: Ermin Street,
Stratton St Margaret, Swindon,
Wiltshire, SN3 4LH
☎ 01793 828227

Wemyss Lodge is a purpose-built home located in a residential area, within easy walking distance of local shops. The home is found three miles from the centre of Swindon. The home produces a monthly newsletter containing details of residents' birthdays, pictures, poems and other interesting material. The home has its own transport and often takes the residents on outings. There is a Catholic Mass held every week and a Christian service takes place on a monthly basis. There are also visits from a mobile library.

Registered places: 10
Guide weekly rate: £415–£585
Specialist care: Respite
Medical services: Podiatry, optician, physiotherapy
Qualified staff: Exceeds standard: 63% at NVQ level 2

Home details
Location: Village location, 10 miles from Marlborough
Communal areas: 2 lounges, dining room, garden
Accessibility: *Floors:* 2 • *Access:* Lift • *Wheelchair access:* Good
Smoking: In designated area
Pets: At manager's discretion
Routines: Flexible

Room details
Single: 10
Shared: 0
En suite: 10
Facilities: TV point, telephone

Door lock: ✓
Lockable place: ✓

Services provided
Beauty services: Hairdressing
Mobile library: ✓
Religious services: Monthly Anglican Communion service
Transport: Car
Activities: *Coordinator:* x • *Examples:* None • *Outings:* x
Meetings: x

West Farm House

Manager: Helen Burnett-Price
Owner: Helen Burnett-Price and
Barry Price
Contact: Collingbourne Ducis,
Marlborough, Wiltshire, SN8 3DZ
☎ 01264 850224

In a quiet village location, West Farm House is an adapted period property that is situated a few minutes' walk from a nearby convenience store. The home has a large walled garden. At West Farm House there is no organised programme of activities, as residents prefer to organise their own time. The home has its own transport and arranges an Anglican Communion service every month.

The Westbury Nursing Home

Manager: Penny Lloyd
Owner: BUPA Care Homes Ltd
Contact: 86 Warminster Road, Westbury, Wiltshire, BA13 3PR
) 01373 825868
@ TheWestburyALL@BUPA.com
www.bupacarehomes.co.uk

The Westbury is situated in a residential area, half a mile away from the town of Westbury. This purpose-built home has been specifically equipped to meet the needs of elderly residents. The home enjoys the benefit of a well-kept garden, patio and conservatory area. Daily activities are arranged, including musical entertainment, reminiscence sessions, gardening and trips out to local places of interest. The Westbury also provides care to people aged 16 and over with physical disabilities, and to those who require palliative or terminal care.

Registered places: 51
Guide weekly rate: Undisclosed
Specialist care: Nursing, palliative care, physical disability, respite, terminal care
Medical services: Podiatry, physiotherapy
Qualified staff: Undisclosed

Home details
Location: Residential area, 0.5 miles from Westbury centre
Communal areas: 2 lounges, dining room, conservatory, hairdressing salon, patio and garden
Accessibility: *Floors:* 2 • *Access:* Lift • *Wheelchair access:* Good
Smoking: ✗
Pets: ✓
Routines: Flexible

Room details
Single: 37
Shared: 7
En suite: 44
Facilities: TV point, telephone point
Door lock: ✓
Lockable place: ✗

Services provided
Beauty services: Hairdressing, aromatherapy
Mobile library: ✓
Religious services: ✓
Transport: ✓
Activities: *Coordinator.* ✓ • Examples: Musical entertainment, quizzes • *Outings:* ✓
Meetings: ✓

The Wingfield Care Home

Manager: Sharon Lewis
Owner: Barchester Healthcare Ltd
Contact: 70 Wingfield Road, Trowbridge, Wiltshire, BA14 9EN
) 01225 771550
@ wingfield@barchester.com
www.barchester-homecare.com

The Wingfield is comprised of two buildings, one catering for elderly residents and the other is a dementia unit. The home is located on the outskirts of Trowbridge, less than a mile from the town centre. There is a bus stop just outside the home. The landscaped garden boasts a pond, sensory pathway and water features. The home employs an activities coordinator who arranges a book club and coffee mornings for the residents. There are also residents meetings held every other month.

Registered places: 89
Guide weekly rate: Undisclosed
Specialist care: Nursing, dementia, respite
Medical services: Podiatry, dentist, optician
Qualified staff: Exceeds standard: 65% at NVQ level 2

Home details
Location: Residential area, 0.8 miles from Trowbridge
Communal areas: 7 lounges, 4 dining rooms, conservatory, garden
Accessibility: *Floors:* 3 • *Access:* Lift • *Wheelchair access:* Good
Smoking: In designated area
Pets: At manager's discretion
Routines: Flexible

Room details
Single: 89
Shared: 0
En suite: 89
Facilities: TV point, telephone point
Door lock: ✓
Lockable place: ✓

Services provided
Beauty services: Hairdressing
Mobile library: ✓
Religious services: Monthly Anglican Communion service
Transport: Minibus
Activities: *Coordinator.* ✓ • *Examples:* Book club, coffee mornings, sensory stimulation • *Outings:* ✓
Meetings: ✓

Registered places: 24
Guide weekly rate: £700
Specialist care: Dementia, respite
Medical services: Podiatry, optician, physiotherapy
Qualified staff: Exceeds standard: 80% at NVQ level 2

Home details

Location: Village location, 8.6 miles from Salisbury
Communal areas: Lounge, lounge/diner, conservatory, garden
Accessibility: *Floors:* 2 • *Access:* Lift and stair lift
    Wheelchair access: Good
Smoking: In designated area
Pets: At manager's discretion
Routines: Flexible

Room details

Single: 21
Shared: 1
En suite: 7
Facilities: TV point, telephone point

Door lock: ✓
Lockable place: ✓

Services provided

Beauty services: Hairdressing
Mobile library: ✓
Religious services: Monthly Communion service
Transport: ✗
Activities: *Coordinator:* ✗ • *Examples:* Exercises, music therapy,
    visiting entertainers • *Outings:* ✓
Meetings: ✓

Woodfalls Care Home

Manager: Patricia Whitston
Owner: Woodfalls Care Ltd
Contact: Vale Road, Woodfalls, Salisbury, Wiltshire, SP5 2LT
☏ 01725 511226
@ woodfallscare@tiscali.co.uk

Located in Woodfalls village, the aptly named Woodfalls Care Home offers easy access to the nearby shop and Methodist church. Salisbury is a nine-mile bus ride away. The garden has a paved path running around it which provides access for the residents. There is also a conservatory for residents to relax in. The home has visits from a mobile library and there is a Communion service once a month. The home arranges outings for the residents as well as internal activities like music therapy.

Useful contacts

Action on Elder Abuse (AEA)

☎ 0808 808 8141
🖱 www.elderabuse.org.uk
Action on Elder Abuse works to protect,
and prevent the abuse of vulnerable
older adults.

Age Concern England

☎ 0808 808 6060
🖱 www.ace.org.uk
Promotes the well-being of older people
by providing services, information
and campaigning on issues like age
discrimination and pensions.

British Red Cross Society

☎ 020 7235 5454
@ www.redcross.org.uk
Offers a range of services including:
home nursing, transport, holidays,
equipment loan for frail elderly people,
home from hospital
schemes, domiciliary and
respite care.

CareAware

☎ 08705 134925
🖱 www.careaware.co.uk
CareAware is a non profit
making public information,
advisory and advocacy service
specialising in elderly care
funding advice in the UK.

Counsel and Care

☎ 0845 300 7585
@ advice@counselandcare.org.uk
🖱 www.counselandcare.org.uk
A national charity providing older people,
their families and carers with advice,
information and financial support.

CSCI (Commission for Social Care Inspection)

☎ 0845 015 0120/0191 233 3323
@ enquiries@csci.gsi.gov.uk
🖱 www.csci.org.uk
Launched in April 2004, the CSCI
is the single, independent inspectorate
for all social care services in England,
set up to regulate social, private and
voluntary health care services.

South-west regional contact team

☎ 0117 930 7110

Elderly Accommodation Counsel (EAC)

☎ 020 7820 1343
@ enquiries@e-a-c.demon.co.uk
🖱 www.housingcare.org
Provides advice on finding and paying
for all types of housing for older people,
including sheltered housing, residential
care, nursing homes and homes which
accept people with mental and physical
disabilities.

Help The Aged

) 020 7278 1114
⏚ www.helptheaged.org.uk
Provides community services and
helps older people to lead independent
lives. They also publish information
on finance, how to stay healthy and
guidance on choosing a care home.

IFA Promotion

) 0800 085 3250
@ contact@ifap.org.uk
⏚ www.unbiased.co.uk
Searches for details of independent
financial advisers close to where you
live or work from around 9,000 IFA
locations UK-wide.

Nursing Homes Fees Agency (NHFA)

) 0800 998 833
@ enquiries@nhfa.co.uk
⏚ www.hsbcpensions.co.uk
NHFA offers advice on financing care,
helping you understand state support
and, if you are self-funding, other
financial products available help you.
⏚ www.careuk.net
A NHFA website with numerous sources
of support, advice and information
available throughout the UK.

NHS Direct

) 0845 4647
⏚ www.nhsdirect.nhs.uk
Provides confidential healthcare advice
24 hours a day.

The Pension Service

) 0845 606 0265
⏚ www.thepensionservice.gov.uk
The government has set up
The Pension Service (part of the
Department for Work and
Pensions) to improve its service
to pensioners or those planning
retirement.

Relatives & Residents Association

) 020 7359 8136
@ info@relres.org
⏚ www.relres.org
Provides support and advice for both
residents of care homes and their
relatives.

Seniorline

) 0808 800 6565
Provides free advice and
information for older people
and their carers. Run by Help
the Aged.

University of the Third Age

) 020 8466 6139
⏚ www.u3a.org.uk
U3A runs learning cooperatives for
older people, providing opportunities
for their members to share learning
experiences in a wide range of
interest groups and to pursue
learning not for qualifications, but
for fun.

Specific care information

Alzheimer's Society

) 0845 300 0336
@ info@alzheimers.org.uk
⌒ www.alzheimers.org.uk
Provides support, information, advice
and local services for those looking
after someone with dementia.

Arthritis Care

) 0808 800 4050
⌒ www.arthritiscare.org.uk
Society for people with arthritis, helping
to promote their health, well being and
independence.

Dementia Information Service for Carers (DISC)

) 0845 120 4048
Advice and information for carers
of older people with dementia.

Diabetes UK

) 020 7424 1000
@ info@diabetes.org.uk
⌒ www.diabetes.org.uk
Works for people with diabetes, funding
research, campaigning and helping
people live with the condition.

Hearing Concern

) 020 7440 9871
@ info@hearingconcern.org.uk
⌒ www.hearingconcern.org.uk
A national charity which provides
support, advice and information for the
deaf and hard of hearing.

Huntington's Disease Association

) 020 7223 7000
⌒ www.hda.org.uk
Local and regional advisers offer
information, support and family visits to
those with Huntington's Disease.

MIND (National Association for Mental Health)

) 0845 766 0163
@ contact@mind.org.uk
⌒ www.mind.org.uk
A mental health charity working for
everyone with experience of mental
distress.

Parkinson's Disease Society

) 0845 608 445
⌒ www.parkinsons.org.uk
Provides help for people with arkinson's
Disease and their relatives.

The Stroke Association

) 0845 3033100
⌒ www.stroke.org.uk
Provides an advisory and information
service for people who have had
strokes, their families and carers.

County contact numbers

BRISTOL

Bristol City Council
) 01179 222 000
⌂ www.bristol.gov.uk

CORNWALL

Cornwall County Council
) 01872 322 000
@ enquiries@cornwall.gov.uk
⌂ www.cornwall.gov.uk

Caradon District Council
) 01579 341 000
@ postroom@caradon.gov.uk
⌂ www.caradon.gov.uk

Carrick District Council
) 01872 224 400
@ comment@carrick.gov.uk
⌂ www.carrick.gov.uk

Kerrier District Council
) 01209 614 000
@ customer.services@kerrier.gov.uk
⌂ www.kerrier.gov.uk

North Cornwall District Council
) 01208 893 333
⌂ www.ncdc.gov.uk

Penwith District Council
) 01736 362 341
@ admin@penwith.gov.uk
⌂ www.penwith.gov.uk

Restormel Borough Council
) 01726 223 300
@ rbc@restormel.gov.uk
⌂ www.restormel.gov.uk

DEVON

Devon County Council
) 01392 382 000
@ info@devon.gov.uk
⌂ www.devon.gov.uk

East Devon District Council
) 01395 516 551
@ eddc@eastdevon.gov.uk
⌂ www.eastdevon.gov.uk

Exeter City Council
) 01392 277 888
⌂ www.exeter.gov.uk

Mid Devon District Council
) 01884 255 255
@ customerservices@middevon.
   gov.uk
⌂ www.middevon.gov.uk

North Devon District Council
) 01271 327 711
⌂ www.northdevon.gov.uk

Plymouth City Council
) 01752 668 000
@ enquiries@plymouth.gov.uk
⌂ www.plymouth.gov.uk

South Hams District Council
) 01803 861 234
  @ customer.services@southhams.
    gov.uk
  ⌐ www.southhams.gov.uk

Teignbridge District Council
) 01626 361 101
  @ info@teignbridge.gov.uk
  ⌐ www.teignbridge.gov.uk

Torbay Council
) 01803 201 201
  @ fss@torbay.gov.uk
  ⌐ www.torbay.gov.uk

Torridge District Council
) 01237 428 700
  ⌐ www.torridge.gov.uk

West Devon Borough Council
) 01822 813 600
  @ info@westdevon.gov.uk
  ⌐ www.westdevon.gov.uk

DORSET

Dorset County Council
) 01305 251 000
  ⌐ www.dorsetforyou.com

Borough of Poole
) 01202 633 633
  @ enquiries@boroughofpoole.com
  ⌐ www.boroughofpoole.com

Bournemouth Borough Council
) 01202 451 451
  @ enquiries@bournemouth.gov.uk
  ⌐ www.bournemouth.gov.uk

Christchurch Borough Council
) 01202 495 000
  @ post@christchurch.gov.uk
  ⌐ www.dorsetforyou.com

East Dorset District Council
) 01202 886 201
  ⌐ www.dorsetforyou.com

North Dorset District Council
) 01258 454 111
  @ customer@north-dorset.gov.uk
  ⌐ www.north-dorset.gov.uk

Purbeck District Council
) 01929 556 561
  ⌐ www.purbeck.gov.uk

West Dorset District Council
) 01305 251 010
  @ communication@westdorset-dc.
    gov.uk
  ⌐ www.dorsetforyou.com

Weymouth and Portland Borough
Council
) 01305 838 000
  ⌐ www.weymouth.gov.uk

GLOUCESTERSHIRE

Gloucestershire County Council
) 01452 425 000
  @ speakout@gloucestershire.
    gov.uk
  ⌐ www.gloucestershire.gov.uk

Cheltenham Borough Council
) 01242 262 626
  @ enquiries@cheltenham.gov.uk
  ⌐ www.cheltenham.gov.uk

Cotswold District Council
) 01285 623 000
  @ cdc@cotswold.gov.uk
  ⌐ www.cotswold.gov.uk

Forest of Dean District Council
) 01594 810 000
  @ council@fdean.gov.uk
  ⌐ www.fdean.gov.uk

Gloucester City Council
- ☎ 01452 522 232
- @ heretohelp@gloucester.gov.uk
- 🖰 www.gloucester.gov.uk

South Gloucestershire Council
- ☎ 01454 868 009
- 🖰 www.southglos.gov.uk

Stroud District Council
- ☎ 01453 766 321
- @ info@stroud.gov.uk
- 🖰 www.stroud.gov.uk

Tewkesbury Borough Council
- ☎ 01684 295 010
- @ generalenquiries@tewkesbury.gov.uk
- 🖰 www.tewkesburybc.gov.uk

SOMERSET

Somerset County Council
- ☎ 0845 345 9166
- @ somersetdirect@somerset.gov.uk
- 🖰 www.somerset.gov.uk

Bath and North East Somerset Council
- ☎ 01225 477 000
- councilconnect@bathnes.gov.uk
- 🖰 www.bathnes.gov.uk

Mendip District Council
- ☎ 01749 648 999
- @ customerservices@mendip.gov.uk
- 🖰 www.mendip.gov.uk

North Somerset District Council
- ☎ 01934 888 888
- @ comments@n-somerset.gov.uk
- 🖰 www.n-somerset.gov.uk

Sedgemoor District Council
- ☎ 0845 408 2540
- @ customer.services@sedgemoor.gov.uk
- 🖰 www.sedgemoor.gov.uk

South Somerset District Council
- ☎ 01935 462 462
- 🖰 www.southsomerset.gov.uk

Taunton Deane District Council
- ☎ 01823 356 356
- @ enquiries@tauntondeane.gov.uk
- 🖰 www.tauntondeane.gov.uk

West Somerset District Council
- ☎ 01643 703 704
- @ customerservices@westsomerset.gov.uk
- 🖰 www.westsomersetonline.gov.uk

WILTSHIRE

Wiltshire County Council
- ☎ 01225 713 000
- @ customercare@wiltshire.gov.uk
- 🖰 www.wiltshire.gov.uk

Kennet District Council
- ☎ 01380 724 911
- @ Kennet@Kennet.gov.uk
- 🖰 www.kennet.gov.uk

North Wiltshire District Council
- ☎ 01249 706 111
- @ customerservices@northwilts.gov.uk
- 🖰 www.northwilts.gov.uk

Salisbury District Council
- ☎ 01722 336 272
- @ thecouncil@salisbury.gov.uk
- 🖰 www.salisbury.gov.uk

Swindon Borough Council
- ☎ 01793 463 725
- @ customerservices@swindon.gov.uk
- 🖰 www.swindon.gov.uk

West Wiltshire District Council
- ☎ 01225 776 655
- @ communications@westwiltshire.gov.uk
- 🖰 www.westwiltshire.gov.uk